# Clinical Ophthalmic Echography

# Clinical Ophthalmic Echography

## A Case Study Approach

Roger P. Harrie, MD

IHC Health Center *and* Clinical Professor, Moran Eye Center, University of Utah,
Salt Lake City, Utah

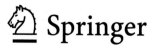 Springer

Roger P. Harrie, MD
IHC Health Center
*and*
Clinical Professor
Moran Eye Center
University of Utah
Salt Lake City, UT
USA

ISBN: 978-0-387-75243-3          e-ISBN: 978-0-387-75244-0
DOI: 10.1007/978-0-387-75244-0

Library of Congress Control Number: 2007943249

# Contents

## Part II   Basic Principles

## Part III   Eye Pain

## Part IV   Blurred Vision

## Part V   Bulgy Eyes

## Part VI   Lumps and Bumps

## Part VII   Echography in Developing Countries

## Part VIII   Orbital Imaging

# Part I
## Indications for Ophthalmic Ultrasound

## Who Really Needs Ultrasound?

There are numerous clinical applications of ocular ultrasound. However, many clinicians complete their training with minimal exposure to echography beyond that for biometry and do not appreciate the value of this technology in their practices. The occasional patient in the general eye practice who is perceived to need an imaging study is referred for computer tomography (CT) or magnetic resonance imaging (MRI) scanning, which are readily accessible in developed countries. The potpourri of diagnostic imaging modalities with insurance coverage is potentially subject to overuse. It is tempting to order MRI scans for headaches, CT scans for pains around the eye, and carotid Doppler duplex scanning for vision disturbances. In many cases, a careful history and physical examination combined with the use of ultrasound can correctly diagnose the problem without the need for more expensive studies.

The general ophthalmologist sees patients on a daily basis who have symptoms related to the eyes or paraocular structures that can be clarified by the use of ultrasound. Common complaints encountered in the clinic include pain in and around the eye; double vision; various forms of flashes, floaters, and geometric shapes such as curves, shadows, and scotomata; bulging eyes; and lumps and bumps around the eyes. Also, ocular examination may reveal problems of which the patient may not be aware, such as iris and posterior segment lesions, elevated optic nerve heads, proptosis, and subtle ptosis.

It is relatively easy in the course of a busy office schedule to put the ultrasound probe on the patient's eye and in a few seconds detect an abnormality that can precisely diagnose the problem or direct the subsequent diagnostic workup. It is not unusual for a patient who has been seen by other medical practitioners with complaints that have been treated with various types of eye drops to be correctly diagnosed by ultrasound. The convenience to the patient of this modality is a major advantage over having to reschedule him/her for expensive radiologic testing. The cost effectiveness of ophthalmic echography is significant compared to other imaging studies. The average cost of a brain MRI is approximately US $1500, brain CT costs approximately US $800, and carotid Doppler costs approximately US $600. In contrast, the average cost of a diagnostic ophthalmic ultrasound examination is about US $300 based on the latest Current Procedural Terminology (CPT®) code 76510 for combined A- and B-scan examination. This cost advantage is illustrated by the following case.

# Case Study 1
## Optic Nerve Drusen

AI was a 10-year-old boy who complained of headaches severe enough to keep him home from school on several occasions for several months. He was taken to his pediatrician and then referred to a comprehensive ophthalmologist, who felt the optic discs were elevated. He was then referred to a neurologist who hospitalized the child and did a complete neurological examination, ordered a CT scan and then an MRI scan and subsequently a cerebral angiogram, and performed a lumbar puncture. This US $20,000 workup proved to be negative for central nervous system pathology. He ultimately was referred for echography, where B-scan quickly demonstrated buried calcified drusen as the cause for the disc irregularity (Fig. 1). A-scan measured the diameter of the optic nerves in the orbit to be within normal limits.

This book uses a case study approach to illustrate how useful echography can be in a typical ophthalmologist's or optometrist's office. This technology gives the clinician another dimension of diagnostic capability. It provides the ability to visualize the posterior segment otherwise obscured by a dense cataract or cloudy cornea. It enables examination of the retrobulbar and orbital structures in a patient presenting with pain or pressure around the eye. It facilitates analysis of visible lesions in the fundus on a level approximating histopathological tissue slices. It fills a niche among all the other powerful imaging technologies by providing information not otherwise obtainable. The clinician proficient in echography experiences a paradigm shift from frustration and inadequacy in dealing with certain types of eye problems to satisfaction in identifying and properly addressing the issue.

The quality of an echographic study is highly examiner dependent so it is essential that the practitioner receive hands-on training with someone skilled in echographic techniques. This is important for the B-scan, but proper use of the A-scan greatly expands one's diagnostic capabilities. The vertical spikes of this modality seem foreign compared to the recognizable anatomic sections of the eye displayed on the B-scan screen, but once understood they increase the diagnostic capacity of the examiner. Many people equate ophthalmic echography with the B-scan unit, which may or may not have a vector A-scan tracing at the bottom of the screen. The diagnostic capability of an instrument that has a separate dedicated A-scan probe is far superior to the single A/B probes. There are excellent combined A- and B-diagnostic echography units on the market that include biometric capability and range in cost from US $20,000 up to US $50,000 for those including an ultrasound biomicroscope (UBM).

A- and B-scan techniques are often used during the same examination for evaluation of the eye and orbit. B-scan is useful for intraocular processes because of its ability to display shape and anatomical relationship to other structures. It is very sensitive to the presence of high reflective material, such as intraocular foreign bodies of various types, and in detecting calcium, such as seen in optic nerve head drusen. Its value in the orbit has largely been supplanted by the continually evolving resolution of computer-linked radiologic technology, such as MRI, CT, and positron emission tomography (PET) scanning. However, B-scan remains clinically useful in the detection of orbital processes, such as

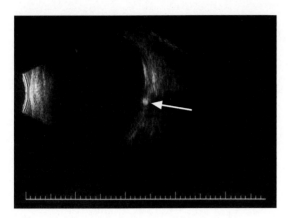

Fig. 1. Small calcified optic nerve drusen (*arrow*)

anterior orbital tumors, subtenon's infiltration by inflammatory or malignant cells, tendon thickening in myositis, and in displaying enlargement of the superior ophthalmic vein in various congestive disorders, such as carotid cavernous or other arteriovenous (AV) orbital fistulas.

The A-scan, on the other hand, fills several orbital niches inadequately covered by B-scan and radiologic scanning techniques. As stated in the American Academy of Ophthalmology Basic and Clinical Science Course, "standardized A-scan is much less aesthetically attractive to the beginner and is more difficult to perform. However, it potentially conveys much more diagnostic information than the B-scan."[1] Its ability to quantitate orbital structures, such as extraocular muscle and optic nerve thickness, can provide very important information not obtainable by other modalities. It is useful in the paraocular examination in such conditions as dacryoadenitis by providing measurements of the lacrimal gland and analysis of its internal structure. It can also provide information about the paranasal sinuses, nasolacrimal system, posterior sclera, and subtenon's space. It is able to provide information about the internal structure of intraocular and orbital tumors that is often highly correlated to the pathological diagnosis.

In the setting of a general ophthalmologic or optometric practice, there are many instances where echography is extremely useful and some in which it can make a major impact on the evaluation and treatment of the patient. Echography is an essential tool and unequalled by other imaging technology in the evaluation of the globe when opaque media precludes an optical view of the intraocular structures. Such abnormalities as corneal opacities, cells in the anterior chamber, lens opacities, and vitreous hemorrhage or inflammation interfere with adequate visualization by the direct or indirect ophthalmoscope. Ancillary tests, such as fluorescein angiography and optical coherence tomography (OCT), are useless in such conditions. The unique ability of high-frequency sound waves to pass through soft tissues without hindrance provides an acoustic window where light is not able to penetrate. The following case illustrates the ability of echography to correctly diagnose a disease process resulting in the application of appropriate therapy.

# Case Study 2
## Intumescent Lens and Angle Closure

MA is a 75-year-old woman who noted the sudden onset of a severe headache with concurrent loss of vision in her right eye. Her left eye was legally blind at the 20/200 level from preexisting macular degeneration, but she had been able to read and watch TV with her 20/40 right eye. She presented at her local emergency room, where a CT scan was performed because of the headache. It was read as normal by the radiologist.

The on-call ophthalmologist who was covering the emergency room that day saw her. He noted vision of bare light perception in her right eye and 20/200 in her left eye. Slit-lamp examination found 2+ to 3+ corneal edema and a poorly seen anterior chamber with 1+ cells and a cataractous lens. Her intraocular pressure was 35 mm left eye (OS) and 23 mm right eye (OD). Gonioscopy was difficult because of the corneal edema, but his impression was a probable closed angle; however, the sudden visual loss was suspicious for ocular ischemia with secondary anterior segment changes. She was started on topical steroids and pressure-lowering agents.

She was seen in his office the next day with markedly reduced pain and a reduction in intraocular pressure to 20 mm. However, her vision remained at the light perception level and she had persistent corneal edema, anterior chamber reaction, and lens opacity. The fundus could not be visualized. He performed a B-scan in his office that revealed a normal posterior segment with a clear vitreous cavity and an attached retina.

She was referred to the neuro-ophthalmology department at the university medical center because of the uncertainty of the diagnosis. A- and B-scan echography was performed and an immersion scan of the anterior segment revealed an intumescent lens and a shallow anterior chamber (Fig. 2). Cataract surgery was performed to improve the visual acuity and reduce the angle closure. The intraocular pressure returned to normal without medications and the corneal edema slowly resolved with improvement of visual acuity to 20/50.

The most common media opacity responsible for reduced vision is opacification of the crystalline lens. Echography is essential in enabling modern cataract surgery both by measuring the axial length of the eye for intraocular lens calculations and to evaluate the posterior pole when the cataract is so dense that the fundus cannot be visualized. Such pathology as vitreous opacities, retinal detachment, and intraocular tumors can be detected prior to lens removal.

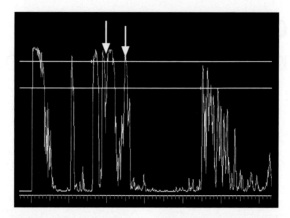

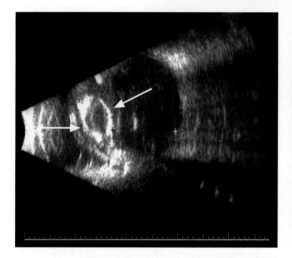 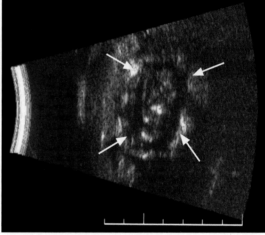

FIG. 2. Top: A scan of lens (*vertical arrows*). Bottom left: Immersion B scan (10MHz probe) of intumescent cataractous lens (*horizontal arrows*). Bottom right: High frequency immersion scan (20 MHz) of lens (*arrows*)

# Case Study 3
## Ciliary Body Melanoma and Sector Cataract

MH is a 73-year-old man who presented to his ophthalmologist with the complaint of reduced vision in his left eye over several months. Examination found visual acuity OD of 20/30 and OS of 20/50. Slit-lamp examination showed mild nuclear sclerosis in both lenses and a dense sectorial cortical cataract in the superior nasal quadrant of the left lens. The fundus could not be seen in this area due to the lens opacity.

B scan showed part of a very peripheral lesion in the vicinity of the superior nasal ciliary body. Immersion scanning confirmed the presence of a ciliary body mass most consistent with a malignant melanoma (Fig. 3). The patient was advised not to undergo cataract surgery because of the potential for disseminating tumor cells via surgical manipulation. It was elected to observe the tumor for growth with serial echography every 3 to 4 months.

Solid and cystic lesions of the ciliary body and iris may go undetected until discovered on a slit-lamp examination as a bulge in the iris. Transillumination can sometimes be helpful in this setting, but the results of this test are often equivocal. This area is best evaluated by an immersion B-scan. The standard 10-MHz probe is adequate to image some of these lesions, but 20 or 50 MHz (UBM) better characterizes smaller ones.

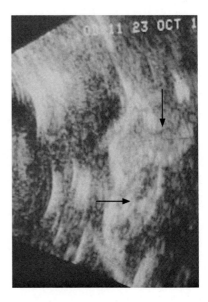

FIG. 3. B-scan of ciliary body melanoma (*vertical arrow*) in contact with crystalline lens (*horizontal arrow*)

# Case Study 4
## Small Ciliary Body Melanoma

NG is a 29-year-old woman who was noted on a routine eye examination to have a pigmented lesion of her left temporal iris root. The same optometrist had checked her in the prior year and this finding had not been noted at that time. Gonioscopy revealed focal involvement of the ciliary body but the adjacent angle was normal. The lesion seemed solid on transillumination.

Immersion scanning using a 20-MHz probe revealed a solid lesion of the anterior ciliary body (Fig. 4). It measured 1.6 mm by 1.5 mm. The finding of a probable ciliary body melanoma was discussed with the patient and she elected to observe

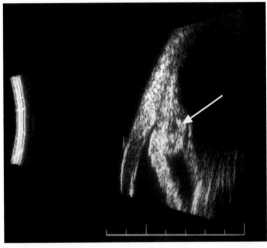

FIG. 5. Immersion scan (20-MHz probe) of iris/ciliary body cyst (*arrow*)

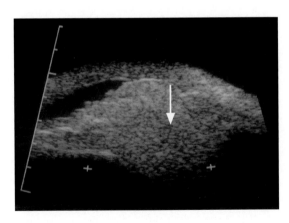

FIG. 4. B-scan of ciliary body melanoma (*arrow*)

it for growth with repeat echography every 4 to 6 months.

Iris and ciliary body cysts are more common than solid lesions and are easily diagnosed on immersion scanning (Fig. 5). Multicystic lesions are not uncommon. It is important to differentiate them from tumors such as melanoma.

The correct diagnosis of anterior segment problems with timely therapy can be facilitated by echographic techniques.

# Case Study 5
## Iris Bombe Around Intraocular Lens Implant

TA is a 62-year-old diabetic with a history of proliferative retinopathy. His right eye had become phthisical after unsuccessful retinal detachment surgery and the vision in his left eye had gradually decreased to the 20/200 level due to a combination of macular pathology and cataract formation. He underwent cataract surgery with the implantation of an anterior chamber intraocular lens implant (IOL) because of zonular dehiscence secondary to previous vitrectomy. His visual acuity improved to the 20/60 level, but he awoke on a Friday morning with a severe headache and marked reduction of his vision.

His ophthalmologist was out of town and a retinal specialist associated with the same group eventually saw him in the afternoon. Examination found vision OS of 20/400, intraocular pressure of 42, and "iris bombe" with iris bulging around the IOL in spite of an apparently patent surgical iridotomy. The patient was urgently referred for echography.

Immersion B-scan with a 20-MHz probe and a scleral shell filled with methylcellulose demonstrated an anterior chamber IOL with bulging of the iris almost to the cornea nasally and temporally, but otherwise the anterior chamber was deep (Fig. 6). This was consistent with trapped pockets of aqueous. A yttrium aluminum garnet (YAG) iridotomy was performed for three spots in the areas of the iris bulge with almost immediate flattening of the iris and relief of the patient's headache. Intraocular pressure was measured at 34 mm and had decreased to 9 mm by the next morning.

Echography is equally important in the evaluation of visible fundus lesions. A-scan provides the unique capacity to characterize the internal structure of intraocular tumors that is highly correlated to the tissue characteristics of the lesion. The quantitative (spike height and regularity) and kinetic (rapid spike movement) criteria described by Ossoinig[2] provide high specificity and sensitivity in evaluation of ocular lesions.

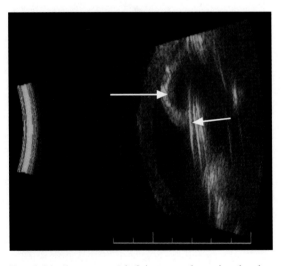

FIG. 6. Iris (*large arrow*) bulging around anterior chamber intraocular lens implant (*small arrow*)

# Case Study 6
## Choroidal Melanoma

MO is a 54-year-old woman who noted a shadow increasing over several months in the lower part of her field of vision in the left eye. She presented to her optometrist, who noted vision OD of 20/20 and OS of 20/30 with some distortion. Fundus examination of the left eye found a lightly pigmented lesion posterior to the superior equator. A visual field examination showed an inferior defect that extended into the lower part of central fixation.

B-scan revealed a solid lesion just above the left macula with basal dimension measurements of 6.2 mm circumferentially and 7.1 mm radially with 2+ spontaneous internal vascularity. A-scan measured thickness of the lesion to be 6.24 mm with medium and regular internal reflectivity (Fig. 7).

These findings were highly consistent with a choroidal melanoma and the patient was referred for radioactive plaque therapy after a systemic evaluation for metastatic melanoma was negative.

The quantitative capability of the A-scan has become essential in the management of intraocular tumors. The last 20 years has witnessed the transition from enucleation as the procedure of choice in the management of intraocular malignant melanoma to observation and radiation in cases of documented growth. A-scan measurements of the thickness of intraocular lesions are integral to this current management paradigm.

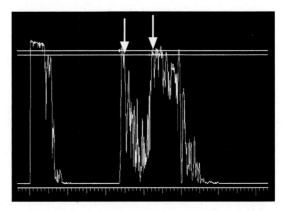

FIG. 7. A-scan of choroidal melanoma. Tumor surface indicated by *first arrow* and sclera by *second arrow*

# Case Study 7
## Small Choroidal Melanoma

GH is a 47-year-old woman who was seen by an ophthalmologist for a routine eye examination. She was found to have an elevated pigmented lesion in her temporal fundus on ophthalmoscopy. A fluorescein angiogram was obtained that showed early hyperfluorescence in the late arterial phase with increasing hyperfluorescence in the late venous phase that persisted after 15 minutes.

B-scan revealed a moderately echodense lesion that measured 5.5 mm in circumferential basal dimension and 6.1 mm in radial basal dimension. A-scan demonstrated a medium reflective lesion that measured 2.76 mm in thickness (Fig. 8). Spontaneous vascularity was not detected. The differential diagnosis included a large choroidal nevus or a small malignant melanoma. It was elected to follow her with repeat echography in 4 months. The lesion has been measured at the same thickness and basal dimensions for 2 years

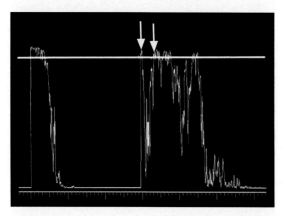

FIG. 8. A-scan of small choroidal melanoma. Tumor surface indicated by *first arrow* and sclera by *second arrow*

with the frequency of examination being extended to one per year.

Echography is an essential tool in the differential diagnosis of intraocular lesions. The echo signal characteristics of the most common choroidal mass lesions are distinctive enough to make an accurate diagnosis in most cases. This list includes malignant melanoma, choroidal hemangioma, metastatic tumors, retinoblastoma, and disease processes that simulate tumors, such as subretinal hemorrhage and disciform scars.

Malignant melanomas are low-to-medium reflective with a regular structure and usually demonstrate spontaneous internal vascularity on A-scan. The B-scan generally demonstrates a dome or mushroom shape (Fig. 9).

Choroidal hemangiomas are medium-to-high reflective with a regular internal structure and do not show spontaneous internal vascularity (Fig. 10).

Metastases to the choroid occur most frequently from primary tumors of the breast in women and the lung in men. Echography shows irregular internal structure with low and high spikes. Spontaneous internal vascularity is usually absent (Fig. 11).

Retinoblastomas are most often found in children at an average age of 2 but have been reported in adults.[3] They are generally calcified, which is readily detectable by echography (Fig. 12).

Subretinal hemorrhage is usually acute in onset and associated with choroidal neovascularization. Echography demonstrates low-to-medium internal reflectivity with regularity of the spikes due to the presence of liquid blood in an acute event versus irregularity in a more chronic process

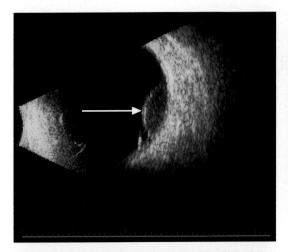

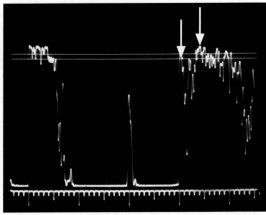

FIG. 11. A-scan of metastatic tumor of the choroid. Tumor surface indicated by *first arrow* and sclera by *second arrow*

with gliotic changes in the subretinal space and choroid (Fig. 13).

Echography is an important tool in evaluation of the retina, which may be hidden by bleeding in the vitreous cavity. Vitreous hemorrhage occurs relatively frequently as a result of neovascularization and vitreoretinal traction in diabetes and other vaso-occlusive disease, such as retinal vein occlusions. It can also occur in patients without underlying vascular disease as a result of traction on the retina in posterior vitreous detachment (PVD). Ultrasound is able to demonstrate an elevated retinal tear or focal retinal detachment that would otherwise go undetected and untreated with the possibility of evolution into a significant retinal detachment.

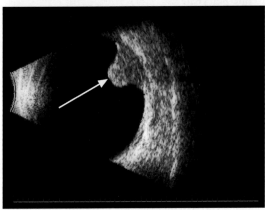

FIG. 9. Top: B-scan of dome-shaped choroidal melanoma (*arrow*). Bottom: B-scan of mushroom-shaped melanoma (*arrow*)

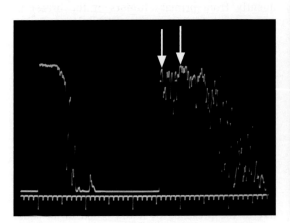

FIG. 10. A-scan of choroidal hemangioma. Tumor surface indicated by *first arrow* and sclera by *second arrow*

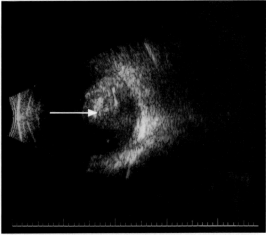

FIG. 12. B-scan of calcium clumps within retinoblastoma (*arrow*)

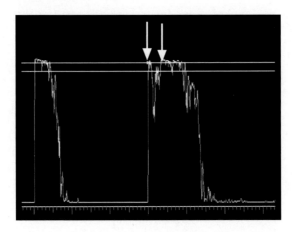

FIG. 13. A-scan of disciform scar (*vertical arrows*)

# Case Study 8
## Posterior Vitreous Detachment and Retinal Tear

NR is a 52-year-old moderately myopic man who noted the onset of flashes of light several weeks prior to presentation at his ophthalmologist's office. He experienced numerous little black floaters and clouding of his vision in the left eye on the morning of the consultation. Examination found vision 20/20 OD and 20/100 OS. Fundus examination was normal in the right eye and no fundus detail could be observed in the left because of a moderately dense vitreous hemorrhage. The patient was advised to stop taking aspirin products, minimize physical activity, and return for follow-up in 2 weeks. However, he was very bothered by the lack of vision in his left eye and sought a second opinion from a retinal specialist.

B-scan demonstrated a moderately dense vitreous hemorrhage and a total PVD with a focal area of vitreoretinal traction inferio-temporally (Fig. 14). The diagnosis of a flap tear with traction was made and the patient was instructed to elevate his head at night and to return the next day for reexamination. The plan was to treat the tear with laser as soon as the blood cleared enough to allow visualization or plan vitrectomy with endolaser if the blood remained and the retina showed evidence of detaching. By the third day the blood had settled enough to allow placement of laser spots around the tear and the retina remained attached.

Detachment of the vitreous occurs commonly in individuals past the age of 40 and 6% to 15% of patients with symptoms of flashes and floaters with a PVD will experience a retinal tear as part of this process.[4] The average practitioner will usually see at least one patient a day with a PVD. These individuals should be examined with indirect ophthalmoscopy and scleral depression and then followed-up within a few weeks. They can be informed that the floater will become less noticeable over time.

A number of people experience only syneresis of the vitreous gel resulting in one or more floaters without a detachment of the vitreous. They sometimes present with complaints of a floater that can be quite concerning to them. Demonstration of the opacity on B-scan and the explanation that it is nonthreatening to the eye can be reassuring to the patient.

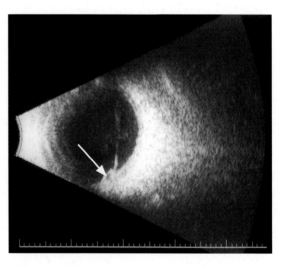

FIG. 14. B-scan of vitreoretinal traction (*arrow*)

# Case Study 9
## Vitreous Syneresis

BG is a 34-year-old man who noted a "shape like a half-circle" in his vision that bothered him constantly. He related this symptom to his primary care doctor who ordered an MRI scan to eliminate intracranial pathology. The scan was normal and the patient was referred to an ophthalmologist. Examination was unremarkable with visual acuity in both eyes of 20/20 and a normal fundus examination. A posterior vitreous detachment was not detected. B-scan demonstrated a small moderately reflective mobile surface in the vitreous that was consistent with condensation and syneresis (Fig. 15). This was demonstrated to the patient and he was given a copy of a photo for his records. He expressed great relief that "there was nothing seriously wrong with the vision" and soon stopped obsessing about the floater.

Some patients can develop a retinal detachment with no or minimal symptoms of a PVD. They may describe a "curved surface or shape" in the peripheral visual field of one eye. If it is a very shallow detachment, ophthalmoscopic examination may not detect it, whereas B-scan is a very sensitive tool with a high sensitivity level to even a slight separation of the retina from the underlying retinal pigment epithelium.

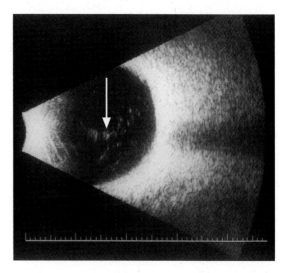

FIG. 15. B-scan of vitreous condensation and syneresis (*small arrow*)

# Case Study 10
## Shallow Retinal Detachment

AH is a 57-year-old Indian woman who presented to an oculoplastic specialist with the complaints of intermittent pain around her left eye. She also mentioned a "curved reflection" noticed intermittently in her upper outer quadrant of vision. Ocular examination including fundus inspection was described as normal. A CT scan was read as normal and she was referred for echography to eliminate myositis or other orbital inflammatory processes.

Orbital A-scan showed only a few low ethmoid sinus signals felt to be most consistent with mild mucous membrane swelling. B-scan detected a shallow inferior nasal retinal detachment (Fig. 16) and she was referred to the retina service for management.

Pain in or around the eyes is one of the most common patient complaints in any ophthalmologic or optometric practice. This symptom is often hard to characterize even after a detailed history is taken and a careful examination is performed. This is especially true if the symptoms are intermittent and not present at the time of the consultation. The practitioner must decide how vigorously to pursue the diagnostic workup. Imaging studies, such as CT and MRI scans, are expensive and often require the patient to take several hours out of a busy schedule to undergo the test. Echography provides a rapid and cost-effective method to efficiently screen for ocular and orbital causes of the pain. Such entities as scleritis, myositis, pseudotumor, superiosteal abscess and hemorrhage, mucoceles, sinusitis, optic neuritis, orbital and lacrimal tumors, and dacryoadenitis are readily detectable by echography.

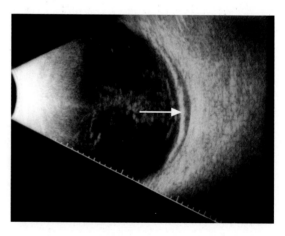

FIG. 16. B-scan of shallow retinal detachment (*arrow*)

# Case Study 11
## Dacryoadenitis

MB is a 25-year-old woman who complained of intermittent aching pain around her left eye over a period of several weeks. Examination was unremarkable with only slight tenderness to palpation of the left superior orbit. A CT scan had been ordered by her primary care doctor and was read as normal by the radiologist. A-scan was performed by the ophthalmologist and demonstrated thickening of the left lacrimal gland of 15.45 mm compared to a normal measurement of 13.2 mm for the right gland. Internal reflectivity was medium reflective compared to the higher reflectivity of the right lacrimal gland (Fig. 17). These findings were most consistent with a low-grade dacryoadenitis and she was given a 2-week course of oral antibiotics with resolution of her symptoms. Remeasurement by A-scan showed reduction in size of the gland to 14.3 mm.

Echography is very useful in the evaluation of the optic nerve. The blurred optic disc is encountered relatively commonly in the course of general ophthalmologic or optometric practice. Many normal discs are somewhat irregular in appearance with blurred margins and this can cause concern for the practitioner about a possible intracranial process, especially in the setting of a patient complaining of headaches. Brain tumors are estimated to occur in a very small percentage of patients, about 1 in 1000.[5] However, in a litigatious society such as the United States, many of these individuals are referred for neuroimaging, which usually turns out to be normal. The wasted time and money spent in such defensive medicine is considerable, and adds to the increasing healthcare portion of the national budget.

The ability of A-scan to quantitate the optic nerve thickness is quite helpful in the evaluation of papilledema. It can assist in answering the question

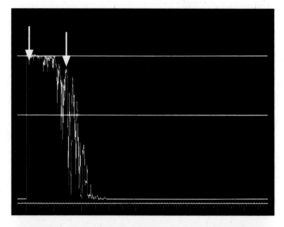

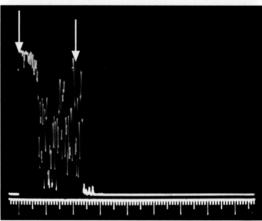

FIG. 17. Top: A-scan of right lacrimal gland (*vertical arrows* define the anterior and posterior surface of the gland). Bottom: A-scan of left lacrimal gland (*arrows*)

of whether an engorged optic nerve head is due to increased fluid in the nerve sheath, as occurs in pseudotumor cerebri, or the result of solid thickening as seen in glioma, meningioma, or cellular infiltration of the nerve sheaths. B-scan gives a very accurate morphological view of the optic nerve head. It is extremely sensitive to calcium deposits such as optic disc drusen.

# Case Study 12
## Optic Nerve Drusen

CJ is a 27-year-old woman who had a long history of migraine-like headaches and had noticed an increase in severity and frequency over the past few months. She was seen by her primary care doctor and told, "everything was normal except for mild hypertension." A low dose of hydrochorothiazide was started, and she was advised to see her eye doctor to eliminate an ocular cause for her symptoms.

An optometrist examined her eyes and documented 20/20 uncorrected vision in both eyes and intraocular pressure of 16 mm in each eye. Pupil reactions were normal with no afferent pupil defect and confrontation visual fields were full. Slit-lamp examination was unremarkable, but the fundus examination documented some irregularity of the optic nerve heads, especially on the right. No spontaneous venous pulsations were appreciated. Humphrey visual field testing was normal except for possible mild enlargement of the blind spots bilaterally. These findings were discussed with the patient and it was suggested that she undergo further workup.

She was referred to a neurologist for an examination followed by an MRI scan. This showed one or two nonspecific white spots in the paraventicular area, but no evidence of a mass lesion. It was assumed that she probably had pseudotumor cerebri and a lumbar puncture (LP) was performed. The opening pressure was borderline so she was started on diamox. She had a severe post-LP headache for several days afterwards, but did experience some relief from her usual headaches with the diamox. She noted increasing side effects from this medication over the next several months.

The nausea and paresthesias became intolerable and she finally stopped the medication. She asked for a second opinion and was referred to a neuro-ophthalmologist. He reviewed the history, examined the optic nerves with ophthalmoscopy, and carefully evaluated the MRI scan. He questioned the diagnosis of pseudotumor cerebri and referred her for diagnostic echography.

A-scan measured the optic nerves to be in a normal range with 2.47 mm OD and 2.5 mm OS (Fig. 18). B-scan showed mild elevation of both discs with small buried calcified drusen bilaterally (Fig. 19). The neuro-ophthalmologist reassured her that she probably had pseudopapilledema and could safely stop taking carbonic anhydrase inhibitors with an annual follow-up examination unless her headaches worsened or new symptoms, such as diplopia, appeared.

Buried optic disc drusen present with disc or peripapillary nerve fiber layer hemorrhage in 2%

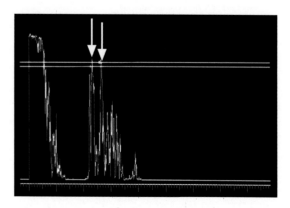

FIG. 18. A-scan of optic nerve sheaths (*vertical arrows*)

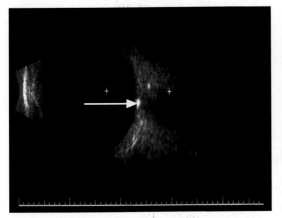 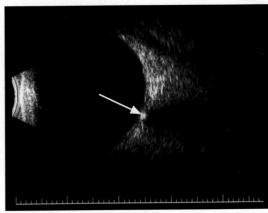

FIG. 19. Left: B-scan of calcified optic disc drusen in the right eye (*arrow*). Right: The left eye (*arrow*)

to 10% of cases.[6] Four types of retinal hemorrhages have been described: (1) splinter nerve fiber layer hemorrhages at the disc; (2) hemorrhages of the optic nerve head extending into the vitreous; (3) deep papillary hemorrhages; and (4) deep peripapillary hemorrhages with or without extension into the macula. Tiny calcifications are easily missed on radiologic studies. Echography is more sensitive than routine CT scans in the presence of faint calcium deposition such as with small buried drusen.

# Case Study 13
## Optic Nerve Druse and Disc Hemorrhage

SF is a 42-year-old woman who was noted on a routine eye examination to have peripapillary hemorrhage just inferior to her left optic disc. Visual field testing showed a focal arcuate defect superior to the blind spot. A fluorescein angiogram did not reveal any subretinal neovascularization.

B-scan demonstrated a tiny druse buried in the optic nerve head (Fig. 20) that was assumed to be the source of the hemorrhage and the patient was told to follow-up in 4 months unless any symptoms of visual loss or distortion occurred.

Echo spikes from calcium within the nerve substance, such as with calcified drusen, stand out in contrast to the relatively lower reflective nerve parenchyma. The same explanation applies to high reflective material within the optic nerve vasculature as sometimes found in central retinal artery emboli. Sergott and colleagues[7] reported that 31% of patients with central retinal artery occlusions were found to have embolic material posterior to the lamina cribrosa on B-scan evaluation with a color Doppler unit. These can also be demonstrated on a standard grayscale B-scan unit.

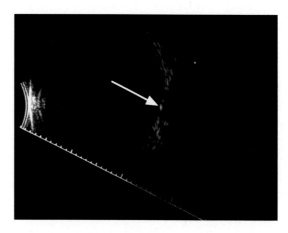

FIG. 20. B-scan of tiny buried druse (*arrow*)

# Case Study 14
## Central Retinal Artery Embolus

CL is a 70-year-old man who presented with the history of marked reduction of vision in his left eye several days ago. Examination found vision 20/30 OD and OS of hand motions at 1 meter. He had a 3+ afferent papillary defect in this eye. Slit-lamp examination was normal and fundus examination found some narrowing of the retinal arterioles and a faint reddish appearance to the central macula. It was assumed that a vascular event had occurred and a workup was done including erythrocyte sedimentation rate, C-reactive protein, complete blood count (CBC) with platelet level, antiphospholipid antibodies, plasma homocysteine, and a carotid duplex scan. These tests were unremarkable except for 50% stenosis of both carotid arteries.

He was referred for orbital color Doppler testing. The grayscale B-scan part of the study showed a small high reflective signal in the optic nerve posterior to the lamina cribrosa in the area of the central retinal artery (Fig. 21). This was consistent with embolic material within the artery most likely originating from an atheromatous plaque in the carotid artery, but a cardiac source could not be ruled out so an echocardiogram was performed and interpreted as normal. A carotid angiogram confirmed an ulcerated atheroma from which the embolus had most likely come. The patient was given the option of medical antiplatelet therapy with aspirin or a surgical endarterectomy.

The sensitivity of echography in detecting intraocular calcification with optic nerve drusen is equally important in the evaluation of leukocoria to eliminate retinoblastoma. The detection of a mass in a small child has ominous implications regarding morbidity and mortality. There is a long differential diagnosis for leukocoria, but the presence of calcium in a mass found within a child's eye is almost pathognomonic for retinoblastoma. However, according to Bullock et al.,[8] it is absent in about 10% of retinoblastomas so any intraocular mass in a child must be viewed with suspicion. CT scans accurately detect calcium when it is present in a moderate amount, but can miss it when only small scattered deposits are present within the tumor. Wilson states, "more than one imaging modality should be used in the evaluation of suspected retinoblastoma, as calcification may be absent on the computed tomography but present on B-mode ultrasound."[9] MRI scans are not able to detect calcium in these tumors.

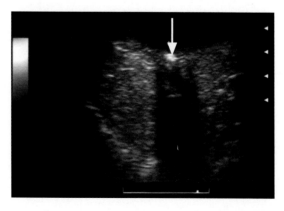

FIG. 21. B-scan of embolic material in central retinal artery (*arrow*). (Photo courtesy of Dr Robert Sergott)

# Case Study 15
## Retinoblastoma with Fine Calcification

TM is a 2-year-old child who was noted by his parents to have a "wandering" left eye that worsened over several months. They consulted with an ophthalmologist who documented an esotropia of 30 prism diopters and found leukocoria on testing the right red reflex. She noted a whitish pink intraocular mass encroaching on the temporal macula on fundus examination. She suspected a retinoblastoma and obtained a CT scan for confirmation. No calcium was detected on the scan (Fig. 22) so she referred the child for echography.

B-scan demonstrated a subretinal mass in the temporal fundus that measured 4.6 mm thick by 8 mm by 7 mm in basal dimensions (Fig. 23). Multiple tiny high reflective signals were seen within the lesion consistent with fine calcification. The diagnosis of retinoblastoma was established and the child was referred to an oncologist for further workup and treatment.

Some pediatric ophthalmologists are now referring children suspected of having retinoblastoma directly for echography and bypassing CT. The optic nerve and brain are then imaged by MRI to rule out intracranial extension of the lesion.[10]

Echography is an excellent screening tool in the office for orbital problems such as proptosis. The most common cause of both bilateral and unilateral proptosis is Graves' disease and echography is a very sensitive and specific modality to evaluate the extraocular muscles. B-scan can demonstrate qualitative muscle enlargement although not to the degree achievable on CT and MRI scans. A-scan adds a quantitative dimension by providing a means to accurately measure muscle thickness. In addition, the analysis of the A-scan spikes within the muscle

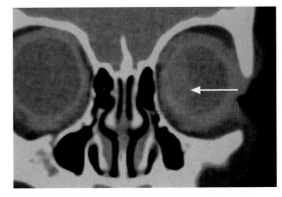

Fig. 22. Computed tomography scan of retinoblastoma (*arrow*)

gives tissue signatures that are characteristic for Graves' as contrasted to other causes of muscle thickening, such as myositis.

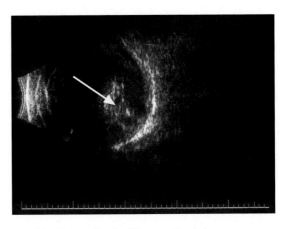

Fig. 23. B-scan of retinoblastoma (*arrow*)

# Case Study 16
## Extraocular Muscles in Graves' Disease

JC is a 32-year-old woman who noted increasing prominence of her right eye over several months. She presented to her primary care doctor, who ordered thyroid tests (TSH and T4) that were normal. He then ordered a CT scan that was interpreted as normal by the radiologist with no mass lesions detected and extraocular muscle thickness "within normal limits." She was referred to an ophthalmologist who documented possible lid lag on the right side and exophthalmometry readings of 19 mm OD and 16 mm OS. She was referred for echography. A-scan revealed several muscles in both orbits that were greater than upper limits of normal for muscle thickness. The internal reflectivity pattern of these muscles was heterogeneous and consistent with Graves' disease (Fig. 24). Thyroid antibody testing was performed and was moderately positive. She was instructed about her disease and how to manage any symptoms that may occur, such as puffy lids and dry, scratchy eyes. She was scheduled for a follow-up examination in 6 months and warned about symptoms of optic nerve compression, and was specifically told to check her color sensitivity to a red object at home.

The extraocular muscles may also be thickened in cases of orbital myositis but the A-scan is quite helpful in viewing the internal structure, which can clarify the differential diagnosis of the enlarged muscle. This capability of internal analysis is especially valuable in cases where the muscle is not abnormally enlarged.

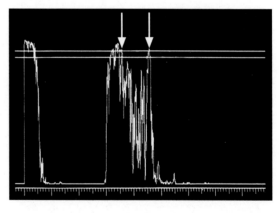

FIG. 24. A-scan of extraocular muscle involved by Graves' disease (*vertical arrows*)

# Case Study 17
## Orbital Myositis

CJ is a 26-year-old man who noted the rapid onset of painful swelling of his right upper and lower eyelids. He was seen at the emergency room and a CT scan was felt to be consistent with mild sinusitis and a preseptal cellulitis and he was given intravenous (IV) antibiotics and sent home on an oral agent. His symptoms improved over several days but then similar symptoms occurred in his left eye. He was seen again at the emergency room and the ophthalmologist on call was asked to come in.

Examination showed slight left upper lid swelling and two prism diopters of left esotropia with some pain on abduction. The CT scan was reviewed and the extraocular muscles appeared subjectively normal in thickness. Echography was later performed and the A-scan measured normal muscle thickness, but the left lateral rectus was low to medium and regular reflective compared to the higher and more irregular reflectivity of the right lateral rectus. This was interpreted as being consistent with inflammatory infiltration (Fig. 25). The patient was started on indomethacin with resolution of his symptoms over the next several weeks.

Orbital tumors usually present with proptosis and/or globe displacement in the vertical plane. Also, the presence of choroidal or retinal folds is sometimes associated with a retrobulbar mass although they are often idiopathic and these patients can be spared unnecessary CT or MRI scanning by a brief screening ultrasound examination in the office.

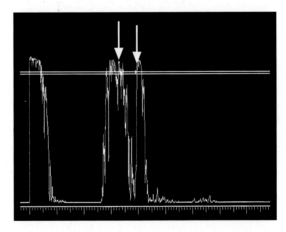

FIG. 25. A-scan of extraocular muscle involved by myositis (*vertical arrows*)

# Case Study 18
## Idiopathic Choroidal Folds

PR is a 26-year-old man who noted some blurring of the vision in his right eye and scheduled an evaluation by his optometrist. Examination found vision 20/25 OD and 20/15 OS. There was mild distortion of the vision in the OD to amsler grid testing. The slit-lamp examination was unremarkable, but the fundus examination showed moderate choroidal folds in the right eye. An orbital tumor was suspected and the patient underwent CT scanning that did not demonstrate a mass and was reported as normal. The patient sought a second opinion from the oculoplastic service at the university medical center.

Ultrasound was performed and no orbital mass was detected by either A- or B-scan. However, there was some subtle flattening of the globe consistent with idiopathic choroidal folds (Fig. 26).

However, choroidal folds can be the result of compression of the posterior wall of the globe by an orbital mass. Such lesions can be detected and characterized at the time of the initial examination with timely referral of the patient for directed follow-up studies and optimal management by a specialist.

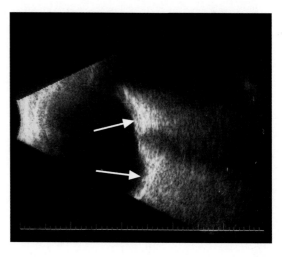

FIG. 26. B-scan of flattening of posterior globe wall (*arrows*)

# Case Study 19
## Choroidal Folds and Orbital Lymphoma

CC is a 34-year-old man who presented to his ophthalmologist with the complaint of "a little distortion of the vision in the right eye." Examination found best corrected vision 20/20-2 OD and 20/20 OS. No afferent pupil defect was noted and the eye appeared normal except for the presence of moderate choroidal folds. Exophthalmometry was not performed. B-scan was performed and a low reflective retrobulbar lesion was immediately detected (Fig. 27). The differential diagnosis included a cystic lesion but lymphoma could not be ruled out. The patient was referred to an orbital surgeon who performed a biopsy with a pathological diagnosis of lymphoma.

The ability of A-scan to display internal structure of orbital tumors is very helpful in the differential diagnosis of such lesions. The most common primary tumor of the orbit in adults is the cavernous hemangioma and the A-scan pattern is almost pathognomonic.

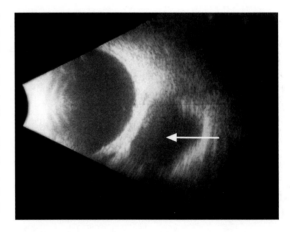

FIG. 27. B-scan of orbital mass (*arrow*)

# Case Study 20
## Cavernous Hemangioma

RJ is a 56-year-old woman who was told by her daughter that her right eye "looked bigger than her left." She consulted her primary care doctor who told her she probably had Graves' disease because of a history of thyroid problems, including treatment for hyperthyroidism with radioactive iodine 131 a number of years ago. An ophthalmologist was consulted who performed an examination and confirmed the presence of 5 mm of proptosis in her right eye. The remainder of the examination was normal including visual acuity in both eyes of 20/20.

B-scan showed an oval encapsulated intraconal mass of over 20 mm in diameter. A-scan demonstrated high internal reflectivity in the anterior part of the lesion with a progressive decrease in spike height towards its posterior aspect (Fig. 28). No spontaneous vascularity was noted and the tumor decreased in size about 20% when moderately firm pressure was applied with the ultrasound probe against the globe. These findings were highly consistent with a cavernous hemangioma and subsequent surgical excision confirmed this diagnosis.

Lacrimal gland enlargement by inflammatory or neoplastic involvement is a relatively common cause of temporal lid swelling in mild cases with inferior displacement of the globe in moderate-to-severe involvement of the gland.

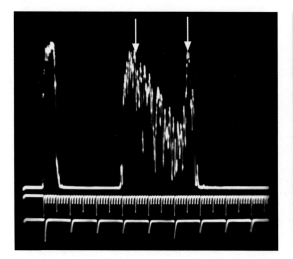 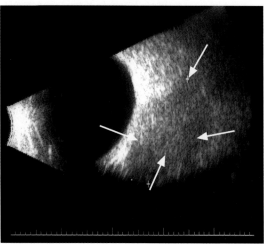

FIG. 28. Left: A-scan of cavernous hemangioma (*vertical arrows*). Right: B-scan of the same lesion (*arrows*)

# Case Study 21
## Pleomorphic Adenoma of Lacrimal Gland

KR is a 28-year-old man who noted some fullness in the outer part of his left upper lid. He thought he could feel some firmness and mild tenderness just below the upper outer rim of the orbital bone. Examination by his ophthalmologist confirmed these findings with inferior displacement of the globe by 2 mm. Echography was performed in the office and showed enlargement of the left lacrimal gland to 18.5 mm and high internal reflectivity, which became lower as the spikes traveled across the gland (Fig. 29). This was suspicious for a benign mixed cell tumor and he was referred for CT scanning and then to an orbit surgeon for an en bloc excision of the lacrimal gland.

Anterior orbital lesions can involve the eyelids with resultant swelling. Echography is a very useful office test to quickly screen for such lesions with some posterior extension back into the orbit. A relatively common tumor in children with such presentation is the infantile or capillary hemangioma.

This can grow rapidly with a doubling time of weeks and must be differentiated from more serious tumors such as rhabdomyosarcoma.

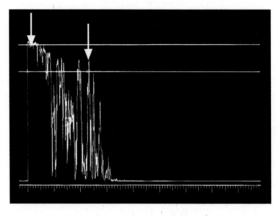

FIG. 29. A-scan of pleomorphic adenoma of the lacrimal gland (*vertical arrows*)

# Case Study 22
## Infantile Hemangioma

SF is a 6-month-old girl who was noted by her parents to have a fullness of her left lower lid that increased when she was crying. This had become more prominent over a few weeks to the point that several relatives had commented on it. The pediatrician was consulted and he ordered a CT scan that showed some nonspecific fullness of the lid but no distinct mass was seen. The child was referred to an ophthalmologist who performed an ultrasound.

A-scan showed a moderately soft lesion measuring 15.5 mm in anterior-to-posterior dimensions with irregular internal reflectivity (Fig. 30). An obstetrical acoustic Doppler unit with a small probe adapted for the orbit demonstrated rapid arterial blood flow within the more central part of the lesion. These findings were highly consistent with an infantile or capillary hemangioma and she was referred to a pediatric ophthalmologist for steroid injection into the tumor.

Echography has the highest specificity of all the imaging studies for the diagnosis of infantile hemangioma. The irregular internal reflectivity on A-scan is a result of the tissue architecture of these lesions with cellular areas (lower reflectivity) interspersed with vascular channels (Fig. 31). They typically demonstrate relatively high arterial blood flow on Doppler studies as opposed to the stagnant venous flow of the cavernous hemangiomas seen in older children and adults. They may be found in the posterior orbit but more commonly present as a "strawberry" lesion visible under the eyelid skin.

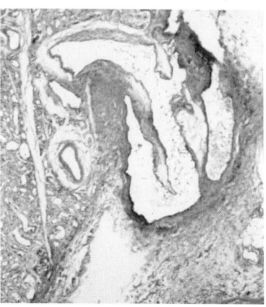

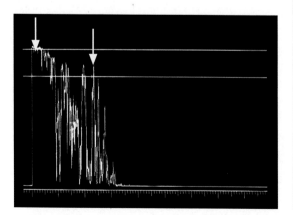

FIG. 30. A-scan of infantile hemangioma (*vertical arrows*)

FIG. 31. Pathology slide of infantile hemangioma

# Case Study 23
## Infantile Hemangioma

MT is a 2-month-old girl who was born with a bluish lesion near her lower right punctum. It grew in size over several weeks and her pediatrician urgently referred her to a pediatric ophthalmologist with the diagnosis of a probable dacriocystocele. The ophthalmologist was prepared to take her to surgery that day to decompress the cystocele but questioned the diagnosis on clinical examination. She was referred on an urgent basis for echography.

A-scan demonstrated a 16.2 mm moderately soft lesion with irregular internal reflectivity of both high and low areas (Fig. 32). Doppler ultrasound revealed diffuse arterial blood flow highly consistent with the diagnosis of infantile hemangioma. Surgery was cancelled and it was elected to watch the lesion with the plan to inject steroids if it grew enough to cause any visual distortion.

The preceding are examples of the value of ophthalmic echography in the clinical setting.

The practitioner who invests the time and effort in learning this technique will realize an immediate benefit in daily clinical practice. This book will provide an in-depth view of this important modality.

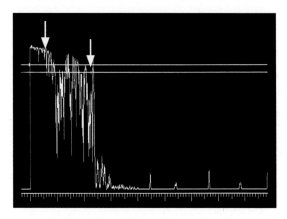

FIG. 32. A-scan of infantile hemangioma (*arrows*)

# Part II
## Basic Principles

The fundamental physical principle underlying diagnostic ultrasound as used in a number of medical disciplines is the generation of sound waves at frequencies above the range of human hearing (greater than 20,000 Hertz or 20 KHz) by the vibration of a thin crystal stimulated by pulses of electric current. The waves of sound then propagate through a medium and are reflected by tissue surfaces back to the resting crystal that is then made to vibrate, generating electrical impulses that are amplified and processed to show a pattern on an oscilloscope screen.

The diagnostic A-scan probe (Fig. 33) has a wafer-thin ceramic crystal near the tip that is stimulated by bursts of electric current to vibrate at a frequency of 8 MHz (8 million cycles per second). The crystal converts this electrical energy into sound energy and then the same crystal receives the reflected sound waves. Its mechanical vibrations are converted to an electric current. This is called the piezoelectric effect, where the same crystal acts as sender and receiver of sound. The transducer transmits sound waves for about 4% of the time. Its vibrations are then damped and it receives the reflected sound waves for the remaining 96% of the time. The returning sound wave is amplified and displayed on a screen as vertical lines of various heights. The amplitude of each spike is related to the strength of the reflection from tissue interfaces from which it is reflected.

The B-scan probe (Fig. 34) uses a transducer similar to that of an A probe, but it sweeps back and forth at an average rate of 25 oscillations per second. It generates sound waves at a frequency of 10 MHz (10 million cycles per second). The returning echoes are processed to display bright dots on a screen which are combined to generate an image. This generates a series of echoes that are processed like pixels on a computer screen to generate an image. The brightness of the image is correlated to the strength of the sound reflection corresponding to the height of the vertical spike on the A-scan image. Current generation B-scan probes are sealed and oil filled, unlike previous versions that had to be injected with distilled water before each use.

Karl Ossoinig pioneered the concept of standardized echography and much of his work concentrated on the A-scan. His criteria for the characterization of numerous intraocular and orbital lesions are based on the use of a standardized A-scan technique, including an S-shaped amplifier in the unit that combines features of linear and logarithmic amplifiers. An examiner cannot take the criteria he developed and use them successfully to diagnose pathology unless an A-scan is used based on these principles. There are several units produced that utilize separate A- and B-scan probes that can be reliably used to evaluate lesions based on the criteria of Ossoinig. Several companies produce excellent ophthalmic ultrasound units that are modular in design with the option to add features to the basic unit as need and budgets allow. It is highly advantageous to have separate diagnostic A- and B-scan probes with individual signal processors.

The history of ultrasound in ophthalmology is a relatively recent one. The principles of ultrasound were understood in the late 1800s and were utilized to develop sonar for submarine warfare in World Wars I and II. During this time, industry adapted the technology for the detection of flaws in materials. The first paper describing the ocular

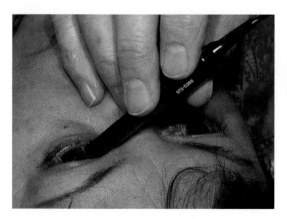

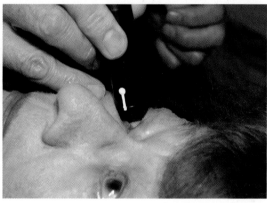

Fig. 33. A-scan probe                              Fig. 34. B-scan probe

use of the "reflectoscope" by Mundt and Hughes appeared in the ophthalmic literature in 1956.[11] They basically described the use of the A-scan to image various ocular structures and abnormalities. An adaptation of the instrument was also used about this time to image gallstones in a patient with cholelithiasis.

Diagnostic echography now has widespread application in medicine, mainly in the specialties of obstetrics and gynecology, cardiovascular disease, peripheral vascular disease, gastroenterology, neurology, and urology. The frequencies used for non-ophthalmic organ systems usually are in the range of 3 to 5 MHz to allow deep penetration into such areas of the body as the abdomen. Higher frequencies than this provide better resolution but poor penetration into the depths required for the examination of most organ systems. The resolution possible in the examination of the eye is much higher than in other parts of the body. The globe is mostly a fluid-filled structure that is ideal for the propagation of ultrasound. The 8 to 10 MHz frequencies used in the examination of all but the more anterior part of the eye allows axial resolution of structures as small as 0.10 mm. The 50 MHz ultrasound biomicroscope (UBM) probe used for anterior segment scans enables resolution on the micron scale (less than 40 μm). Such imaging capability allows the diagnosis of lesions on almost a histopathologic level and is reflected in the 99.7% diagnostic accuracy for choroidal melanoma as reported in the Collaborative Ocular Melanoma Study (COMS).

Ophthalmic echography has advantages over other imaging techniques in the clinical practice of ophthalmology. An instrument that is readily available, portable, cost effective, and provides rapid and accurate diagnosis of intraocular and orbital pathology can be an invaluable aid to the practicing clinician. The use of diagnostic ultrasound reached a zenith in the 1970s, when it was the major imaging modality for the eye and orbit. Plain film x-rays were only of use within the globe to diagnose metallic foreign bodies and within the orbit to image processes that affected the bone. However, the preference for echography as the imaging technique of choice proved to be short lived as computer technology was applied to radiologic imaging. Computed tomography (CT) scanning has progressed from requiring hours to gather the raw data for a single scan to current generation scanners that can reconstruct an image from millions of points of data in 1 second. This ability of increasingly powerful computers to process masses of data has resulted in the incredible anatomical images possible today. CT imaging was challenged in the mid-1980s by magnetic resonance imaging (MRI) technology based on different principles but just as dependent on computer processing.

Magnetic resonance imaging scanning doesn't use x-rays or nuclear energy to image. The original name for this process was NMR (nuclear magnetic resonance), but the public aversion to anything "nuclear" prompted the name change to MRI. This technology uses very powerful magnets to affect the spin of protons and records the emitted radio signals as the protons return to their baseline state. The most commonly imaged proton is the one in the hydrogen nucleus. The rapidly advancing computer graphic capabilities pioneered in CT scanners were adapted to this modality and MRI is now the procedure of choice for most soft tissue imaging. Functional MRI (fMRI) is a recent application of magnetic resonance imaging. A baseline MRI scan is taken of the brain and then multiple scans are taken during different patient activities. Other evolving MRI techniques include diffusion-weighted MRI, magnetic resonance spectroscopy, and MR dynamic color mapping. MRI technology followed and in many ways has surpassed CT technology. Another rapidly developing area of medical imaging technology is that of radionuclide imaging including PET (positron emission tomography) and SPECT (single photon emission computed tomography).

This technology utilizes the uptake of specially prepared radioactively tagged molecules (most commonly glucose but sometimes water or ammonia) to image physiologic processes as they occur in the living organism. Glucose is metabolized throughout the normal body, but is utilized more by rapidly dividing cancer cells. These areas appear brighter on the PET scan. These scanners are combined in a CT to localize the anatomical locations of the "hot spots" (Fig. 35). The potential for the ability to image pathology at the biochemical level is the latest step in an incredible diagnostic imaging journey that started just over 30 years ago. PET/CT scanners are beginning to make their appearance in major medical centers. The next imagers will surely address the genetic revolution now occurring in medicine. The ability to study disease and image function at the level of the gene will be the tools of future generations of doctors and technicians.

These radiologic advances have largely replaced B-scan ultrasound as the procedure of choice for the orbit and some clinicians suggest its usefulness in the study of intraocular pathology is also threatened. High-resolution MRI scans can demonstrate intraocular tumors, retinal detachments, and vitreous hemorrhage. Because most communities have several MRI and CT scanners available, the impetus is strong to utilize these modalities for ophthalmic diagnosis. Only a few university medical centers have dedicated ocular ultrasound departments with technicians skilled in the use of diagnostic echography.

In many areas the practice of ocular ultrasound is now mostly confined to A-scan biometry in comprehensive ophthalmology practices and the

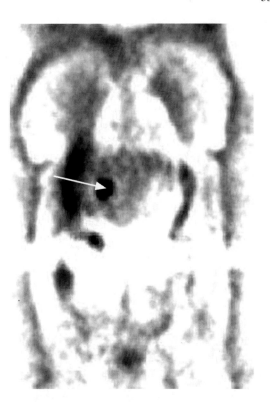

FIG. 35. Positron emission tomography (PET) scan of foci of metastatic tumors (*arrow*)

use of B-scan by retina specialists. Ophthalmic biometry units are relatively inexpensive, which has allowed most ophthalmologists who perform cataract surgery to purchase their own. Eye techs are generally trained only in biometry and intraocular lens implant (IOL) calculations and not diagnostic ultrasound. Retinal specialists use their B-scan units mostly to aid in preoperative and postoperative evaluations of vitreous hemorrhage and retinal detachments. A few ocular oncologists utilize them in the evaluation of ocular tumors.

Most ophthalmologic ultrasound units are sold primarily for the B-scan capability. Practitioners are generally most comfortable with B-scan images because of the recognizable topography displayed on the screen, as opposed to the unfamiliar vertical spikes of the A-scan. This is especially true for a generation familiar with the imaging capabilities of CT and MRI scans. These modalities "cut" radiologic sections through structures and the medically trained mind is comfortable mentally reconstructing the entire lesion from a compilation of these slices. Three-dimensional (3D) imaging is evolving that does such reconstruction with computer graphics, but most CT scans are currently displayed as a series of tissue slices. The ultrasound B-scan is based on the same principle of image processing, although by acoustic instead of radiologic sectioning. An A-scan acts more like penetrating tissue with a needle to take a "core" sample for biopsy versus "slicing" sections of the tissue with the B-scan.

An example of the A- versus B-scan dichotomy is the familiar mushroom shape of a choroidal melanoma as it breaks through Bruch's membrane that is immediately evident to the untrained eye on the B-scan but displays only a series of vertical internal spikes on the A-scan (Fig. 36). However, the diagnostic information contained in all of those "dancing" lines on the A-scan is the major reason for

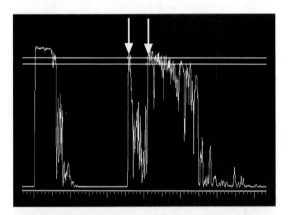

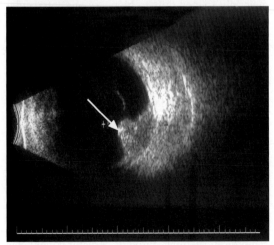

FIG. 36. Top: A-scan of malignant melanoma of the choroid. Bottom: B-scan of the tumor (*arrows*)

the 99.7% accuracy of the diagnosis of melanomas reported in the recently completed COMS study.

The A-scan displays the reflected signals as vertical lines. It is like freezing the B-scan transducer so it does not oscillate and recoding the signals from that point as a line instead of a grayscale dot. The height of the vertical line is a function of the reflectivity of the interface as is the brightness of the B-scan dot. The physical basis for the intensity of the reflected signal is impedance. The equation, $Z$ (impedance) = sound velocity ($v$) × tissue density ($d$) is the physicist's way of saying that the greater the difference in impedance between two different media the higher the A-scan spike or the brighter the B-scan dot. The result of this principle is that there is greater reflection of sound waves when they are traveling through tissue at a specific velocity and then spread through a different tissue at a different velocity unique to that tissue. This change in velocity results in sound reflection from the interface between the two tissues; the greater the change in velocity, the stronger the reflection.

The interface between the vitreous (sound velocity 1532 m/s) and a densely cellular tumor, such as malignant melanoma (1550 m/s), with a relatively smooth surface results in strong sound reflection. When the sound beam is directed perpendicular to the tumor, it is reflected back directly into the probe. A large percentage of the returning sound energy is then amplified to give a steeply rising echo spike. When the beam is angled more obliquely to the surface, some energy is lost due to reflection away from the probe and the echo spikes are lower in amplitude and less steeply rising (Fig. 37). This effect is based on Snell's law of reflection, which he derived for light rays but is equally applicable to sound. His equation stating that the angle of incidence equals the angle of reflection gives the result of maximal reflection from the surface reflecting the wave.

It is common for ophthalmic ultrasound equipment to have a vector A-scan superimposed on the screen with the B-scan image. The same probe is utilized for both and the signal is processed by the same unit to display the B-scan in the center of the screen and a small A-scan tracing at the bottom. The A-scan tracing is derived from the B-scan vector envelope and is not a stand-alone signal. A vector (line) can be displayed to cut through a given section of the B-scan image and the corresponding A-scan display can theoretically be analyzed for internal

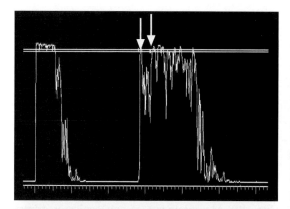

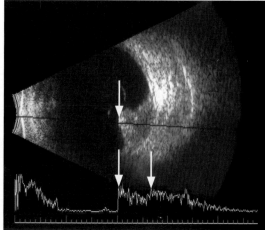

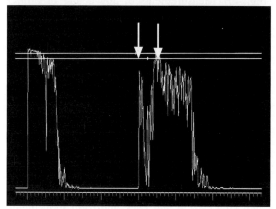

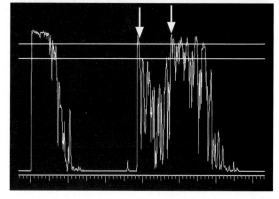

FIG. 37. Top: A-scan obtained when sound beam is perpendicular to the tumor surface (*vertical arrows*). Bottom: A-scan when sound beam is oblique to the surface (*vertical arrows*)

FIG. 38. Top: B-scan with superimposed vector A-scan of choroidal melanoma (*vertical arrows*). Bottom: Standardized A-scan of the same tumor demonstrating typical internal reflectivity (*vertical arrows*)

frequency characteristics. This seems advantageous in principle, but in practice the quality of the A-scan is such that meaningful information about the internal characteristics of any lesion is suboptimal. Figure 38 illustrates the difference in diagnostic usefulness between a dedicated A-scan image and one derived from an A/B vector. This type of A-scan is not useful in evaluation of the orbit.

One possible exception to the disadvantage of a superimposed vector A-scan is its use in measuring the axial length of an eye with a posterior staphyloma. It is difficult to be certain that the sound beam of an A-scan biometer is congruent with the fovea on the sloping side of a staphyloma. However, with a combined A-and B-scan unit, the B-scan can be used to image the macula and then the vector A-scan superimposed on it (Fig. 39). Roldivar states that the accuracy of this technique is questionable as the

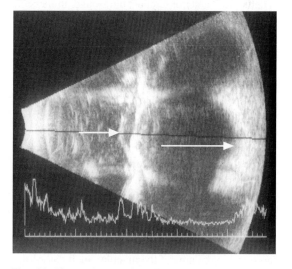

FIG. 39. Vector A-scan through staphyloma (*horizontal small arrow* at cornea and *large arrow* at macula)

fovea's location in the depths of the staphyloma is difficult to determine exactly.[12] Experienced echographers feel that by aligning the beam with the double-peaked cornea, anterior and posterior lens, and retina spikes a reasonable estimate of the anatomic axial length can be obtained. In addition, many A-scan biometry probes have a fixation light in the tip that enables the measurement of the true visual axis in those patients capable of fixation on the light.

The authors of the Current Procedural Terminology (CPT®) code book in the United States have struggled with this superimposed vector A-scan problem for years, and in 2005 published a new code (76510) that is defined as "[o]phthalmic ultrasound, diagnostic; B-scan and quantitative A-scan performed during the same patient encounter."[13] In other words, this code can only be used if a separate A-scan (quantitative or nonvector) and B-scan are used to examine a patient. The definitions of the old codes have been modified. Code 76511 is "quantitative A-scan only" and 76512 is "B-scan (with or without superimposed non-quantitative A-scan)." The examiner can elect to perform only an A-scan examination (code 76511) or only a B-scan examination (76512) and bill for either as opposed to performing them both. Medicare, and, therefore, most insurance carriers will not pay for both of these codes at one examination setting. If separate A- and B-scan examinations are performed during the same patient encounter then code 76510 must be used. Code 76513 is used for immersion scanning and is defined as "anterior segment ultrasound, immersion (water bath) B-scan, or high resolution biomicroscopy." This procedure can be done in conjunction with any of the other three codes (76511, 76512, or 76510) and both will be paid. Code 76514 is used for corneal pachymetry. The ultrasound biometry codes are 76516, defined as "[o]phthalmic biometry by ultrasound echography, A-scan," and 76519, defined as "with intraocular lens power calculation."

A-scan biometry units utilize probes optimally focused for measuring from the anterior corneal surface to the retinal surface. Such a probe could detect an abnormality such as a tumor only if a systematic examination of the eye was performed. The standard axial measurement of the globe could only display a lesion such as a tumor if it were large and in the area of the macula. Such pathology would usually result in difficulty in obtaining axial measurements and not be diagnostic of a tumor.

Diagnostic A- or B-scan would be required to characterize the lesion. There are a number of reported cases of intraocular tumors that were not detected until after the removal of a cataract.[14] Preoperative biometry failed to alert the examiner to the presence of the lesion.

The axial length of the eye is most accurately measured when the sound beam is directed perpendicular to the corneal surface. The screen displays a double-peaked corneal spike, steeply rising and highly reflective anterior and posterior lens spikes, and a steeply rising maximally high retinal spike (Fig. 40). Measurements of any ocular or orbital structure are most accurate when the sound beam is maximally perpendicular to the surface. This is theoretically possible in the orbit because of sound beam refraction even though the probe applied to the globe must be angled obliquely to the optic nerve or extraocular muscles. Refraction of the sound beam by orbital tissue bends it in a direction that is perpendicular to the structure being examined, such as the optic nerve sheath.[14]

The examiner monitors the perpendicularity of the sound beam to the structure being examined by constantly watching the screen while making small side-to-side and back-and-forth movements with the probe. Once the structure being examined is identified, this coordination of what is seen on the screen with the small movements of the probe insures maximal perpendicularity to its surface. This technique, as with any motor skill, will improve with practice. It is advisable to start with examination of the normal eye. The probe is placed so that the sound beam is directed perpendicular to

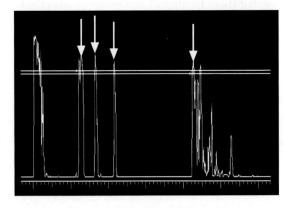

FIG. 40. A-scan axial length (*arrows* at cornea, anterior and posterior lens, and retina)

the retina and the globe is systematically scanned in 8 quadrants (45° sections), which results in a complete scan of the posterior segment. The anterior segment of the eye from the pars plana forward can only be viewed echographically when some sort of immersion technique is used to move the probe away from direct contact with the eye.

The initial spike on the echogram results from the reverberation of the crystal in the tip of the probe. This creates the initial spike on the echogram that obscures the 3 to 5 mm part of the globe that is in direct contact with the probe (Fig. 41). This is related to the speed of the sound wave and the distance it travels before it is reflected back to the crystal in the tip of the probe. This creates an acoustic "dead zone" where information is not obtainable unless the probe is moved several millimeters back. This hidden area is "moved into the view" of the probe by the use of various immersion techniques.

Coleman described a water bath apparatus in the late 1960's where plastic drapes were positioned over the patient's eyes, fixed to the skin with adhesive, and suspended by a metal frame.[15] This reservoir was filled with water and the tip of the probe immersed in it. This technique allowed wide-angle views of the entire globe. However, it was logistically cumbersome and many patients became claustrophobic during the examination. The contact B-scan pioneered by Bronson has generally replaced this method.[16] However, the water bath technique continues to be used in a few centers specializing in ocular oncology.

A modification of the water bath method has evolved with the development of various types of plastic shells. They fit between the eyelids and are filled with a conducting medium such as methylcellulose (Fig. 42). The probe tip is placed within the shell and this allows scanning of anterior structures. A set of these shells can be obtained from Hanson Ophthalmic Labs in Iowa City, Iowa. An alternate technique is to cut off the finger of a latex examination glove and fill it with water. The B-scan probe is placed about ½ to ⅔ depth within the glove containing the liquid and this creates an enclosed immersion chamber for examination of the anterior structures of the eye as the glove finger tip is placed in contact with the globe; because the probe itself is removed from the ocular surface, this part of the eye is moved out of the probe's dead zone, allowing visualization of an otherwise inaccessible area.

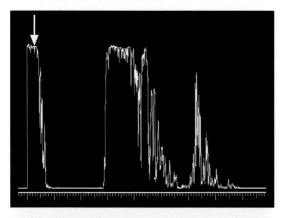

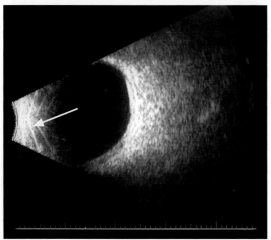

FIG. 41. Top: Dead zone of A-scan probe (*arrow*). Bottom: B-scan probe (*arrow*)

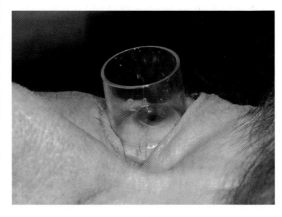

FIG. 42. Scleral shell for immersion scanning

Contact biometric A-scan probes are built with the piezoelectric crystal recessed deeply into the probe. A small fluid chamber is built into the tip of the probe to allow it to contact the cornea directly and still be able to display the cornea on the screen for axial length measurements.

Ophthalmic echography is a more interactive process with the patient than other imaging techniques such as MRI and CT scanning. Once the patient is positioned in the MRI "tunnel" or on the CT table, the technician sits in a separate room and manipulates the controls to direct the scanning process. The series of scan sections are saved and reviewed by a radiologist who may request more views of a particular area or terminate the examination when he is satisfied that sufficient information has been obtained.

Ultrasound of the eye involves a hands-on approach. The patient can be questioned during the examination in a dialogue that may direct the examination itself. He may remember historical points about his problem that he had forgotten to include in the initial history. The probe is gently pressed against the globe or lids and the patient is asked if he feels pain or tenderness in a particular spot. He is asked to look in different directions to enable scanning of otherwise inaccessible areas of the eye. His head can be positioned in different positions to move an intraocular gas bubble around to allow visualization of the fundus after vitrectomy with fluid–gas exchange. He can be asked to perform a valsalva maneuver to expand an orbital varix that would otherwise be undetectable. This dynamic interaction between the examiner and the patient often yields clinical information that would otherwise be missed.

It is important to examine the eye and orbit in a systematic way. It is tempting to point the probe "where the action is," such as at an enlarged lacrimal gland or an intraocular tumor, but other pathology can be overlooked with such an approach. Both the globe and the orbit should be examined in a consistent and repetitive manner for each patient. Each examiner needs to ultimately decide which system is best for her, but it should be standardized for each examination setting.

# Case Study 24
## Choroidal Melanoma

JC is a 60-year-old man who presented to his ophthalmologist with the complaint of recently decreased vision in his right eye. Examination with the ophthalmoscope showed a swollen optic nerve head with some engorgement of the retinal vessels consistent with a central retinal vein occlusion. Echography was performed and the optic nerve was found to be thickened on A-scan examination with a moderate degree of fluid within the nerve sheath (Fig. 43). The examiner approached the patient systematically and scanned the opposite eye and incidentally found a peripheral choroidal tumor that was highly consistent with a malignant melanoma (Fig. 44).

The same stepwise approach can be used for either A- or B-scan. The examining chair is reclined almost horizontally and the patient is asked to look directly towards the ceiling. She is informed that echography is a safe, harmless

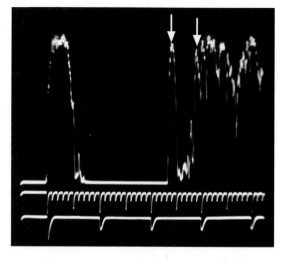

FIG. 44. A-scan of choroidal melanoma (*first vertical arrow* at tumor surface and *second vertical arrow* at sclera)

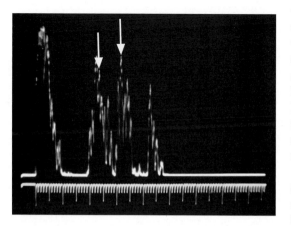

FIG. 43. Thickened optic nerve (*vertical arrows* at nerve sheaths)

test and is based on the same principle as the ultrasound used on the abdomens of pregnant women to image the baby. She is reassured that the methylcellulose is just a thick artificial tear solution. It will not harm the eye, but things will be blurry for a few minutes after the examination. It can be gently washed out with irrigating solution or wiped away with moist tissues. Women are advised to not wear makeup when they come for the examination.

A drop of topical anesthetic is placed in the eye and the probe is placed at the 6:00 limbus with the eye open. It is advisable to first scan the 12:00 meridian with the A-scan probe at the 6:00 limbus because it is smaller and less intimidating to the patient than the B-scan probe. The B probe can then be used to scan the rest of the globe. If a patient is especially anxious or is a small child, the examination can be performed through closed eyelids. This makes orientation within the globe a little more difficult, but the optic nerve shadow is used as a landmark to localize the area being scanned. An accurate differential diagnosis of a pathological process can sometimes be influenced by proper localization.

# Case Study 25
## Retinoblastoma

TM is a 2-year-old child who had been examined by her local ophthalmologist and suspected to have an intraocular tumor on indirect ophthalmoscopy. She was referred to a pediatric ophthalmologist for an examination under anesthesia and echography. Ultrasound was performed through closed lids and the initial impression was that of a small irregularly reflective lesion that was in the extreme inferior periphery near the ciliary body. The differential diagnosis included a dyktioma (medulloepithelioma) because of this apparently anterior location. Indirect ophthalmoscopy using a cotton tip applicator to rotate the globe was then performed and the lesion was seen to be just inferior to the equator. This immediately made the diagnosis of dyktioma untenable and retinoblastoma much more likely. The child had a marked Bell's phenomenon while asleep and the eye had rotated superiorly, which rotated the lesion quite inferiorly, resulting in the erroneous localization by echography (Fig. 45).

The probe is held between the thumb and the forefinger much like a pen is held when writing. The display is continually watched as the probe is gently angled to display the retinal spike as steeply rising and as high as possible. This insures perpendicularity to the retina and allows for the detection of subtle abnormalities. The gain for the A-scan is set at tissue sensitivity. This setting is available in several models of ultrasound units. It requires the use of a "tissue model" supplied by the dealer with which to calibrate the A-scan probe for optimal sensitivity in scanning the globe for pathology. A few drops of water are placed on the surface of the tissue model and the top of the probe is placed into it. A horizontal reference line is then selected on the screen and the gain is adjusted until the area occupied by the signal is the same above and below the line (Fig. 46). This probe calibration in combination with certain internal adjustments inside the unit before the unit leaves the factory is an important part of standardized echography as described by Ossoinig. Once a lesion is detected the gain can be reduced for measuring purposes (Fig. 47), or it can be increased to demonstrate mild vitreous opacities, such as in early endophthalmitis (Fig. 48).

The probe at the 6:00 limbus is then slowly slid along the globe towards the inferior fornix of the lid while trying to keep it as perpendicular to the inner wall of the eye as possible. The screen is watched and slight adjustments are made with the hand to keep the retinal spike maximally high while the probe is moved posteriorly. This allows scanning of the fundus more and more anteriorly as the probe is moved. The limit of the scan is reached when the fundus signal starts to drop away and perpendicularity cannot be maintained as evidenced by a retinal spike that becomes lower in height and is jagged instead of steeply rising (Fig. 49). This maneuver is then repeated every 1.5 clock hours around the globe. For example, it is moved from the 6:00 position to the 7:30 position on the limbus and moved posteriorly along the globe in this quadrant. It is then moved to the 9:00 position, the 10:30 position, and so on until it is back at the 6:00 position. This succession of probe positions will allow a complete scan of the globe except for its most anterior part beginning at the ciliary body.

An A-scan of the orbit is performed at globe expansion as indicated on the designated setting on the instrument control panel and then repeated at orbit expansion while the examiner's attention is

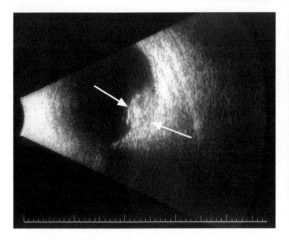

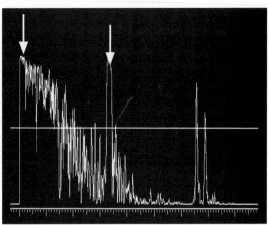

FIG. 45. Retinoblastoma (*first arrow* at tumor surface and *second arrow* at sclera)

FIG. 46. Calibration of the A-scan probe (*arrows*)

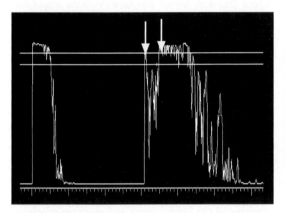

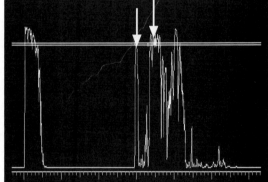

FIG. 47. Left: A-scan of lesion (*vertical arrows*) Right: Reduced gain for measuring (*vertical arrows*)

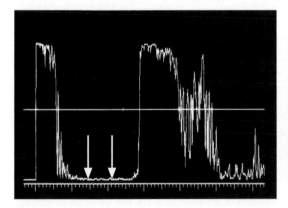

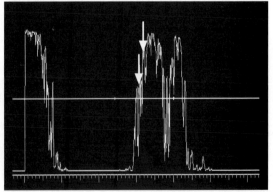

FIG. 48. A-scan of vitreous opacities (*vertical arrows*) demonstrating increased amplifier gain of 6 decibels

FIG. 49. A-scan demonstrating the breakdown of signals towards the peripheral retina (*vertical arrow*)

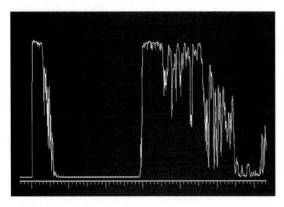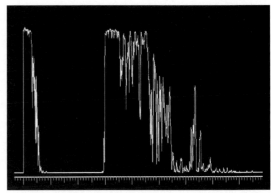

FIG. 50. Left: A-scan of globe expansion. Right: A-scan of orbital expansion of screen

directed towards the orbital structures. This latter setting simply compresses the image on the screen and brings the right edge towards the center so that the orbital portion is more visible (Fig. 50). Most of the orbit can be scanned in this manner except for the more anterior part, which is best examined with a paraocular approach. In this view the probe is placed directly against the lid and directed so the globe is not included in the scan (Fig. 51). The probe is angled inferiorly to superiorly along the lid, which allows a scan of that part of the orbit. This maneuver is repeated every 1.5 clock hours, resulting in the anterior orbit being completely scanned.

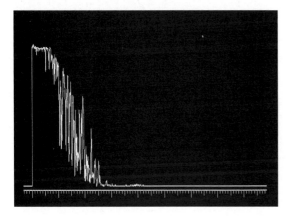

FIG. 51. Paraocular A-scan

This system of probe positioning may seem complicated and tedious at first but is accomplished in only a couple of minutes as the examiner becomes more comfortable with practice. If steps of the process are left out, it is possible to miss pathology that sometimes is more important than the presenting complaint.

# Case Study 26
## Shallow Retinal Detachment

MK is a 49-year-old Indonesian woman who presented with the complaint of pain around her right eye. There was moderate tenderness to palpation of her superior orbit and mild episcleral injection was noted in the deep superior fornix when she looked inferiorly with maximal effort. Echography was performed with particular attention to the superior orbit but no abnormality was noted. However, a thorough 8-quadrant B-scan of the globe revealed a shallow nasal retinal detachment that would have been missed if such a systematic approach had not been used (Fig. 52).

The systematic examination of areas of the globe and orbit not directly related to the patient's complaints can detect significant pathology.

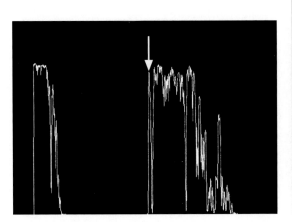 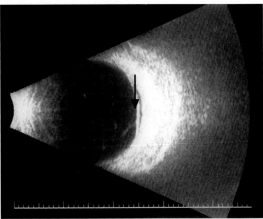

FIG. 52. Left: A-scan of shallow retinal detachment (*vertical arrow*). Right: B-scan of the detachment (*vertical arrow*)

# Case Study 27
## Pleomorphic Adenoma of Lacrimal Gland

SS is a 72-year-old woman who experienced inter-mittent tearing of her left eye for several months. She was given a prescription for antihistamines by her primary care doctor without relief of her symptoms. She consulted an optometrist who referred her to an oculoplastic surgeon for surgical correction of the problem. He diagnosed a partial nasolacrimal duct obstruction and recommended surgery. However, she was reluctant to undergo an operation and decided to wait with the hope that the situation would spontaneously improve. Her symptoms worsened and she was referred to another ophthalmologist while visiting her sister in another city.

He took a careful history and elicited the symp-tom of some aching around her eye for over a year. Physical examination was unremarkable except for mild cataracts. A-scan was performed and a 17-mm mass was noted in the area of the left lac-rimal gland. Internal reflectivity was typical for a pleomorphic adenoma (benign mixed cell tumor) of the lacrimal gland (Fig. 53) and a CT confirmed a lacrimal mass with no bone destruction. She was referred to an orbital surgeon for an en bloc exci-sion of the tumor.

It is important to use liberal amounts of a con-ducting medium such as methylcellulose while performing A- and B-scans. This allows optimal conduction of ultrasound energy and minimizes artifacts. It also enables the probe to be angled more anteriorly while still on the globe to visualize anterior lesions without the need to do an immer-sion scan. However, attention should be directed to the probe as it is angled towards the anterior globe and orbit. If it is angled so much that the leading part of it loses contact with the globe, then artifacts

can be induced on the screen (Fig. 54). A helpful technique at this point is to apply more methylcel-lulose beneath the tip of the probe as it is starting to angle up to the point of losing contact with the surface. This may be enough to extend the visu-alization of more anterior structures and cancel out artifacts.

As the globe is scanned with the A-scan, the examiner watches the vitreous cavity for any spikes above baseline while simultaneously watching the surface of the fundus for any devia-tion from the normal high reflective and smooth retinal surface. Such a change from the normal is usually quite apparent with a lower reflective lesion such as a malignant melanoma as it grows towards the vitreous cavity (Fig. 55). It can be more difficult with a high reflective lesion such as a nevus or small hemangioma (Fig. 56), which can be relatively hidden adjacent to the high reflective retina, choroid, and sclera. Ossoinig has recommended the globe be scanned at tis-sue (normal) sensitivity and again with the gain reduced by 24 decibels to detect such high reflec-tive lesions (Fig. 57).

The B-scan is more sensitive in detecting small high reflective lesions and should be used to scan the globe and orbit in a similar manner to the A-scan. There is not a tissue sensitivity setting for the B-scan. The gain and brightness controls should be adjusted to display an image of medium gray-scale (Fig. 58). Foreign bodies or calcified lesions are best seen with reduced gain on the B-scan (Fig. 59). Any abnormality of the normal gently curving concave inner surface of the globe is reason to stop and image the area in different probe directions (Fig. 60). A small lesion such as a choroidal nevus

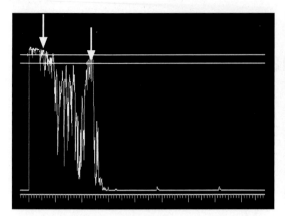

Fig. 53. A-scan of pleomorphic adenoma (*vertical arrows*)

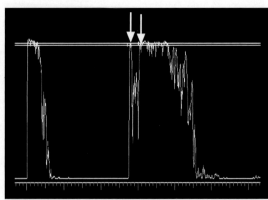

Fig. 55. A-scan of minimally elevated fundus lesion (*arrows*)

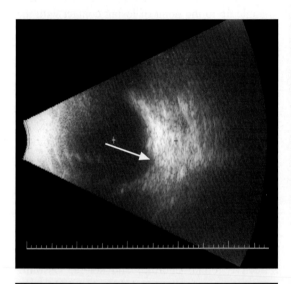

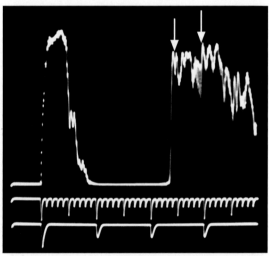

Fig. 56. A-scan of high reflective lesion (*arrows*)

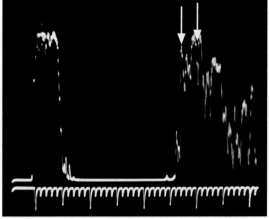

Fig. 54. Top: B-scan of artifacts caused by lack of contact of probe with globe (*arrow*). Bottom: A-scan of artifact by partial probe contact (*arrows*)

Fig. 57. A-scan of choroidal hemangioma at reduced gain (*arrows*)

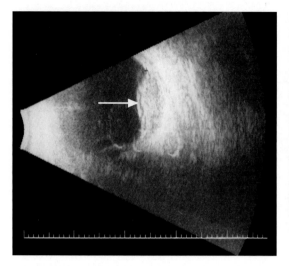

FIG. 58. B-scan of lesion demonstrating grayscale (*arrow*)

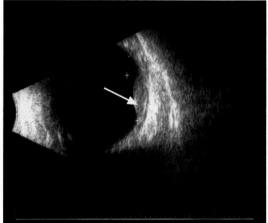

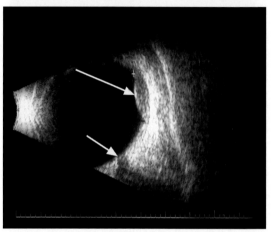

FIG. 60. Top: B-scan of lesion using transverse probe position (*arrow*). Bottom: B-scan of lesion using longitudinal probe position (*long arrow*). Optic nerve (*short arrow*)

can be difficult to image by A-scan even after having been detected by the B-scan. In such cases it is helpful to go back and forth between the two modalities. The patient is told to maintain her eye position while the location of the lesion is determined by the B-scan. Then the A-scan is aimed at the same location and moved in tiny back-and-forth and side-to-side movements until the lesion is detected. The surface spike is maximized and the greatest thickness is measured. In some cases of very flat nevi less than 1.0 mm in thickness, the B-scan will detect them but the A-scan will not unless directed by the B-scan (Fig. 61).

Once the lesion is characterized topographically, the A-scan is directed in that location to character-

ize internal structure. The pattern of reflectivity on A-scan (height and regularity) is correlated to the microscopic anatomy of the tissue with significant accuracy in generating a reasonable differential diagnosis. The combined use of A- and B-scan characterizes a lesion respecting size, shape, and internal structure.

The A-scan is also extremely useful in the quantification of intraocular and orbital structures. Thickness measurements are accurate to 0.1 mm. Such sensitivity is essential when suspected intraocular tumors are followed over time for the detection of growth. The decision to treat a lesion is often based on the documentation of such growth. Thickness measurements are more accurate than basal dimensions as determined by the B-scan because lesions often partially invade the

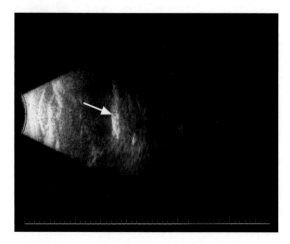

FIG. 59. B-scan showing calcification (*arrow*)

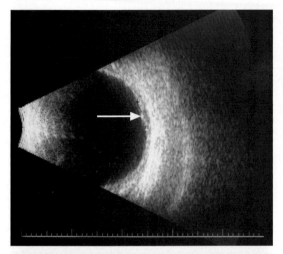

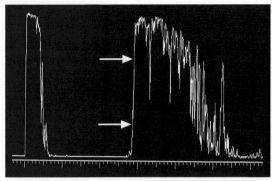

Fig. 63. A-scan showing nodes (*horizontal arrows*)

choroid so the division between the pathological and normal tissue can be very difficult to distinguish on the echogram (Fig. 62).

The lesion is imaged with the A-scan and the probe is manipulated in incremental movements back and forth and side to side until the surface of the lesion is maximally displayed. The surface echo spike should be steeply rising and smooth without nodes, which are tiny bright dots on the vertical spike (Fig. 63). It should be as high as the initial spike (Fig. 64) and the thickness of the lesion should be taken at its maximal value. At least 3 measurements should be taken and they should be within 0.2 mm of each other. Such accuracy is relatively easy with a lesion in the nasal or superior fundus because the probe can be placed on the temporal or inferior globe and aimed nasally across the eye. There is ample room to angle the probe and obtain good repeatable measurements.

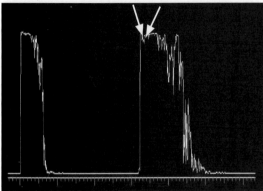

Fig. 61. Top: B-scan of small choroidal lesion (*vertical arrows*). Bottom: A-scan of lesion (*arrows*)

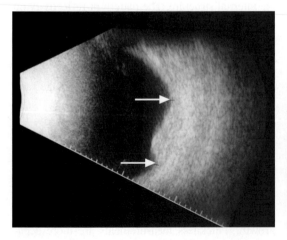

Fig. 62. B-scan of lateral extension of choroidal tumor (*horizontal arrows*)

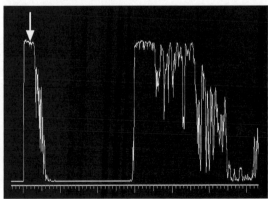

Fig. 64. Initial signal on A-scan echogram (*arrow*)

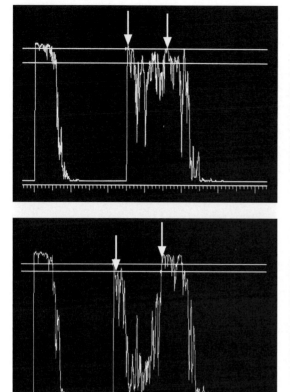

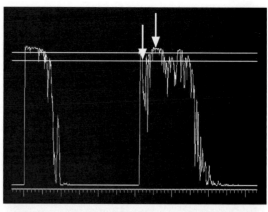

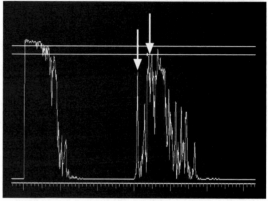

FIG. 65. Top: A-scan of internal reflectivity of choroidal hemangioma (*arrows*). Bottom: A-scan of internal reflectivity of choroidal melanoma (*arrows*)

FIG. 66. Top: A-scan of lesion demonstrating perpendicularity (*arrows*). Bottom: A-scan of lesion misdiagnosed by failure to be perpendicular (*arrows*)

It is more difficult when the lesion is in the temporal or inferior fundus because a prominent nose or brow makes it difficult to direct the probe. This is especially true for more peripheral lesions.

A-scan provides essential information about the internal structure of various lesions. Choroidal melanomas are generally low-to-medium reflective versus choroidal hemangiomas which are high reflective (Fig. 65). However, the characterization of internal structure is not reliable unless the probe is perpendicular to the surface of the lesion. This is insured when the surface spike is at the same height as the initial spike and steeply rising. If it is not, then the internal spikes are not truly representative of the pathology (Fig. 66).

One of the harder concepts for beginning echographers to grasp is the relationship between the B-scan probe position and the orientation of the echographic image on the screen. All B-scan probes have a small white dot on one side of the probe near the tip (Fig. 67). This indicates within which plane the transducer is sweeping back and forth. It also marks the orientation of the image on the screen so that "up" on the screen always corresponds to the position of the white dot. The examiner can verify this by activating the B-scan probe and gently pushing repeatedly on the membrane next to the white dot while watching the image on the screen. The upper part of the image will jiggle corresponding to the frequency of membrane depressions by the finger.

No matter in what direction the probe is placed on the eye, the upper part of the echographic image on the screen corresponds to the location of

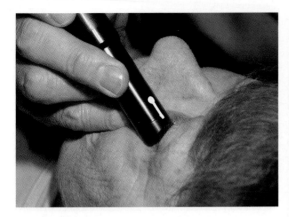

FIG. 67. B-scan probe with white dot

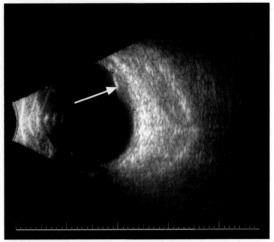

FIG. 69. Horizontal axial scan of lesion (*arrow*)

the white dot. A helpful example is to consider a growth at the 12:00 equator of the right globe. The probe is placed at the 6:00 limbus and turned so the white dot is at the top. This tells the examiner that the transducer is sweeping up and down in the vertical plane displaying a vertical section of the lesion. The image of the growth on the screen will be displayed at the 12:00 equator with the image on the screen corresponding to the vertical orientation of the lesion in the eye (Fig. 68). In this same eye, if the probe remains at the 6:00 limbus but is rotated horizontally so that the white dot is towards the nose, the transducer is now sweeping side to side in the horizontal plane and the image on the screen is a nasal–temporal section through the tumor with the image on the screen being electronically

rotated in space so that its nasal pole is now up on the screen (Fig. 69). This orientation would be reversed if the probe was rotated 180°, placing the white dot temporally. The top of the image on the screen would then correspond to the temporal part of the lesion and the bottom to the nasal part.

The best way to understand the B-scan probe orientation is to examine a patient with a visible fundus lesion. Practice imaging it with the probe rotated with the white dot in different directions and think about what part of the lesion corresponds to the top, bottom, right, and left side of the image on the screen. Just as in indirect ophthalmoscopy the brain will automatically compute the proper orientation as the examination becomes routine with practice. The A-scan probe does not require such orientation because the sound beam is emitted as a single wave and not as a compilation of separate waves generated by an oscillating B-scan probe.

The screen image orientation of a lesion is thus determined by the rotation of the B-scan probe as dictated by the location of the white dot. A related key concept in B-scan examination is the position of the lesion in the eye in relation to the overall anatomy of the globe. The optic nerve is usually the best point of reference. The example of the tumor at the 12:00 equator in a right eye will help in explaining this concept. The probe is placed on the cornea and rotated so

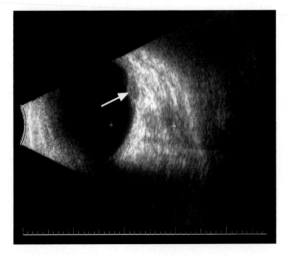

FIG. 68. Vertical B-scan of lesion (*arrow*)

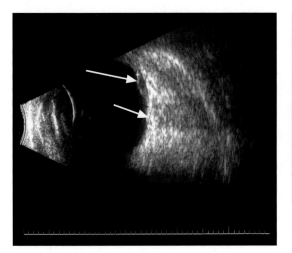

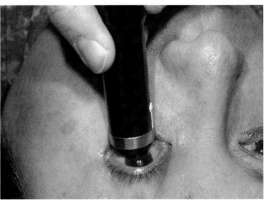

FIG. 72. B probe parallel to limbus (transverse)

FIG. 70. Vertical B-scan of lesion (*large arrow*) with optic nerve inferiorly (*small arrow*)

that the white dot is at the top. The lesion will be seen on the upper part of the screen and the optic nerve below it (Fig. 70). This is because the transducer in the probe is sweeping up and down (superior–inferior) and the nerve is in this plane as it sweeps inferiorly. This would be called a vertical axial scan at the 12:00 equator. The measurements of the lesion in this orientation are recorded as its vertical dimensions. The probe by convention is then rotated so the white dot is nasal and the probe is aimed towards the lesion in a horizontal axial view. The optic nerve will

not be seen in this view because the transducer is sweeping from right to left (nasal to temporal) above the plane of the nerve (Fig. 71). The measurements of the lesion in this orientation are recorded as its horizontal dimensions. Fundus lesions are traditionally imaged by the B-scan in these two views as the transducer sweeps vertically over the lesion with the white dot on the superior pole of the probe and then with the white dot directed nasally as it sweeps horizontally. Transverse views are always obtained with the probe parallel to the limbus (Fig. 72).

A very useful probe orientation is with the probe held perpendicular to the limbus, giving a longitudinal view (Fig. 73). This is especially helpful for more peripheral lesions. Here, the probe is directed in the same axis as the lesion with the white dot pointed towards the pathology. The image on the screen will therefore always be displayed with the

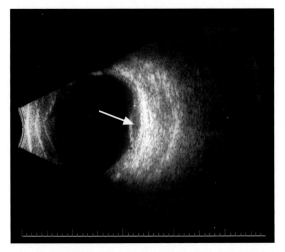

FIG. 71. Horizontal B-scan of lesion above plane of optic nerve (*arrow*)

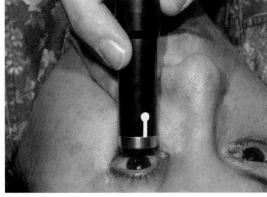

FIG. 73. B probe perpendicular to limbus (longitudinal)

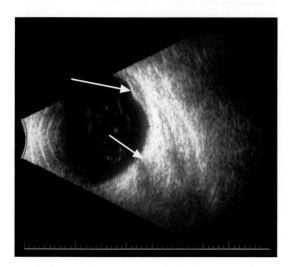

FIG. 74. Longitudinal B-scan of peripheral lesion (*large arrow*) with optic nerve shadow at bottom (*small arrow*)

optic nerve shadow inferior to the lesion (Fig. 74). For a tumor at the 12:00 position anterior to the equator, such a probe orientation would be called a longitudinal scan at 12:00 anterior to the equator abbreviated as L12AE. Longitudinal probe positions are always perpendicular to the limbus. For example, a lesion in the right eye at 9:00 anterior to the equator would be scanned in the longitudinal view by placing the probe on the globe nasally to the cornea with the white dot pointing towards the growth. This would be labeled an L9AE view. A transverse image of this lesion would be obtained by rotating the probe while keeping it on the nasal globe, but it would now be parallel to the limbus with the white dot superiorly. This would be labeled a transverse or T9AE view. Any fundus lesion can thus be localized by scanning in both a longitudinal view (probe perpendicular to the limbus) and a transverse view (probe parallel to the limbus).

These B-scan maneuvers result in the lesion being characterized as to its size and position in the globe. This is very important for staging a lesion such as a malignant melanoma. The size and position of these tumors have been correlated in various studies with the prognosis for metastasis and mortality. Meaningful follow-up of a lesion over time is only possible with accurate size and position measurements.

Most ocular and orbital pathology is optimally evaluated by A- and B-scan during the same patient encounter. The preferred approach is to use the B-scan to detect abnormalities and obtain a gestalt of the general shape and structural relationships. Reclining the examination chair to a horizontal position and asking the patient to look straight towards the ceiling to begin the examination. The globe is quickly scanned in the 8 meridians while the patient is asked to look in those directions, for example, "roll your eye up towards the top of your head, move your eye up and to the right," etc. The patient is then asked to look straight ahead at the ceiling while vertical and horizontal (axial) scans are taken of the posterior pole. This part of the examination directly over the cornea may be done with the eyes closed to minimize patient apprehension and avoid any injury to the cornea. Generally, the cornea will not be abraded with a smooth ultrasound probe and the liberal application of methylcellulose, but it is advisable to minimize direct contact with the corneal surface unless needed to better characterize a lesion posterior to the equator of the globe. However, the image obtained in this manner will be degraded slightly by the sound beam passing through the lids and the crystalline lens in a phakic patient.

The vitreous cavity is observed for sound reflections above the baseline while simultaneously watching the fundus for irregularities of the normal smooth convex shape. Any abnormalities detected during the initial screening are then studied in greater detail using the longitudinal and transverse B-scan positions. The A-scan is then applied to the eye and a brief screening scan may be performed in the 8 meridians as a double check on anything that may have been missed on the B-scan. This step is not essential, however, and it is usually sufficient to direct the A probe to the abnormality detected on the B-scan examination. It is very important to maximize perpendicularity to the lesion with the A-scan and adequate time and effort should be expended until this is accomplished.

All of the published ultrasound criteria for the optimal differential diagnosis of an intraocular lesion are dependent upon useful information obtained from good echographic images. It is common for beginning echographers to leap to diagnostic conclusions based on insufficient and inadequate information. The excitement of detecting a lesion and then recording A- and B-scan images of it can override the need for meticulous attention to detail in adequately scanning. If the proper information is obtained while scanning and documenting the pathology, the differential diagnosis follows logically. Just as in clinical examination of the eye by the slit-lamp or ophthalmoscope, the echographer is best advised to not jump to a diagnosis based on initial cursory impressions, but to describe what is seen. The systematic description of a lesion includes the B-scan criteria of shape, location, and relation to intraocular structures. The A-scan criteria are then added, including the characteristics of height, surface mobility, and the internal features of reflectivity including regularity, spike height, and spontaneous vascularity. These echographic descriptors have been developed by Ossoinig.[17]

Echography is sometimes useful in detecting associated clues that may assist in the diagnosis of an abnormality. The echographic analysis of adjacent structures can be helpful in identifying a specific pathologic process. For example, subretinal neovascularization with hemorrhage and disciform scarring is often macular in location. Careful examination of the opposite eye with B-scan at high gain may detect subtle macular thickening that supports the diagnosis of the "wet" form of macular degeneration.

# Case Study 28
## Subretinal Hemorrhage

BJ is a 68-year-old man who presented with complaints of a sudden decrease in vision in his right eye. Vision in that eye was 20/200 and in the left eye was 20/20-2. Clinical examination found a large subretinal hemorrhage. A malignant tumor such as choroidal melanoma could not be ruled out. The other eye was found to have some subtle macular pigment changes but no grossly detectable thickening.

Echography was performed with B-scan demonstrating an elevated echodense macular lesion with an irregular surface (Fig. 75). A-scan revealed irregular internal structure with moderate vascularity (Fig. 76). Careful inspection of the opposite eye by high-gain B-scan showed some irregular slight macular thickening that was suggestive of mild macular degeneration (Fig. 77). This weighted the differential diagnosis towards subretinal neovascularization of the right eye with acute hemorrhage as opposed to a tumor. Echography was repeated in a

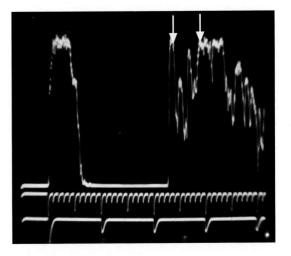

FIG. 76. A-scan of the same lesion (*arrows*)

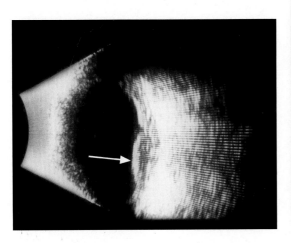

FIG. 75. B-scan of subretinal disciform lesion (*arrow*)

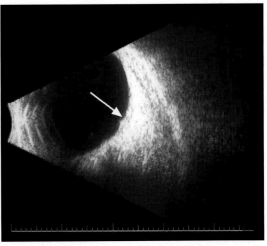

FIG. 77. B-scan of macular thickening (*arrow*)

month and demonstrated reduced thickening of the submacular process and higher reflectivity consistent with gliotic scarring (Fig. 78). These changes continued over several months and serial echograms documented the progressive decrease in thickness.

Other ocular conditions that can be diagnosed with the examination of associated structures by echography include inflammatory processes such as posterior scleritis. This entity can simulate a neoplasm but there will usually be infiltration of other tissues, such as subtenon's space or adjacent extraocular muscle tendons, that would be very unlikely with a focal choroidal malignancy.

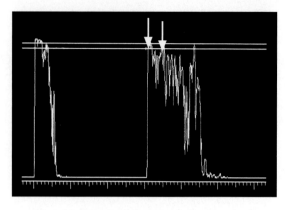

FIG. 78. A-scan of gliotic subretinal scar (*arrows*)

# Case Study 29
## Posterior Scleritis

MH is a 21-year-old man who complained of pain behind his left eye and reduction in vision. Examination found a slightly elevated lesion temporal to the macula. A malignant tumor was included among the diagnostic possibilities. B-scan revealed choroidal and lateral rectus tendon thickening (Fig. 79). This picture was felt most consistent with posterior scleritis with involvement of the lateral rectus tendon and the patient responded rapidly to a tapering dose of prednisone.

Suspicious conjunctival lesions can sometimes be associated with intraocular or orbital processes.

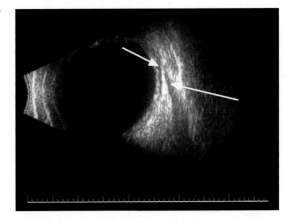

FIG. 79. B-scan of subtenon's lucency (*short arrow*) with adjacent lateral rectus tendon thickening (*long arrow*)

# Case Study 30
## Lymphoma of Extraocular Muscle

AA is a 75-year-old woman who presented with a fleshy temporal conjunctival lesion that had been enlarging over several months. It was initially diagnosed as a pterygium, but echography was performed and revealed low reflective thickening of the lateral rectus muscle (Fig. 80). The differential diagnosis included orbital lymphoma that was confirmed on biopsy.

Malignant processes can be associated with subtle abnormalities in other areas of the eye. Vitreous seeding can occur adjacent to the lesion with opacities detectable on A- and B-scan (Fig. 81). Multiple tumors can occur with the spread of metastatic lesions and these can be difficult to see clinically, but echography may detect them (Fig. 82). The other eye should be carefully scanned to detect clinically occult metastatic tumors.

Such helpful clues may be subtle and only discovered because a methodical and systematic approach has been used in the echographic examination.

The examination of the orbit by echography is the converse of the intraocular examination. Instead of watching for reflectivity above the baseline level of the vitreous gel, the orbit is observed for reflectivity lower than the adjacent reflective orbital tissue. The normal orbit contains many different tissue interfaces because of the different structures present. These include orbital fat that has a septate microstructure, extraocular muscles, blood vessels, the optic nerve and its sheaths, and connective tissue. This multiplicity of tissue interfaces results in strong reflection of the sound waves so that much of the normal orbit is quite highly reflective with maximally high spikes on the A-scan and echodensity on the B-scan (Fig. 83).

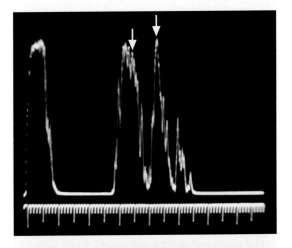

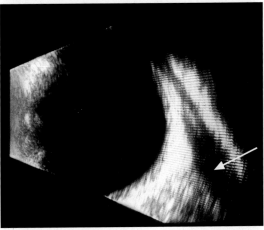

FIG. 80. Top: A-scan of lymphoma of lateral rectus muscle (*arrow*). Bottom: B-scan of muscle (*arrows*)

The extraocular muscles are more homogenous in internal structure than the surrounding orbital tissue so the echo reflectivity becomes relatively

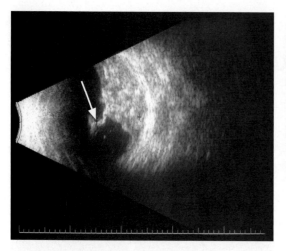

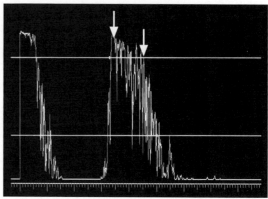

FIG. 83. A-scan of normal orbital tissue (*arrows*)

FIG. 81. B-scan of vitreous opacities adjacent to intra-ocular tumor (*arrow*)

lower (Fig. 84). These muscles are best examined sequentially by A-scan in a transocular view. Placing the probe at the 6:00 limbus and directing it towards the superior orbit image the superior rectus. It is aimed at the 12:00 position just behind the superior orbital rim and moved side to side and back and forth in small movements. When the reflectivity begins to become lower than normal orbital tissue, the probe is kept in that same horizontal plane and angled posteriorly while attempting to display the anterior and posterior muscle sheaths by maximizing their height. The muscle is followed posteriorly until the two steeply rising

maximally high spikes begin to drop off towards the apex of the orbit. The anterior tendinous part is imaged by angling the probe anteriorly towards the orbital rim and watching the space between the two muscle sheaths become narrower and closer to the globe (Fig. 85). It is often difficult to visualize the tendon in a normal muscle, but demonstrating it is an important differential point in distinguishing inflammatory myositis from other causes of muscle thickening, such as Graves' disease. The tendon is usually thickened in myositis and not the other myopathies (Fig. 86).

The B scan can be especially helpful in imaging the tendon near its attachment to the globe, whereas the tendon can "get lost" near the high reflectivity of the sclera on the A-scan. The B-scan can image

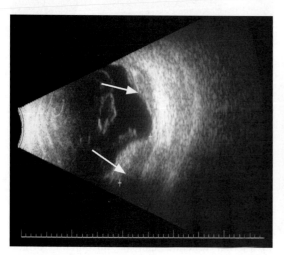

FIG. 82. B-scan of multiple tumors (*arrows*)

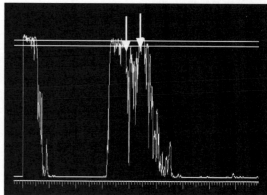

FIG. 84. A-scan of normal rectus muscle (*vertical arrows*)

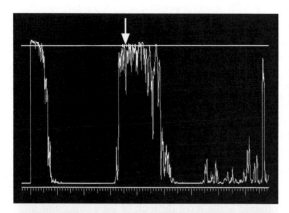

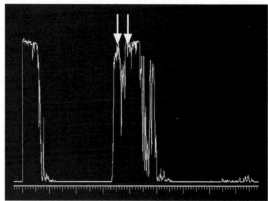

FIG. 86. A-scan of thickened extraocular muscle tendon (*vertical arrows*)

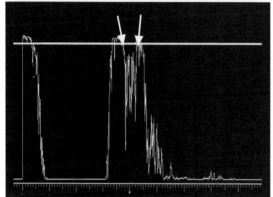

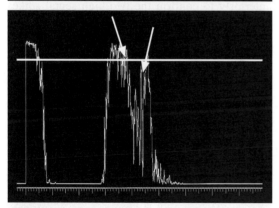

FIG. 85. Top: A-scan of normal rectus tendon (*arrow*), Middle: Muscle in mid-orbit (*arrows*), Bottom: Apex (*arrows*)

the extraocular muscles both in a longitudinal (long section) and in a transverse (cross-section), as seen in Fig. 87. The gain should be reduced to increase the contrast between the lesser echodensity of the muscle and the surrounding more echodense orbital tissue (Fig. 88).

A major advantage of the A-scan versus CT and MRI is the ability to quantitate the width of the extraocular muscles (Fig. 89). The muscle is followed back into mid-orbit and the two sheath spikes are maximized respecting height and smoothness of the spike. A measurement is taken at this point and recorded. It is important to take the measurement at the maximal width of the muscle both to compare it to normograms of normal extraocular muscle dimensions and for follow-up over time to document increase in width such as in Graves' disease. There are several published tables of values for normal extraocular muscle thickness.[18–20]

The following is a compilation of these reports with some modification of the values based on the author's personal experience:

The imaging of the other extraocular muscles is continued around the globe in either a clockwise or counterclockwise direction, but systematically for each eye. The superior and medial recti are usually the easiest to image with ample room to angle the probe when it is placed inferiorly for the superior rectus and laterally to view the medial rectus. The inferior and lateral recti are more difficult to image in the transocular view as a direct function of the degree of prominence of the brow or nose. Placing the probe against the eye in the inferotemporal quadrant and aiming towards the trochlea at the superior nasal orbital rim enables a view of the superior oblique tendon. The superior oblique hugs the bone as it is followed toward the apex, unlike the rectus muscles

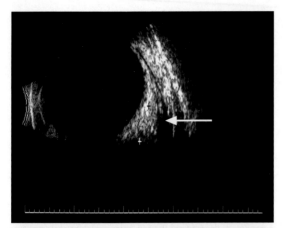

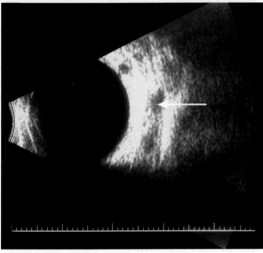

FIG. 87. Top: Longitudinal B-scan of extraocular muscle (*arrow*). Bottom: Transverse B-scan of the same muscle (*arrow*)

| Superior rectus | 5.0 to 6.0 mm |
|---|---|
| Medial rectus | 4.0 to 5.0 mm |
| Inferior rectus | 2.5 to 3.5 mm |
| Lateral rectus | 3.0 to 4.0 mm |
| Superior oblique | 1.5 to 2.5 mm |

FIG. 89. Compilation of values for A-scan measurements of normal extraocular measurements

that angle away from the orbital bone towards their origin in the posterior orbit (Fig. 90). The inferior oblique is the most difficult of the extraocular muscles to image because of its very anterior position in the orbit as it slings from the nasal to the temporal side. It can best be seen in the paraocular view if it is enlarged by infiltration, such as in inflammation or malignancy.

The probe should constantly be moved side to side incrementally as it is angled more posteriorly into the orbit. It is relatively easy to get lost in apical structures, such as the superior and inferior orbital fissures, and mistake nonmuscular tissues for the muscle being followed. To reorient oneself the probe should be angled slightly anteriorly to confirm the two high septal spikes bordering the relatively lower reflective muscle. Once this is confirmed the probe is then directed posteriorly again while minimizing its lateral movement in an attempt to stay within the plane of the muscle.

Imaging the optic nerve requires the same constant probe "minimovements" as the nerve is

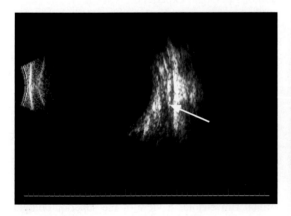

FIG. 88. Reduced gain on B-scan to demonstrate extraocular muscle (*arrow*)

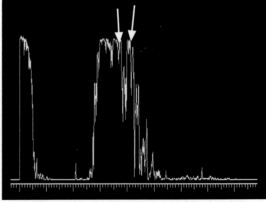

FIG. 90. A-scan of superior oblique muscle (*arrows*)

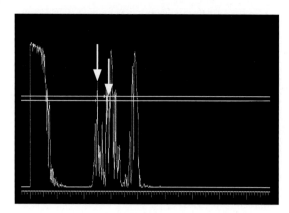

FIG. 91. A-scan of normal optic nerve (*vertical arrows*)

The optic nerve is formed as the one million nerve fibers originating from the retinal inner nerve fiber layer. It then leaves the eye and travels through the posterior orbit, exits through the optic foramen, and joins fibers from the contralateral nerve at the optic chiasm just above the pituitary gland. The same dural sheath that envelops the brain encases it. The dura fuses with the sclera as the nerve exits the eye through the fibrous matrix called the lamina cribosa. There is a potential space between the pia layer that covers the nerve substance and the dura that contains a very thin layer of cerebrospinal fluid (CSF).

In some cases of papilledema the CSF is increased around the nerve and is detectable on the A-scan. Ossoinig described the "sheath sign"[21] that is present when this space is identifiable (Fig. 92). The 30° test consists of first measuring the sheath-to-sheath distance in primary gaze and then having the patient abduct the eye about 30°. The intersheath distance is then remeasured and it is concluded that excess CSF is present if this measurement decreases by more than 20% from that in primary gaze. This is probably due to a compressive thinning of the intrasheath fluid as the nerve is put on stretch in abduction.

followed from its exit behind the globe towards the optic foramen. The probe is first placed on the temporal globe and directed towards the medial rectus muscle and medial orbital wall. The medial rectus is used as a reference point and the optic nerve is seen lateral to it (closer to the globe on the screen). The steeply rising twin sheath spikes of the optic nerve are detected as the probe is angled up and down and side to side (Fig. 91). The nerve is followed posteriorly until the sheath spikes drop away near the apex. The same orientation techniques applied to the extraocular muscles are used where the probe is angled posteriorly and slightly superiorly/inferiorly to insure that that the nerve is being imaged and not confused with adjacent structures. The widest dimension of the nerve is found and this location is selected to measure the sheath-to-sheath width.

The ease of imaging the optic nerve is highly dependent on how it curves as it goes through the orbit. In some patients the nerve is seen almost as soon as the probe is placed on the temporal globe and is easily followed along its course posteriorly towards the apex. In others it can be very difficult no matter how the probe is manipulated. In these patients it is advisable to try placing the probe on the nasal globe and aiming it temporally. The nerve may be more easily seen from this position. If it is still difficult to image the nerve, the patient is asked to adduct or abduct the eye a little. This maneuver will sometimes rotate the nerve into a position where it is more readily seen.

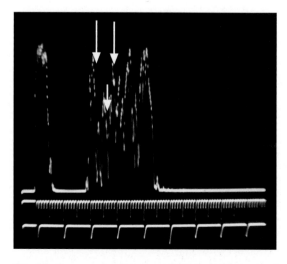

FIG. 92. A-scan of optic nerve "sheath sign" (*vertical arrows*). Optic nerve parenchyma (*small arrow*)

# Case Study 31
## Optic Nerves in Pseudotumor Cerebri

AC is a 25-year-old woman with a history of head-aches that had worsened in the past few months. She was moderately obese but otherwise had a normal medical history. Examination revealed moderate optic disc elevation bilaterally. An MRI scan was reported as normal. She refused lumbar puncture and was therefore referred for echography to quantitate the optic nerve. A-scan measured the sheath-to-sheath diameter of the right optic nerve to be 4.5 mm and the left as 4.8 in primary gaze. The right nerve was remeasured in abduction to be 3.5 mm and the left to be 3.6 mm (Fig. 93). She was diagnosed with pseudotumor cerebri on this basis and begun on oral diamox and a program of weight reduction.

Thickening of the nerve from solid pathological processes, such as optic nerve glioma, meningioma, or cellular infiltration as in lymphoma, results in unchanged sheath-to-sheath measurements on the 30° test.

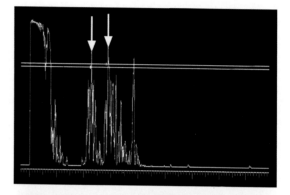

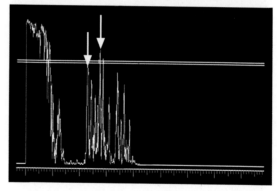

FIG. 93. Top: A-scan of thickened optic nerve sheath in pseudotumor cerebri (*vertical arrows*). Bottom: After 30° test (*vertical arrows*)

# Case Study 32
## Lymphoma of the Optic Nerves

SJ was a 75-year-old man who had a history of non-Hodgkins lymphoma that had been in remission for several years after completing a course of chemotherapy. He presented to his oncologist with rapid vision loss in both eyes and was noted to have bilateral optic disc edema. Ophthalmic examination found vision of 20/200 OD and 20/400 OS. Bilateral disc swelling and some venous engorgement was noted.

Computed tomography scan showed moderate thickening of both optic nerves. A-scan measured the right optic nerve thickness to be 6.2 mm and the left to be 5.8 mm in primary gaze (Fig. 94). A 30° test was performed and there was insignificant change in the thickness of both nerves. This was felt to be consistent with solid infiltration of the nerves with the differential, including lymphatomous invasion of the nerve sheaths. A lumbar puncture was performed and monoclonal B-cell lymphocytes were found in the spinal fluid. The diagnosis of central nervous system (CNS) lymphoma was made. A course of radiotherapy was initiated and the patient responded with dramatic improvement in his vision to the 20/25 level bilaterally. He expired from his disease within 6 months but maintained functional vision until his death.

B-scan examination of the optic nerve is most useful at the intraocular portion anterior to the lamina cribrosa, while measurements of the nerve diameter behind the globe are less accurate than those of the A-scan.[22] An elevated nerve head is easily seen by this modality and the presence of calcium deposits (optic nerve head drusen) are readily detected. Calcified drusen give a high foreign body–like spike (100% compared to the initial spike) on the A-scan (Fig. 95). Occasionally there

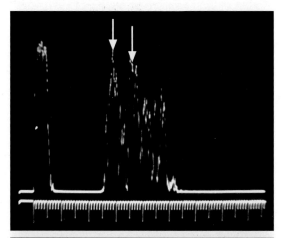

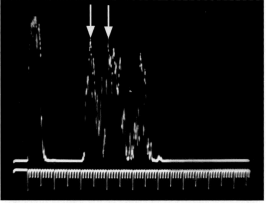

FIG. 94. Top: A-scan of solid thickening of optic nerve (*vertical arrows*). Bottom: After 30° test (*vertical arrows*)

is the false impression of calcified optic nerve head drusen in a particular probe position. It is essential to image the nerve in other probe positions to verify this diagnosis (Fig. 95). Occasionally, retrobulbar calcium or other echolucencies are seen such as in a phlebolith of the central retinal vein

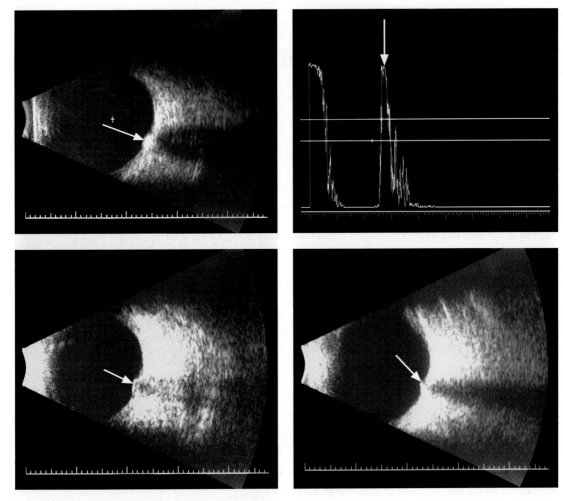

FIG. 95. Upper left: B-scan optic nerve drusen (*arrow*). Upper right: A-scan of drusen (*arrow*). Lower left: B-scan of pseudo-drusen in transverse view (*arrow*). Lower right: B-scan of the same nerve in horizontal view (*arrow*)

(Fig. 96) or an embolus in a central retinal artery occlusion (Fig. 97).

The optic nerve shadow on the B-scan (Fig. 98) can appear narrower or wider as the gain is increased and decreased. Small children will sometimes have a bulbous appearance to the optic nerve shadow behind the globe (Fig. 99). This appearance can simulate increased nerve thickness caused by a solid tumor or increased nerve sheath cerebrospinal fluid as in optic nerve hygroma. Such pathology can be ruled out by imaging the retrobulbar nerve with the A-scan and measuring the sheath-to-sheath diameter (normally under 2.5 mm).

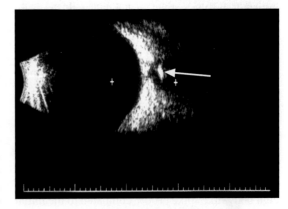

FIG. 96. B-scan of phlebolith of central retinal vein (*arrow*)

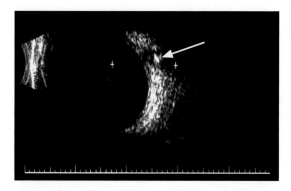

FIG. 97. B-scan of embolic material in central retinal artery (*arrow*)

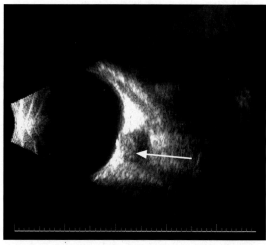

FIG. 99. B-scan of bulbous optic nerve shadow in an infant (*arrow*)

Echography allows a noninvasive study of normal and abnormal tissues at high resolution. Systematic examination techniques insure that most pathological processes will be imaged providing unique information that is not obtainable by CT and MRI scans. The ability of the A-scan to quantitate and display internal features of structures in the globe and orbit is a powerful addition to the topographical display of the B-scan.

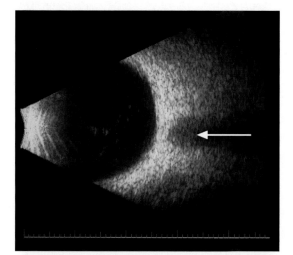

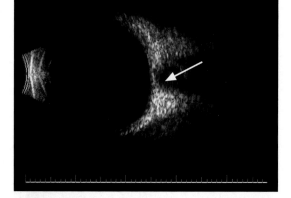

FIG. 98. Top: B-scan of normal optic nerve shadow (*arrow*). Bottom: B-scan of nerve shadow at reduced gain (*arrow*)

# Part III
## Eye Pain

One of the most common patient complaints in a general ophthalmic practice is pain in or around the eye. The starting point in the evaluation of this symptom is a thorough history. The patient must be given time while the examiner attentively listens to the narrative. A careful physical examination is then performed with detailed attention to ocular and periocular structures as directed by the history. The examination starts with an overview of the whole patient. Non-ocular clues, such as acne rosacea or vitiligo (patches of depigmented skin), can aid the diagnosis. The slit lamp is an indispensable tool to evaluate the anterior segment for a multitude of conditions causing pain from the superficial punctuate keratopathy of keratoconjunctivitis sicca to a chronic smoldering iritis. The ophthalmoscope (direct and indirect) is equally useful in the inspection of the posterior segment from the optic nerve head to the pars plana. The addition of echography to the clinician's armamentarium greatly expands the ability to determine the source of the patient's pain.

The ciliary body, ciliary sulcus, orbit, and posterior periocular area are hidden from the examiner's view and a long differential diagnosis is generated based on the patient's description of symptoms. It is vital for the practitioner to be able to correctly diagnose the cause of the complaints of pain. Only then can proper therapy be instituted. Sometimes the symptoms are the tips of significant systemic icebergs, such as potentially lethal Wegener's granulomatosis or malignant tumors, which makes a correct diagnosis even more imperative. General categories of eye pain include trauma, increased intraocular pressure and neoplasms such as adenocystic carcinoma of the lacrimal gland, and invasive sinus carcinomas. The "itis" are in the largest group, which includes inflammatory conditions such as iritis, scleritis, and myositis. This general grouping also contains infections such as sinusitis and ketatitis. Echography plays a role in the diagnosis of many of these conditions.

# Case Study 33
## Retinal Tack

GA is a 29-year-old woman with a long history of problems with her right eye. She was born with a severe optic nerve coloboma ("morning glory syndrome") and had two episodes of retinal detachment in that eye. The scleral buckle placed in the first retinal surgery began to extrude after 10 years and caused moderate discomfort. This element was removed but the retina redetached after a year and she underwent another operation with the injection of silicone oil into the eye. The retina remained attached and she later underwent removal of the oil with a concurrent cataract surgery with intraocular lens implantation. She did well until about 5 months before presentation at the ophthalmologist's office with the complaints of pain and tenderness in that eye. Examination was unremarkable for a cause of the pain with a quiet eye noted on slit-lamp and ophthalmoscopic examination. A head and orbital computed tomography (CT) scan was read as normal.

Echography revealed a colobomatous optic nerve and an attached retina. The patient complained of significant tenderness when the A-scan probe was placed in the superior temporal quadrant. A strong foreign body signal was generated with multiple signals originating from a focal area in the wall of the globe (Fig. 100). Multiple signals are echographic articrafts resulting from the reverberation of sound waves between interfaces. The previous retinal surgeon was contacted and asked to review the surgical record. He found that titanium retinal tacks had been placed at the time of the initial buckling surgery and had not been removed. These were postulated to be eroding against the sclera and were the source of her pain. They were subsequently removed and her symptoms substantially improved.

Academic centers are often the tertiary stop on the patient's search to find the cause of life-impacting ocular pain. They generally utilize the full armamentarium of an impressive array of diagnostic testing, which increasingly includes sophisticated and expensive radiologic modalities. It is very advantageous in terms of time and money if the patient's first contact with the medical system results in a correct diagnosis with the institution of proper therapy. The gatekeeper comprehensive ophthalmologist has the opportunity to intervene at an early stage and start the patient on the road to recovery.

However, many of the symptoms under the general classification of eye pain (aching, throbbing, pressure, etc.) ultimately cannot be found to have a cause by current diagnostic technology. This may change as advances occur in techniques. For example, the diagnosis of orbital myositis was rarely made before the application of echographic and, later, CT in the mid-to late 1970s. The exclusion of treatable pathology is almost as important as its detection. Patients with chronic complaints of a mostly subjective basis can consume valuable and limited medical resources as they move from doctor to doctor and undergo multiple diagnostic workups. Echography in the primary eye care setting can provide reassurance to both clinician and patient that there is nothing seriously wrong and there is not a need to pursue other tests unless the symptoms become more specific for a disease process.

It is important to follow a systematic approach in the evaluation of a patient with eye pain. The basic principles of a careful history and physical examination are as important now as they were in the days of Hippocrates. The over-reliance on diagnostic technology is a trap into which many

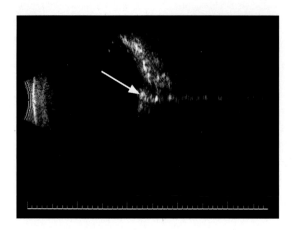

FIG. 100. B-scan of retinal tack (*arrow*)

students of the medical sciences fall. The pressures on the practitioner to see a large number of patients a day in managed care settings make it seem easier to order a test or send for a specialty consultation than to give full attention to the patient and really listen to what he is saying. One study found that the average patient is interrupted every 16 to 18 seconds by the doctor as the history is being elicited.[23] If the patient is allowed to tell his story, it generally takes less than a couple of minutes and valuable insights may be gained that otherwise would not be appreciated.

Ocular pain should be analyzed as to its character, location, onset, intensity, and duration. This approach is generally applicable to any body system and it directs the subsequent examination in the appropriate direction. A helpful open-ended question is: "What do you think is causing your pain?" The patient has usually thought about it long enough to add some important insight as to etiology. Pain characterized by scratchiness or dryness is usually localized to the anterior surface of the eye. Posterior segment and orbital pathology more often cause pain of an aching or boring type. It is best to let the patient describe the pain in her own words. She should be encouraged to be as specific as possible.

The exact location of the pain can be more difficult to describe, but patients with an orbital source have a sense that it is "deep" or "behind the eye," as opposed to the foreign body feeling that occurs with irritation of the cornea or conjunctiva. Ophthalmic pain associated with adjacent non-ocular areas can indicate a process, such as the neuralgia of herpes

zoster with tingling and burning of the scalp or the tender temporal artery of giant cell arteritis. The paranasal sinuses are a frequent source of pain around the eyes. These patients often complain of a pressure feeling that is made worse when bending over or bearing down. The absence of drainage from the sinuses into the nose or throat does not rule out sinus disease. Blocked sinus ostiae can result in fluid buildup resulting in pressure pain. Echography provides a rapid office screening test for sinus disease.

The onset of pain defines the acuteness of the problem. A sudden onset is more typical of an acute inflammatory process than a slowly growing orbital tumor. Many patients describe sharp, shooting pains that last only a few seconds and come sporadically. This symptom often has no detectable cause after a clinical examination. The patient can be invited to return to the office if the duration of the pain increases enough to allow examination during the time of its occurrence. Pain that is increasing in severity and duration over time is more concerning and merits a second look by the practitioner.

The patient is also asked to grade the pain on a 1-to-10 scale. The 10 of posterior scleritis is generally much more severe than the 4 or 5 of retrobulbar neuritis. It is helpful to ask a family member for input. The wife of the stoic rancher will contradict his dismissal of a "little aching" and volunteer that it is a severe problem that keeps him awake half of the night. The mother of the incessantly complaining teenager may interject that "she suffers from the princess and the pea syndrome" and complains about every little ache and pain.

The duration is correlated to the yield of diagnostic testing. Pain that occurs off and on for years often results in negative or equivocal results after diagnostic testing versus discomfort that is more recent and less episodic. With less severe and more chronic pain, it is helpful to ask a spouse or other family member how long the patient has complained about the pain. Old medical records should be obtained. If the patient has had the same discomfort for 5 years instead of the several months that he remembered in the history, it suggests less severe disease.

The examination of structures including the posterior sclera is certainly more dependent on ancillary testing than those anteriorly, but diagnostic clues can be gathered by careful inspection and palpation. For example, the patient is instructed to look as far inferiorly as possible and the upper lid is elevated to reveal the anterior aspect of processes involving the lacrimal gland or superior rectus and superior oblique tendons. The palpating finger is gently pressed into the area of the lacrimal sac to check for a firm nodule suggestive of a tumor as the cause for the patient's symptoms of epiphora.

This area of the body is unique with its anatomic and physiologic interconnections of nerves, muscles, and optical structures. Eye pain can be one of the most severe types of discomfort in the human body because of its exquisitely sensitive afferent fifth nerve supply. This distress is amplified by a very real psychological overlay. Many people view sight as the most precious of the body's senses and the fear of its total or even partial loss can be overwhelming.

# Case Study 34
## Mild Sinusitis

SH is a 52-year-old woman with a history of shooting pains around her left eye for several years. She stated that the episodes lasted 10 to 20 seconds and occurred several times a day. She felt they were increasing over the past few months and was quite concerned about them especially because she "had a sister who went blind from something wrong with the nerves to her eyes." She had been to several doctors regarding this complaint over the past year and had undergone CT scanning with no diagnosis being offered. She had been given various eye drops to try, including artificial tears, various anti-inflammatory agents, and antibiotic drops with no reduction of her symptoms. Examination was unremarkable with 20/20 uncorrected vision and normal slit-lamp and fundus examination.

Echography was performed and demonstrated only a few signals from the ethmoid sinus complexes, suggestive of mild mucous membrane swelling (Fig. 101). The patient was informed that this may be the cause of some of her symptoms and she was begun on steroid nasal sprays. More importantly she was reassured that there was no detectable serious cause of her symptoms and she was not going blind like her sister. She seemed greatly relieved by this explanation and a follow-up call to her in 6 months found that the level of her ocular symptoms had decreased.

Headache complaints are so common in ophthalmologic practice that a systematic approach must be taken to avoid overutilizing expensive radiologic techniques. A careful history is essential. Questions are directed to duration and severity of the complaint with special attention to a recent change in pattern. Headaches that wake

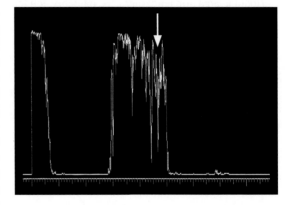

FIG. 101. A-scan of thickened mucous membranes (*arrow*)

up the patient at night or are present first thing in the morning are more concerning than those that appear after hours on the computer or on an especially stressful day at work. Increasing severity and frequency of headaches are associated with serious pathology in a significant number of cases. Such entities as compressive mass lesions, intracranial aneurysms, and dangerously high blood pressure must be considered.

High blood pressure can be immediately eliminated as a cause of headache and ocular pain at the time of the office visit. Every eye practitioner should have a blood pressure cuff and stethoscope readily available. A good clinician will discover several cases of uncontrolled high blood pressure a year. These patients commonly report that "I am in good control with my blood pressure medications" or even deny having high blood pressure during the history, but report being on blood pressure medications when asked about their medication list. Some will state "I just checked my blood pressure last week at the grocery store and it was okay." The American Heart Association recently lowered the criteria for the definition of normal blood pressure to an upper limit of 120/80. This is not just an arbitrary definition to make life harder for patients, but is based on epidemiological evidence that blood pressure higher than this value puts the patient into a hypertensive suspect group and leads to an increased risk of cardiovascular disease such as heart attack and stroke.[24]

Other simple office tests in the evaluation of headaches include palpation around the eye and periocular area for tenderness. A palpably tender temporal artery is suspicious for temporal arteritis in an individual aged 70 years or older with a history of significant headaches, jaw claudication, and amaurosis fugax. Tenderness in the area of the lacrimal gland is suggestive of inflammation or malignancy. One of the causes of a tender eyeball can be the ocular ischemic syndrome. In this entity subtotal occlusion of the external carotid or common carotid artery can result in ischemia to the globe with pain and tenderness.

The optic disc should be carefully evaluated for papilledema. Obscuration of vessels on the disc with engorgement and splinter hemorrhage is highly suspicious for increased intracranial pressure. Echography is a test that can easily be performed in the office to evaluate the optic nerve head for calcified drusen and the retrobulbar nerve for increased sheath fluid. In the 30° test the nerve is measured in the primary position and remeasured as the patient abducts the eye 30°. A reduction of more than 20% in thickness is suggestive of increased fluid around the nerve consistent with papilledema. The most common cause of such increased nerve sheath fluid is pseudotumor cerebri.

# Case Study 35
## Optic Nerves in Pseudotumor Cerebri

JB is a 42-year-old woman with a history of obesity and increasingly severe headaches over several months. She also complained of transient gray-outs of vision in her right eye when she stood up. These had increased over a month to several times a day and lasted 15 to 25 seconds at a time. Examination by an ophthalmologist documented mild elevation of the right optic nerve more than the left and blurring of both disc margins.

Echography was performed and no calcified drusen were detected. The right optic nerve measured 5.4 mm in primary gaze with a reduction to 3.8 mm on the 30° test (Fig. 102). The left nerve measured 4.5 mm with a borderline change to 3.7 mm on the 30° test. This was felt to be consistent with pseudotumor cerebri (idiopathic intracranial hypertension or ICH) and the patient was referred for neurological evaluation. A spinal

tap found increased opening pressure and this coupled with a normal MRI scan supported the diagnosis of ICH.

Headaches and pains around the eyes are not infrequently related to various kinds of sinus disease. The close proximity of the paranasal sinuses to the orbit and the relatively thin bones that separate the sinus cavities from the orbital tissue can result in sinus abnormalities causing the patient's complaints. The classic symptoms and signs of sinusitis include pressure pain around the eyes that is made worse on bending over or bearing down, and focal tenderness directly over the involved sinus. There can be atypical variations, however, with eye pain as the main complaint. Occasionally sinus disease is related to such painful orbital conditions as myositis or optic neuritis.

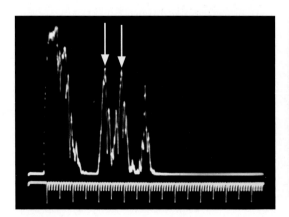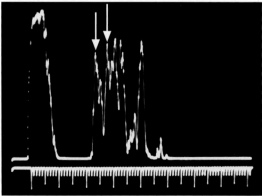

FIG. 102. Left: A-scan of thickened optic nerve (*vertical arrows*). Right: Reduction in thickness after 30° (*vertical arrows*)

These cavities in the head are normally air filled, which blocks the penetration of the high-frequency sound waves generated by the A-scan. The detection of signals on A-scan examination indicates something in the sinus besides air, such as mucous membrane swelling, fluid, or polyp formation, although it is relatively common to see one or two spikes from the area of the ethmoid sinus in normal individuals with no other evidence of sinus disease. This is probably from a nondiseased ethmoid air cell that reflects the signal because of its size or orientation with respect to the sound beam (Fig. 103). Sinus pathology can be further evaluated by CT scanning after detection by the A-scan if it is extensive.

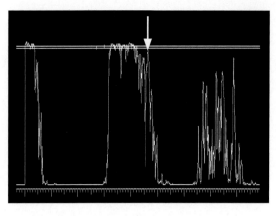

FIG. 103. A-scan of ethmoid sinus air cell (*arrow*)

# Case Study 36
## Sinus Polyp

CL is a 23-year-old woman who experienced intermittent aching around her left eye for several months. It had recently become more constant and was severe enough to wake her from a sound sleep on two occasions. Her primary care doctor had ordered a set of sinus x-rays that were reported as normal. He prescribed pain pills and suggested she consult an eye doctor if her symptoms worsened. She continued to have symptoms and was evaluated by an ophthalmologist who performed a complete eye examination with no objective findings to explain her pain.

He performed an A-scan in the office that revealed moderate left maxillary sinus signals most consistent with a solid lesion, such as a polyp, and mild ethmoid signals suggestive of mucous membrane swelling (Fig. 104). She was put on a course of antibiotics and decongestants and referred for a CT scan. Her symptoms improved and the CT confirmed a polyp in the left maxillary sinus. She was told to make an appointment with an ear, nose,

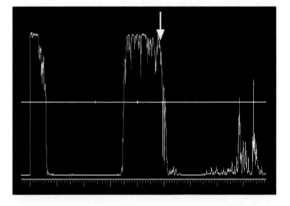

FIG. 105. A-scan of lamina papyracae (*arrow*)

and throat (ENT) doctor for surgical removal of the polyp if her symptoms recurred and were bothersome to her.

The paranasal sinuses can be seen on both transocular (through the globe) and paraocular (bypassing the globe) ultrasound examination. The ethmoid sinus complex is most easily examined by transocular A-scan. The probe is placed temporally on the globe, usually with the eyelids closed. This position provides unimpeded access to the sinus without interference from the brow or nose. The eye acts as an acoustic window to allow excellent transmittance of the signal. Normally the thin medial wall of the sinus, the laminae papyracae, is displayed as a high reflective spike (Fig. 105) and the air-filled sinus that it bounds serves as a barrier to the penetration and propagation of high-frequency sound.

Abnormalities of these sinuses can also be detected on the paraocular examination. For the ethmoids, the A-scan probe is placed medial to the globe and directed towards the ethmoid complex.

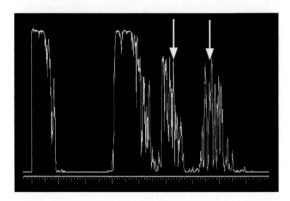

FIG. 104. A-scan of maxillary polyp (*first arrow*). Multiple signals (*second arrow*)

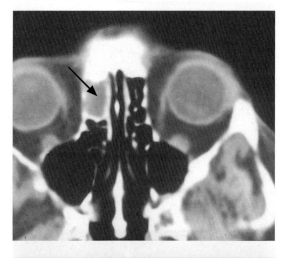

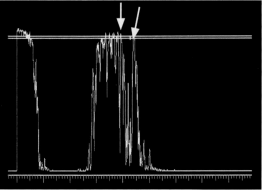

FIG. 106. Top: CT scan of ethmoid opacity (*arrow*). Bottom: A-scan of orbital bone (*first arrow*) and ethmoid sinus signals (*second arrow*)

is to visualize this sinus in a paraocular view by gently inserting the probe below the globe inside the inferior orbital rim and aiming towards the sinus. The thin bone of the orbital floor will allow the transmission of the ultrasound beam and reflect signals when the sinus is not completely air filled. Significant abnormalities in this sinus can also be detected by placing the A-scan probe on the cheek under the eye with a liberal application of methylcellulose and watching for echo spikes coming from within.

The frontal sinus is rarely displayed because of its smaller size and the thick frontal bone that encloses it. It is best seen in pathological conditions by placing the probe directly over the frontal sinus just above the brow and aiming into the sinus.

Significant sinus disease usually demonstrates multiple high-amplitude A-scan signals with a decreasing amplitude, as there is some loss of sound energy as the spikes are generated more deeply within the sinus cavity (Fig. 107). In milder cases of sinusitis, a lesser number and lower height of signals is probably the result of mucous membrane swelling within the sinus, which is often clinically nonsignificant. The advantage of echography as a screening method is the ease of use and the rapidity of diagnosis.

When a patient is diagnosed with mild-to-moderate sinus disease based on A-scan criteria, it is reasonable to offer a trial of oral decongestants and nasal sprays for a week to see if the symptoms resolve.

The probe is swept in small movements back and forth (anterior to posterior) and up and down (superior to inferior), watching for any spikes that may occur. The presence of spikes correlates to the mucous membrane swelling, fluid, or solid lesions, such as polyps or, rarely, malignancy. The A-scan findings generally correlate to the presence of abnormalities as found on CT (Fig. 106), but radiologic studies are more specific for the extent and type of pathology.

The non-air-filled maxillary sinus can also be seen on A-scan. The probe is placed superiorly on the globe and aimed downward towards the cheek, although a prominent brow can make it somewhat difficult to aim the sound beam directly into the sinus as it passes through the eye. An alternative

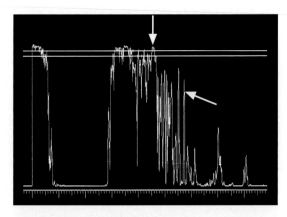

FIG. 107. A-scan of orbital bone (*first arrow*) and significant ethmoid spikes (*second arrow*)

# Case Study 37
## Moderate Sinusitis

MC is a 13-year-old girl who had recurring head-aches and complained of some aching around her eyes when she exerted herself. She was noted to have a mild violaceous swelling around her eyes. A-scan revealed several prominent spikes from the ethmoid–maxillary complex (Fig. 108). She was started on antibiotics, decongestants, and nasal sprays and improved over a few days. Repeat examination showed a reduction in the number and height of the spikes. Further imaging studies were not felt to be necessary because of the clinical response.

More severe disease as evidenced by the severity of symptoms and numerous high echo signals usually requires ENT consultation and sinus CT study.

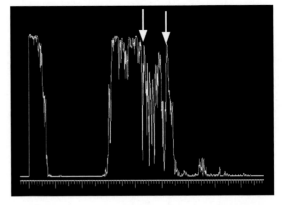

Fig. 108. A-scan of orbital bone (*first arrow*) marked ethmoid/maxillary spikes (*second arrow*)

# Case Study 38
## Ethmoid Sinusitis

AB is a 70-year-old man who had chronic pain around his left eye. He described this pain as an aching with some intermittent pressure component. He had been seen by several ophthalmologists with diagnoses ranging from allergy to dry eye. Clinical examination was basically unremarkable and a plain film sinus x-ray had been read as normal.

Echography was performed and revealed a large number of high reflective signals from the left ethmoid complex that decreased in height toward the posterior wall of the sinus (Fig. 109). This was interpreted as a non-air-filled sinus. He was referred for ENT evaluation but the examination was normal and plain film sinus x-rays were reviewed by the otolaryngologist and said to be

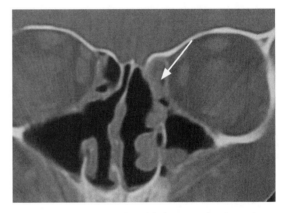

Fig. 110. CT Scan of ethmoid sinus opacity (*arrow*)

unremarkable. Finally, a sinus CT scan was performed and verified the presence of ethmoid sinus opacification (Fig. 110).

The ultrasound spikes are nonspecific and only a CT scan can distinguish a mass in the sinus versus other pathology. Rarely, malignancy can originate in the sinuses or invade them secondarily. Such pathology would be suspected on A-scan by the intensity of signals and their depth into the sinus. There is often bone destruction with malignant processes and this effects the A-scan by allowing deeper penetration of the sound beam into the sinus cavity than is normally detected when the bone is intact.

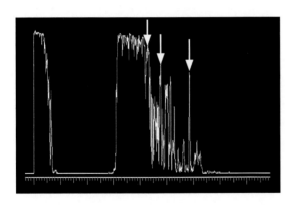

Fig. 109. A-scan of ethmoid sinusitis (vertical *arrows*)

# Case Study 39
## Sinus Melanoma

TA was an 80-year-old woman who presented with complaints of pain around her left eye. Examination found a normal right eye and a pseudophakic left eye with vision of 20/25 and lateral displacement of this eye by 3 mm. There was mild edema of the nasal lid on examination and some tenderness to palpation. She was treated with antibiotics and decongestants, but returned in 2 weeks with worsening of her symptoms.

Echography demonstrated multiple high reflective spikes originating deeply within the ethmoid complex (Fig. 111). CT scan was consistent with a mass in the sinus with bone destruction (Fig. 112) and she was referred to ENT for biopsy. The pathology report stated that a primary sinus malignant melanoma had invaded the orbit. The tumor proved unresponsive to therapy and she died from metastatic melanoma within a few months.

Bone destruction is not always a result of a malignant process. Sinus mucoceles can erode into

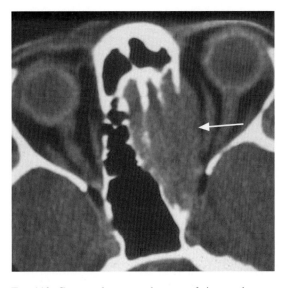

FIG. 112. Computed tomography scan of sinus melanoma (*arrow*)

the orbit from the sinus with the creation of a bony defect. These are most common in the superior nasal orbit and originate from the frontal ethmoid complex. The patient may be minimally aware of the lesion in the early stages of development, but later might experience a dull aching pain as the mucocele grows in size and eventually causes inferomedial displacement of the globe. This malposition often occurs slowly enough that diplopia is not recognized. Palpation may reveal a firm lesion with a gritty texture to it. This is due to a thin shell of bone that encapsulates the lesion as it expands into the orbit.

A-scan usually demonstrates a low to low-to-medium reflective lesion depending on the amount of mucous that it contains. It is quite well

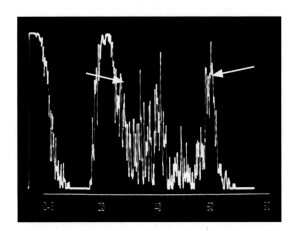

FIG. 111. A-scan of sinus melanoma (*arrows*)

outlined as the rim of bone creates a highly reflective interface. A characteristic finding of an orbital mucocele is a bony defect detected as the A-scan probe is angled over the lesion. This appears as a sudden dropout of the medial orbital bone spike with the appearance of another deeper signal that comes from the wall of the sinus. This creates the so-called zig-zag sign as described by Ossoinig, wherein the orbital bone and sinus wall spikes seem to jump up and down as the probe moves across the bone defect. This is not pathognomonic of a mucocele because other processes that erode bone can give a similar picture. A CT scan is then recommended to further evaluate the extent of the process. Rarely an orbital mucocele can enter the intracranial cavity as it grows medially.

# Case Study 40
## Frontal Ethmoidal Mucocele

TA was a 72-year-old sheepherder who had not received any medical care for a number of years. He presented with complaints of a deep aching pain and double vision. Examination revealed vision in the left eye of 20/40 and 5 mm of proptosis with 4 mm of left globe displacement inferolaterally. His referring ophthalmologist suspected Graves' disease.

Echography demonstrated a large lesion in the superior nasal left orbit with a prominent bone defect (Figs. 113 and 114). The posterior sinus wall spike was quite deep. Signals from the other paranasal sinuses were detected and the diagnosis of a mucocele and pansinusitis was made. CT scan showed a huge mucocele with erosion intracranially bordered by a thin rim of bone (Fig. 115).

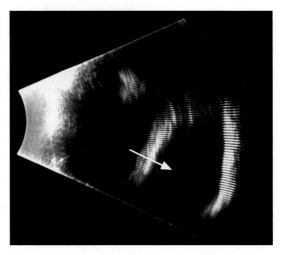

FIG. 114. B-scan of lesion (*arrows*)

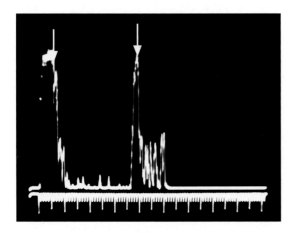

FIG. 113. A-scan of mucocele (*arrows*)

The nasolacrimal system can also generate A-scan signals if there are abnormalities. When the probe is angled medially and somewhat inferiorly in the direction of the lacrimal sac, it can often be displayed along with the nasolacrimal duct in the normal individual, although the anatomy of this system is better appreciated on immersion B-scan and the course of the duct from the nasolacrimal fossa to the inferior meatus of the nose can sometimes be followed. Multiple A-scan spikes from this area are suggestive of abnormality. Dacriocystitis will result in swelling of the lacrimal sac that can be appreciated on echographic examination. The presence of mucus, stones, polyps, and, rarely, malignant tumors will result in multiple spikes coming from the sac.

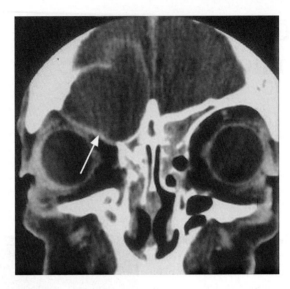

FIG. 115. Computed tomography scan of large mucocele (*arrow*)

# Case Study 41
## Foreign Body in Nasolacrimal Duct

CB is a 34-year-old woman who had undergone LASIK refractive surgery 6 years prior to presentation. She experienced symptomatic dry eyes afterwards and punctal plugs were placed in the lower punctae bilaterally with improvement in her symptoms. For the past several months she experienced intermittent tearing and pain in the left eye. There was some tenderness to palpation in the area of the left lacrimal sac. A punctal plug was visible in the right lower punctum but not in the left.

Echography was performed and immersion B-scan using the saline-filled finger of a glove over the probe detected a possible foreign body signal in the area of the nasolacrimal osteum in the inferior outlet of the sac (Fig. 116). This was consistent with migration of the plug with a ball valve obstruction of the nasolacrimal system. A dacriocystorhinostomy (DCR) was performed and the plug was removed.

Chronic aches and pains around the eyes are quite common with sinus disease as the culprit in many patients, but there are other causes detectable by echography. It is not uncommon for the lacrimal glands to be involved by infectious, inflammatory, or malignant processes.

The probe should be placed in the superotemporal area of the orbit and angled from the orbital rim towards the globe. This procedure should be performed from about the 12:00 position over to 10:30 for the right orbit and 12:00 to 1:30 for the left to encompass the entire lacrimal gland. Normally a medium-to-high reflective structure is seen measuring 9 to 14 mm in the anterior to posterior dimension (Fig. 117).

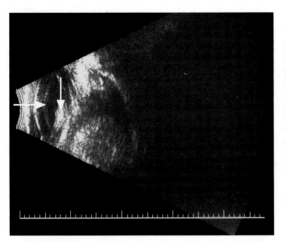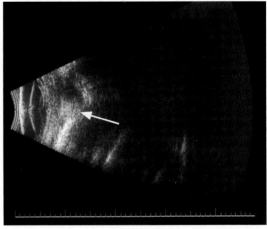

FIG. 116. Left: Immersion B-scan of foreign body (*vertical arrow*) in lacrimal sac (*horizontal arrow*). Right: B-scan of foreign body at junction of lacrimal sac and nasolacrimal duct (*arrow*)

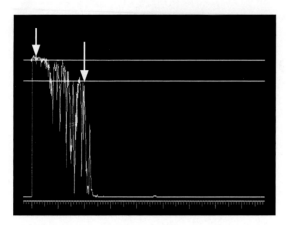

FIG. 117. Normal lacrimal gland (*arrows*)

Abnormalities should be suspected if the gland is much larger than this, if there is more than 2 to 3 mm asymmetry between the right and left side, or if internal reflectivity is low or low to medium on the A-scan. Also any complaints of tenderness as gentle pressure by the probe is applied supports an abnormality of the lacrimal gland as being causative in the patient's complaints of orbital pain.

Various inflammatory cells can invade the lacrimal gland as part of an orbital pseudotumor. With modern imaging techniques, the general designation of pseudotumor is usually directed to the specific orbital structure that is involved: myositis with extraocular muscles, dacryoadenitis with the lacrimal gland, optic neuritis with the optic nerve, and posterior scleritis. There may be involvement of one or more of these structures and there are sometimes collections of inflammatory cells in other parts of the orbit giving a masslike effect in the case of an orbital pseudotumor.

The question of lacrimal gland infection versus nonspecific inflammation can only be resolved by biopsy and microscopic study with growth of an organism on culture. It is more practical to document thickening of the gland by echography or CT scan and start the patient on a course of antibiotics. The clinical response then directs further diagnostic and therapeutic efforts.

According to Wright, about 50% of lacrimal infiltrative processes are inflammatory or infiltrative and the other half are due to epithelial tumors, with half of these being malignant epithelial lesions, although other authors[25] suggest a higher ratio of nonepithelial processes such as lymphoma. A-scan reflectivity can provide important clues to these entities.

# Case Study 42
## Dacryoadenitis

YU is a 65-year-old woman who presented with complaints of chronic pain around her left eye. Examination revealed some tenderness to palpation in the area of the left lacrimal gland. A-scan showed slight enlargement of the gland and the reflectivity was low to medium in the central part (Fig. 118). The diagnosis of probable dacryoadenitis was made and she was given a course of oral antibiotics for a week with resolution of her symptoms and some reduction in size of the lacrimal gland on follow-up echography. She was followed with serial clinical and echographic examinations over a year without recurrence of her symptoms and was demonstrated to have further reduction in the size of the gland.

Lid tics and blepharospasm are very common in clinical practice. Inflammation of the lacrimal gland can sometimes be the cause of these symptoms.

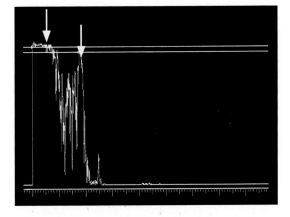

FIG. 118. A-scan of lacrimal gland involved by dacryoadenitis (*vertical arrows*)

# Case Study 43
## Dacryoadenitis

CN is an 18-year-old man who was noted by his parents to "blink excessively" on the left side. He stated that he had only a slight vague discomfort on that side and was not certain why he was repetitively blinking. A-scan examination revealed a lacrimal gland enlarged to 15.35 mm on the left versus 13.2 mm on the right (Fig. 119). It had a medium reflective area and was mildly tender to compression by the probe. He was diagnosed with dacryoadenitis and given a course of antibiotics with resolution of his symptoms over several weeks, although repeat echography revealed slight residual thickening of the gland of 14.4 mm. He was instructed to return for follow-up in 4 months.

Sjögren's syndrome is relatively common and lacrimal gland dysfunction is correlated to an invasion of the tissue by inflammatory cells. A-scan examination of the lacrimal gland in these patients can be helpful in demonstrating thickening and areas of low reflectivity within the gland. However, the gland in more mild cases of Sjögren's syndrome often appears unremarkable on echographic evaluation.

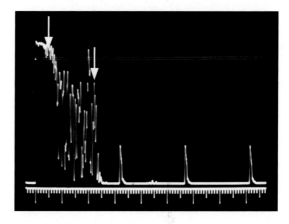

FIG. 119. A-scan of inflamed lacrimal gland (*vertical arrow*)

# Case Study 44
## Dacryoadenitis and Rheumatoid Arthritis

DA was a 42-year-old woman with a history of rheumatoid arthritis. She complained of scratchy, red eyes and used artificial tears sporadically. A-scan revealed a borderline thickened lacrimal gland with some irregular reflectivity with a central medium reflective area (Fig. 120). The situation was discussed with her and she increased her use of artificial tears and was started on Restasis with resultant reduction of inflammation in the gland with increased tear production.

Sarcoidosis can involve the lacrimal gland and may be difficult to diagnose because of its varied clinical presentations. It is stated that about 8% of patients with sarcoidosis will have lacrimal gland involvement.[25a] It affects the eye and orbit in about 20% of cases and can result in episcleritis, scleritis, iritis, vitritis, retinal vasculitis, and optic neuritis. The incidence of paraocular involvement is less well defined as the symptoms can be subtle and orbital imaging studies are not often performed.

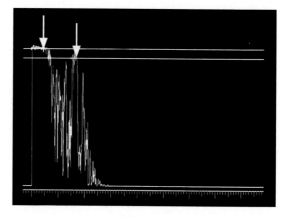

FIG. 120. A-scan of lacrimal gland in Sjögren's syndrome (*vertical arrows*)

A-scan can supply helpful diagnostic information by demonstrating lacrimal gland enlargement with low-to-medium areas of internal reflectivity.

# Case Study 45
## Dacryoadenitis and Sarcoidosis

CS is a 54-year-old woman who had a history of uveitis 8 years previously. She had a mild chronic cough and had a "normal" chest x-ray in the last year. A-scan examination of the lacrimal gland showed bilaterally enlarged lacrimal glands with areas of medium internal reflectivity (Fig. 121). Sarcoidosis was included in the differential diagnosis and she was referred for a chest CT that revealed enlarged perihilar lymph nodes consistent with sarcoidosis. A bronchial endoscopic biopsy confirmed the diagnosis.

Benign mixed cell tumors or pleomorphic adenomas are responsible for about 25% of epithelial tumors of the lacrimal gland. These tumors are not truly benign because of the fact that they can be converted into locally invasive and potentially lethal malignancies by incomplete biopsy. An en bloc excision must be performed with the removal of all the involved part of the lacrimal gland. A-scan is quite helpful in this situation by alerting the surgeon to the possibility of a pleomorphic adenoma and the

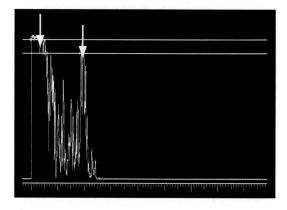

FIG. 121. A-scan of lacrimal gland in sacrcoidosis (*vertical arrows*)

need to plan an appropriate surgical approach. The reflectivity pattern is medium-to-high reflective with a decrease in the average internal spike height from the anterior to the posterior part of the lesion (angle kappa) as described by Ossoinig.

# Case Study 46
## Pleomorphic Adenoma of Lacrimal Gland

SS noted some prominence of her right eye with mild discomfort over several months. Examination found 2 mm of proptosis on the right side and mild inferior displacement of the globe. A-scan demonstrated a medium-to-high reflective, well-outlined lesion in the superior temporal orbit. A significant angle kappa was demonstrated with the initial part of the lesion noted to be high reflective, which uniformly decreased to medium height in the mid- to posterior part of the tumor (Fig. 122). It was rather firm and nontender upon compression by the probe. There was some molding of the bone but no bone defect was detected. A diagnosis of probable benign mixed cell tumor of the lacrimal gland was made and an en bloc excision later confirmed this.

These tumors can be confused on A-scan with cavernous hemangiomas of the orbit. The reflectivity pattern is cavernouslike (alternating high and

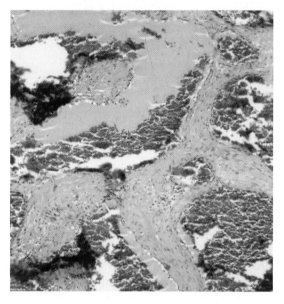

FIG. 123. Microscopic structure of cavernous hemangioma

low-medium spikes) in both lesions. In cavernous hemangiomas this is due to the cystic spaces filled with stagnant blood with minimal flow (Fig. 123). The sound beam strikes the septae between blood-filled cavities and becomes high reflective. It starts to decrease in height of reflectivity as it passes through the homogenous blood, but soon hits other septae and becomes high again. This repetitive pattern of high and low spikes as it passes through the tumor gives a characteristic honeycomb or cavernous A-scan pattern (Fig. 124).

A similar pattern is seen in benign mixed cell lacrimal tumors because of the tissue structure of solid homogeneous populations of cells with con-

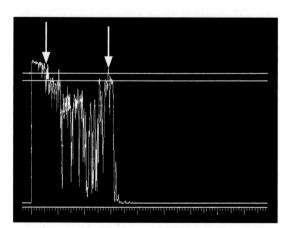

FIG. 122. A-scan of pleomorphic adenoma (*arrows*) kappa (*arrows*)

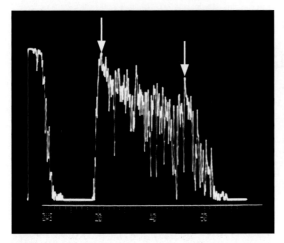

FIG. 124. A-scan of cavernous hemangioma (*vertical arrows*)

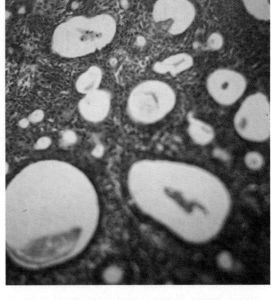

FIG. 125. Microscopic structure of pleomorphic adenoma

nective tissue pseudoseptae interspersed among them (Fig. 125). This tissue structure results in an A-scan pattern of high spikes separated by low areas (Fig. 126). A key differential point is the usual anatomic location of cavernous hemangiomas in the muscle cone compared to mixed cell lacrimal tumors that are located in the superior temporal orbit. Lacrimal tumors are usually detectable on the paraocular examination because of their more anterior location, while cavernous hemangiomas are not because of their deeper position in the orbit.

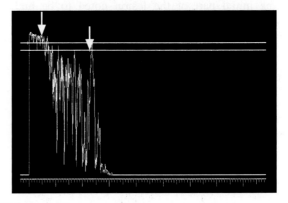

FIG. 126. A-scan of pleomorphic adenoma of lacrimal gland (*vertical arrows*)

# Case Study 47
## Pleomorphic Adenoma of Lacrimal Gland

RA complained of mild aching behind his right eye for about a year. He could feel some firmness when he pressed just under his outer brow on the left side. Clinical examination verified firmness to palpation in the lacrimal gland area.

A-scan demonstrated a medium reflective lesion in the superior temporal orbit with a cavernouslike structure and a positive angle kappa (Fig. 127). It was very similar to a cavernous hemangioma but the location was consistent with a benign mixed cell tumor. Excisional en bloc biopsy later confirmed this.

Adenocarcinomas of the lacrimal gland are responsible for about 25% of nonepithelial tumors in this structure. They usually present clinically with a more rapid onset than benign mixed tumors and there is often significant pain associated with them due to perineural infiltration. The prognosis for survival is less than 50% after 5 years.[26] They tend to invade the orbital bone relatively early in their course and this is best demonstrated on CT

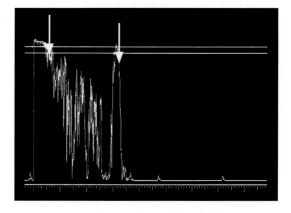

FIG. 127. A-scan of pleomorphic adenoma of lacrimal gland (*vertical arrows*)

scan with bone windows. A-scan demonstrates a firm gland with irregular internal reflectivity. The lesion borders are often ill defined, especially with bone involvement.

# Case Study 48
## Adenocystic Carcinoma of Lacrimal Gland

LL was a 56-year-old man with complaints of a deep aching around his right eye for several weeks. Examination found a firm, somewhat tender mass in the area of the lacrimal gland. A- and B-scan revealed a poorly defined lesion with high and low areas with the appearance of a cystic pattern in some parts of the tumor (Fig. 128).

Computed tomography scan showed bone destruction with extension of the lesion posteriorly into the orbit. Biopsy of the lacrimal gland confirmed an adenocystic carcinoma. He later underwent orbital exenteration.

The superior orbit is frequently a source of complaints of pain and tenderness. The patient is instructed to look as far inferiorly as possible and the examiner carefully inspects the superior fornix for clinical findings such as conjunctival injection, lid edema, or other signs of inflammation. With the exception of disease of the lacrimal gland, echographic and radiologic studies are often unremarkable in the examination of this area and the patient can be reassured that there is no significant disease process. The cause of the pain is usually nondetectable with current imaging techniques because CT and MRI are also interpreted as unremarkable.

An exception to the low diagnostic yield in the superior orbit is the entity of trochleitis with superior oblique tendonitis, which can be readily detected on A-scan. The tendon is best imaged by placing the probe on the inferior temporal sclera and aiming towards the superior nasal orbit in a transocular approach. The probe should then be moved in small back-and-forth and side-to-side movements to maximally image the tendon. It runs along the medial wall of the orbit until it joins the superior oblique muscle and arches toward the orbital apex. It is thickened and lower reflective than the opposite superior oblique tendon when inflamed. The trochlea is best seen by imaging the superior oblique tendon in a transocular view and then looking at the orbital tissue just temporal to this area.

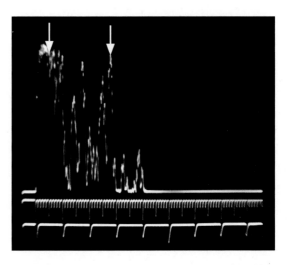

FIG. 128. A-scan of adenocystic carcinoma of lacrimal gland (*vertical arrows*)

# Case Study 49
## Superior Oblique Tendonitis

NB is a 26-year-old man who complained of pain and pressure around his left eye. It was aggravated somewhat when he looked down. A-scan measured the left superior oblique tendon to be 3.59 mm compared to 2.1 mm on the right (Fig. 129). There was thickening of the trochlear area (Fig. 130) and the patient experienced some tenderness when gentle pressure was applied with the probe at this point. The diagnosis of superior oblique tendonitis and trochleitis was made and steroid was injected into the area of the trochlea with marked relief of his symptoms after several days.

Superior oblique tendonitis is in the subcategory of orbital myositis under the more general category of orbital pseudotumor. Idiopathic inflammation of any of the extraocular muscles can result in severe pain behind the eye that is aggravated by movement. Usually the discomfort is most severe when

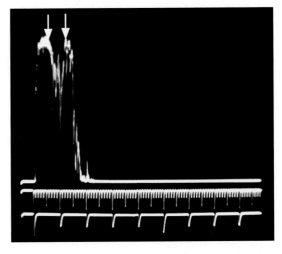

FIG. 130. A-scan of thickened trochlea (*vertical arrows*)

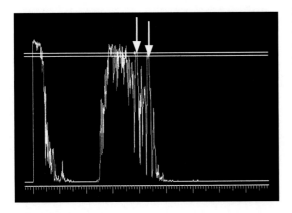

FIG. 129. A-scan of inflamed superior oblique muscle (*vertical arrows*)

the patient looks in the opposite direction to the involved muscle. In other words, myositis of the left medial rectus would result in increased pain on abducting the left eye because of the stretch on the inflamed muscle.

The systemic workup of orbital myositis is usually unrewarding. The inflammatory process is generally confined only locally to the orbit and is not part of other inflammatory conditions in the body. Echography is quite sensitive in the diagnosis of myositis and is a valuable technique to follow the patient over time to document the progress of the condition. A single extraocular muscle is most commonly involved, but other muscles on the same side or in the opposite orbit may also be affected. The muscle tendon is not uncommonly by myositis and shows low reflective thickening on A-scan and echoluceny up to its attachment to the globe on B-scan. Other causes of extraocular muscle thickening, such as Graves' disease usually do not involve the tendon and this is an important differential feature.

# Case Study 50
## Orbital Myositis

TH is a 9-year-old boy who was picked up from day care by his mother when she noted that his right eye was quite red with prominent swelling and redness of the eyelids. He was somewhat uncomfortable so she proceeded directly to the emergency room. An ophthalmologist was called to examine the child and his differential diagnosis included orbital cellulitis and rhabdomyosarcoma. The operating room was notified and the boy was tentatively scheduled for orbital exploration and biopsy, but he was referred for echography prior to surgery.

A-scan demonstrated marked thickening of the right lateral rectus muscle measuring 10.0 mm compared to 3 mm for the left lateral rectus (Fig. 131). Internal reflectivity was quite low and regular. The tendon was noted to be thickened. The diagnosis of orbital myositis was made and the patient was given a loading dose of prednisone and the surgery was delayed for 24 hours. He showed marked improvement by the next day and the steroids were tapered over the next 2 weeks, with resolution of the process as documented on repeat echography.

Orbital myositis may be a chronic disease with initial response of the condition to anti-inflammatory treatment, but later flare-ups require reinstitution of therapy. Echography is an easy and effective method to monitor these patients over time.

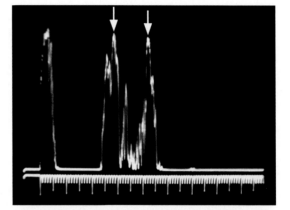

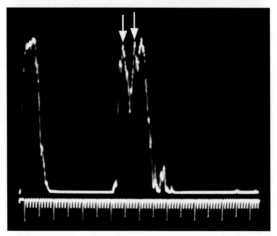

FIG. 131. Top: A-scan of inflamed lateral rectus muscle (*vertical arrows*). Bottom: A-scan of lateral rectus tendon (*arrows*)

# Case Study 51
## Low-Grade Orbital Myositis

JH is a 35-year-old woman who noted the sudden onset of pain behind her left eye. Her symptoms worsened on left gaze and she noted some diplopia when looking in that direction. A CT scan was equivocal regarding thickening of the left lateral rectus muscle.

Echography revealed low reflectivity on A-scan and echolucency with tendon thickening on B- scan (Fig. 132). The diagnosis of left lateral rectus myositis was made and the patient was started on indomethacin and gradually improved over a week. However, repeat ultrasound at that time revealed only a slight reduction in the thickness of the muscle. The patient suffered a recurrence of her symptoms several times over the next 2 years. Because of the persistence of the condition, a biopsy of the lateral rectus was performed with the pathological diagnosis of low-grade inflammatory infiltration.

Orbital myositis is not uncommonly associated with sinus disease. The close proximity of the ethmoid sinuses to the medial rectus and the maxillary sinus to the inferior rectus may be the source of the extraocular muscle inflammation by the infected sinus. If prednisone is prescribed for these patients, it is advisable to cover them with concurrent treatment by oral antibiotic therapy.

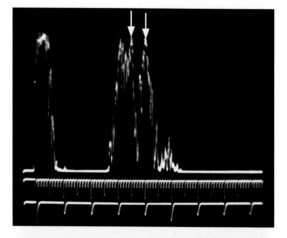

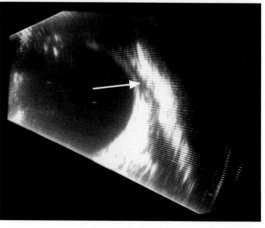

FIG. 132. Top: A-scan of chronically inflamed extraocular muscle (*arrows*). Bottom: B-scan of tendon (*arrow*)

# Case Study 52
## Orbital Myositis and Sinusitis

AA is a 45-year-old woman who complained of chronic pain and aching around her left eye. She self-treated with over-the-counter decongestants and nasal sprays with adequate control of her symptoms. She had seen an otolaryngologist 1 year previously and a set of plain sinus x-rays had been read as normal.

She presented with complaints of an exacerbation of her symptoms for the previous 2 weeks and noted some pain on looking to the right. Echography demonstrated thickening of the right medial and superior rectus muscles with low-to-medium internal reflectivity. Moderate signals were detected in the right frontal ethmoid sinus complex consistent with sinusitis (Fig. 133). She was referred for sinus CT scanning, which demonstrated opacification of the ethmoid and maxillary sinuses. She was started on indomethacin for the myositis and referred to ENT for definitive sinusitis therapy.

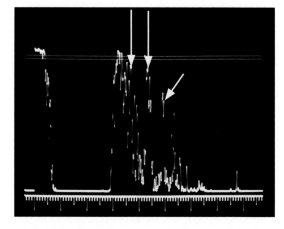

FIG. 133. A-scan of sinusitis (*small arrow*) adjacent to an inflamed extraocular muscle (*large arrows*)

Occasionally processes other than idiopathic myositis can cause muscle thickening and low reflectivity.

# Case Study 53
## Eosinophilic Myositis

LT is a 32-year-old man who complained of pain around both eyes for several weeks. Movement of the eyes in multiple directions aggravated his symptoms. There was mild edema and erythema of the eyelids bilaterally. MRI scanning revealed borderline thickening of several extraocular muscles but this was felt to be nonspecific.

Echography demonstrated extraocular muscle measurements within normal limits but internal reflectivity was low reflective in all of them (Fig. 134). This presentation was felt to be atypical for orbital myositis so the patient was referred for biopsy. The diagnosis of eosinophilic myositis was made. A complete blood count revealed normal serum eosinophils. He responded to treatment by oral prednisone with resolution of the ocular symptoms within several weeks.

The tendonitis component of orbital myositis is often accompanied by an inflammation of the sclera contiguous to the area of tendon insertion. This may be a secondary reaction to the primary myositis. Conversely, there may be inflammation of the adjacent extraocular muscle tendon in posterior scleritis. This can give a picture much like myositis, wherein there is pain when the patient moves the eye especially in the opposite direction to the inflamed tendon.

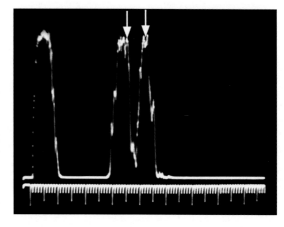

FIG. 134. A-scan of eosinophilic myositis involving an extraocular muscle (*vertical arrows*)

# Case Study 54
## Orbital Myositis and Scleritis

MK is a 32-year-old woman who complained of redness and discomfort of her right eye for several days. Her pain was worse when she looked to the left. Clinical examination demonstrated focal injection over the area of the medial rectus tendon. A- and B-scan showed thickening and low reflectivity of this tendon. The medial rectus muscle belly appeared to be of normal thickness and internal reflectivity. The adjacent sclera was slightly thickened with increased echoluceny of subtenon's space (Fig. 135). She responded to an oral anti-inflammatory with resolution of her symptoms over several weeks.

Scleritis may present as a deep boring pain in the eye. The B-scan is often useful in the demonstration of focal scleral thickening with typical inflammatory edema of the adjacent subtenon's space, which appears as echolucency on the scan. The A-scan correlates with high-to-medium reflective thickening of the sclera and low reflectivity in the retrobulbar space.

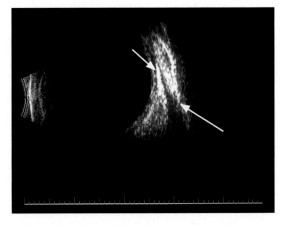

FIG. 135. B-scan of focal scleritis (*small arrow*) adjacent to an inflamed extraocular muscle (*large arrow*)

139

# Case Study 55
## Posterior Scleritis

ST is a 21-year-old man who complained of an intermittent chronic throbbing pain behind his eye. There was only mild temporal conjunctival injection on clinical examination. B-scan demonstrated posterior scleral thickening with echolucency of subtenon's space (Fig. 136). A-scan quantitated the thickness of the sclera to be 2.1 mm and revealed an adjacent low reflective area in the orbit. He had no associated systemic symptoms and was started on an oral nonsteroidal anti-inflammatory with gradual improvement of his symptoms over 2 weeks. Repeat echography showed resolution of the scleral edema.

Posterior scleritis can be difficult to diagnose clinically if there is not an anterior component to the characteristic conjunctival injection and scleral edema. It has sometimes been misdiagnosed as a choroidal tumor on the intraocular examination when the inflamed sclera causes edema of the adjacent choroid.

Benign reactive lymphoid hyperplasia is another entity that can be misdiagnosed as a tumor. These patients are found to have focal echoluceny of subtenon's space with thickening of the involved choroid. There is a nodular type of thickening of subtenon and this correlates pathologically to a focal collection of inflammatory cells. The process usually causes only mild discomfort unlike the deep pain of scleritis and the sclera is generally of normal thickness.

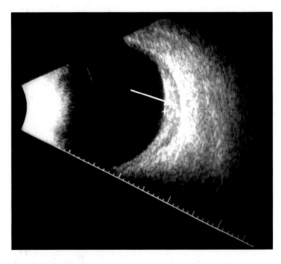

FIG. 136. B-scan of posterior scleritis with scleral thickening (*arrow*)

# Case Study 56
## Benign Reactive Lymphoid Hyperplasia

KE is a 43-year-old woman who presented with the complaint of several weeks of blurred vision in her left eye. She gave a history of a mild aching feeling intermittently during that time period. Examination found visual acuity of 20/20 OD and 20/50 OS. The slit-lamp examination was unremarkable, but fundus examination of the left eye found a creamy yellowish choroidal thickening of the temporal posterior pole.

Echography revealed choroidal thickening on A- and B-scan with a focal low reflective lesion in the retrobulbar space (Fig. 137). The sclera was of normal thickness and reflectivity. The differential diagnosis included a neoplastic process such as lymphoma, but was suggestive of benign reactive lymphoid hyperplasia because of the nodular area in subtenon's space. The process improved over several weeks and systemic workup was negative for malignancy.

Other disease processes can invade subtenon's space. Various types of lymphoma can involve this space with a cellular infiltrate that will give echolucency on B-scan and low reflectivity on A-scan indistinguishable from inflammatory edema.

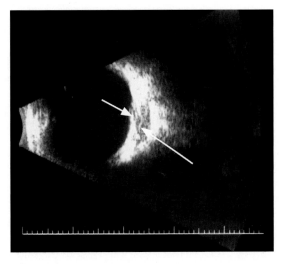

FIG. 137. B-scan of choroidal thickening (*small arrow*) with adjacent subtenon's lucency (*large arrow*)

# Case Study 56
## Benign Reactive Lymphoid Hyperplasia

# Case Study 57
## Orbital Large Cell Lymphoma

MA was a 55-year-old man who presented with recent reduction of vision in his right eye and some mild discomfort. Clinical examination found swelling in the posterior pole of the fundus and mild papilledema.

Echography was performed and demonstrated diffuse lucency in subtenon's space and mild thickening of the retrobulbar optic nerve. The posterior globe wall and adjacent subtenon's tissue was thickened (Fig. 138). He was felt to have an inflammatory process and started on high-dose oral steroids. He initially improved with resolution of his pain and recovery of his vision to 20/25. However, a month later his ocular symptoms recurred and he became systemically ill with an enlarged liver and spleen. He died shortly thereafter and autopsy discovered systemic large cell lymphoma.

The Vogt–Koyanagi–Harada (VKH) syndrome is another disease entity that can occasionally present

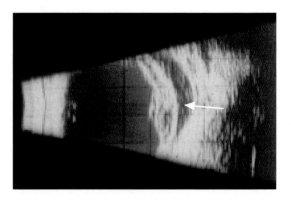

FIG. 138. B-scan of subtenon's infiltration by large cell lymphoma (*arrow*)

with inflammatory infiltration in subtenon's space. The choroid may demonstrate characteristic low-to-medium reflectivity with increased scleral thickness.

# Case Study 58
## Choroiditis and Vogt-Koyanagi-Harada Syndrome

DR was a 27-year-old man of Middle Eastern extraction who complained of severe headaches and some neck pain. He had noted several patches of depigmentation on his skin and some whitening of eyelashes. He also mentioned blotchy vision worsening over the past several weeks. Clinical examination found subretinal fluid inferiorly in the right eye. B-scan demonstrated choroidal thickening and mild echolucency in subtenon's space (Fig. 139). There was medium internal reflectivity on A-scan (Fig. 140).

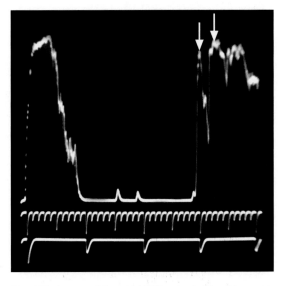

FIG. 140. A-scan of choroidal infiltration in Vogt-Koyanagi-Harada (*arrows*)

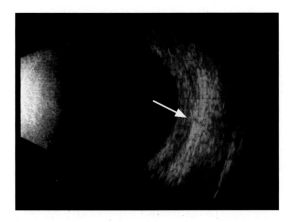

FIG. 139. B-scan of choroidal infiltration in Vogt-Koyanagi-Harada syndrome (*arrow*)

Graves' disease can sometimes be shown to have luceny of subtenons. This finding can be present in several retrobulbar inflammatory conditions. It may occur in Graves' patients who have an acute inflammatory process with the rapid onset of chemosis, lid edema, and some degree of ocular discomfort. Pathologically, inflammatory cells involving both the extraocular muscles and orbital connective tissue and fat infiltrate the orbit diffusely. This infiltration with accompanying edema can involve the retrobulbar area and give the echographic picture of echolucency.

# Case Study 59
## Myositis and Graves' Disease

BD is a 76-year-old man who presented at the emergency room with a picture resembling orbital cellulitis. His right orbit appeared congested with marked chemosis, lid edema, and he had limitation of ocular movement. These findings combined with a significant degree of pain prompted the ER doctor to initiate antibiotic intravenous therapy. First-generation CT scanning showed only diffuse orbital opacification thought to be consistent with cellulitis. A-scan was later obtained and demonstrated enlargement of all of his extraocular muscles with massive low reflective thickening of the superior rectus. Increased echolucency in subtenon's space was noted (Fig. 141). The diagnosis of acute inflammatory Graves' disease with concurrent myositis was made and he was started on high-dose steroids with rapid improvement in the inflammatory symptoms.

Echography is especially helpful in the evaluation of various extraocular muscle disorders. The quantitative capacity of A-scan allows for the measurement of muscle thickness to an accuracy of 0.5mm. Serial comparisons of muscle thickness over time is possible by measuring the thickness at the greatest dimension. The measurement of an extraocular muscle at its maximum dimension allows for a reproducible measurement of that muscle over time. This provides a major advantage over other imaging modalities by providing quantitation of muscle thickness, which is of great importance in diagnosing and treating different conditions affecting these muscles.

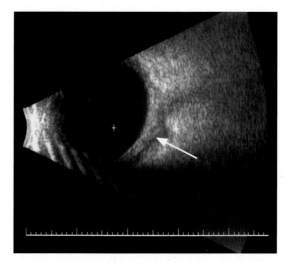

FIG. 141. B-scan of subtenon's lucency in inflammatory Graves' disease (*arrow*)

149

# Case Study 60
## Myositis and Graves' Disease

DH is a 55-year-old man who was diagnosed with acute inflammatory myositis of his right superior rectus muscle based on CT scan findings of thickening of that muscle with other extraocular muscles (EOMs) appearing of normal thickness. His initial symptoms of pain and marked swelling were greatly relieved by high-dose prednisone treatment. However, he continued to have signs of orbital congestion with some degree of exophthalmos. Echography was obtained and the other extraocular muscles were measured to be of thickness greater than the upper limits of normal on a normogram. Their internal reflectivity on A-scan was consistent with Graves' disease. The internal spikes were medium-to-high reflective (Fig. 142). His thyroid workup found a borderline low thyrotropin with the presence of antithyroid antibodies. He was referred for management of the thyroid to his internist. His ophthalmologist followed his ocular status with a plan for radiation therapy or decompressive surgery if his Graves' orbitopathy worsened.

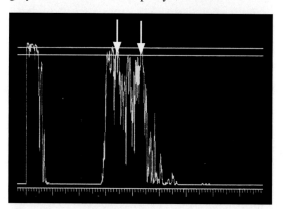

FIG. 142. A-scan of typical Graves' muscle (*vertical arrows*)

Another cause of thickened extraocular muscles with low-grade orbital pain is the venous congestion that occurs from low-flow arteriovenous fistulas such as is found in a dural–sinus fistula. This originates from an abnormal connection between the arterioles of the intracranial dura and the cavernous sinus. Such a connection can occur after head trauma or, more commonly, spontaneously. The extraocular muscles in these patients are generally not as thick as in patients with Graves' disease but may be above the upper limits of normal muscle diameter. This thickening is due to the venous congestion of the orbit due to the stasis of outflow.

The spontaneous occurrence of a dural–sinus fistula without a history of trauma is most often found in middle-aged women who present with chronic complaints of aching around either one or both eyes and who are found on examination to have corkscrew conjunctival and episcleral vascular injection with elevation of the intraocular pressure. They may have blood in Schlem's canal as viewed on gonioscopy.

Echography may reveal enlargement of the superior ophthalmic vein with rapidly moving spikes consistent with arterial blood flow. In many cases, however, the flow is low grade and the dilated superior ophthalmic vein is imaged by B-scan without the detection of rapid arterial flow. However, orbital color Doppler can often detect the superior ophthalmic vein in such patients (Fig. 143) and demonstrate reversal of flow (the vein is displayed with red color instead of blue) with pulse wave forms quantitatively diagnostic of arterial flow.

A relatively common cause of orbital pain is inflammation of the optic nerve as occurs in optic neuritis. These patients usually present with mild-to-severe pain made worse on movement of

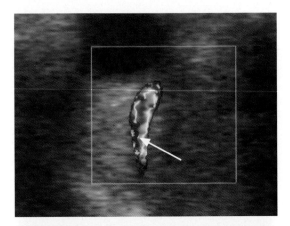

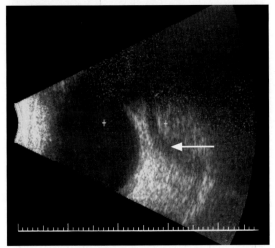

FIG. 143. Top: Color Doppler of arterialized superior ophthalmic vein (*arrows*). Bottom: B-scan of superior ophthalmic vein

within the optic nerve sheath tends to spread out on abduction of the eye and results in a thinning of the sheath-to-sheath diameter. This test is usually most helpful in cases of pseudotumor cerebri with papilledema, but can sometimes be useful in the setting of optic neuritis.

Measurement of the optic nerve by A-scan is based on the same principles as that of the extraocular muscles. The nerve is usually visualized by placing the probe on the temporal globe and directing it nasally. Otherwise, the opposite placement (nasally) should be tried if the nerve is difficult to image. The probe is angled to display the nerve just posterior to its exit from the globe and then is followed into the posterior orbit. As postulated in the measurement of the extraocular muscles, refraction of the sound beam enables it to be maintained in a perpendicular direction to the nerve sheaths. The spike of each sheath is maximized in height and smoothness of the ascending limbs. The maximal thickness of the nerve is noted and this is taken as the nerve dimension.

Optic neuritis sometimes causes mild thickening of the optic nerve, but the 30° test is usually negative or equivocal at best. It is postulated that the nerve parenchyma is swollen due to the inflammation and there is a minimal increase in the perineural optic sheath cerebrospinal fluid. This is more suggestive of thickening of the nerve substance as it resists compression on the 30° test. A-scan measurements do not change appreciably in primary gaze versus those taken on abduction of the globe by 30°.

the eye. Optic neuritis is often associated with reduction of visual acuity and a central scotoma. The process may be idiopathic, but is commonly part of a demyelinating disease such as multiple sclerosis.

Echography is often unremarkable in these cases, whereas MRI scanning will show enhancement of the optic nerve sheath consistent with inflammation. However, the B scan will sometimes demonstrate the T sign as the edema associated with inflammation results in a retrobulbar echolucency connecting with the optic nerve shadow (Fig. 144). The optic nerve may be thickened on A scan and demonstrate a mildly positive 30° test. In this technique, the patient is instructed to look about 30° temporally and the optic nerve is remeasured and compared to the measurement in primary gaze. Increased fluid

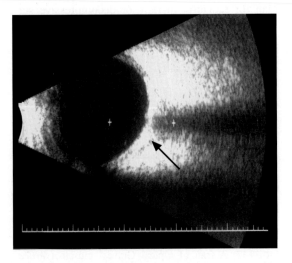

FIG. 144. B-scan of subtenon's lucency in optic neuritis (*arrow*)

# Case Study 61
## Retrobulbar Neuritis

MD is a 32-year-old woman who presented with pain behind her left eye and loss of central vision. The pain worsened on looking horizontally in either direction. Examination revealed visual acuity in that eye of 20/200, a positive afferent pupil defect, and a normal-appearing optic disc. The presumed diagnosis of retrobulbar neuritis was made based on the clinical setting.

Echography was performed and A-scan measured the right optic nerve to be 3.2 mm in greatest diameter and the left nerve 3.88 mm (Fig. 145). The 30° test was negative with a nonsignificant reduction to 3.74 mm on abduction of the left eye. B-scan showed mild echolucency of subtenon's space posterior to the left globe. These findings were consistent with optic nerve edema secondary to retrobulbar neuritis.

Most cases of optic neuritis are the result of demyelinating disease, but there are rarely other causes such as sarcoidosis. These patients usually

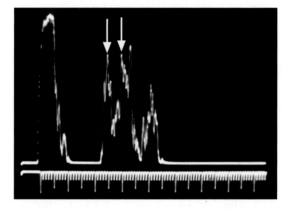

FIG. 145. A-scan of mild optic nerve thickening in optic neuritis (*vertical arrows*)

present with a chronic course with fluctuating vision and low-grade pain over time. They may have other areas of ocular inflammation such as iritis, panuveitis, vitritis, and retinal vasculitis.

# Case Study 62
## Sacroid Optic Neuritis

KD is a 43-year-old woman who had a history of recent cough and shortness of breath, a nodular rash on her legs, and reduced vision in her left eye with mild aching. Examination revealed some sheathing of the mid-peripheral retinal vessels, and moderate edema of the optic disc with several disc hemorrhages.

Echography demonstrated thickening of the optic nerve to 4.5 mm on A-scan and some increased lucency of subtenon's space by B-scan at the globe/optic nerve junction (Fig. 146). The 30° test was negative with no significant change in nerve diameter on abduction of the globe. Later workup included a chest CT, serum angiotensin-converting enzyme levels, and a parotid gland

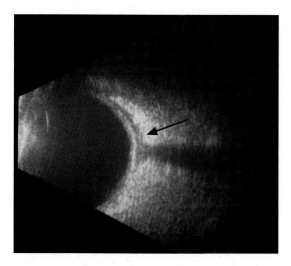

FIG. 146. B-scan of sarcoid involvement of optic neuritis with increased subtenon's lucency (*arrow*)

biopsy that demonstrated noncaseating granulomas. The patient was referred for bronchoscopy, which supported the diagnosis of sarcoidosis.

Rarer causes of optic neuritis include herpes simplex and herpes zoster, syphilis, Lyme disease, and other infectious etiologies. Pain accompanies these entities to varying degrees. There is usually some degree of visual loss and clinical examination reveals a spectrum of optic disc swelling from a normal appearance in purely retrobulbar neuritis to fulminant papilledema. Echography is useful in the workup of inflammatory optic nerve processes by revealing the presence of one or a combination of the following: fluid around the nerve, parenchymal edema, and solid infiltration of the nerve. It can also assist in identifying causes of pseudopapilledema, such as optic disc drusen or analomous disc morphology.

Orbital pain can be due to pathology of the subperiosteal space, such as infection or inflammation. Acute sinusitis may respond initially to antibiotic treatment but the patient may not fully recover after several weeks, which should alert the clinician to the possibility of a subperiosteal abscess. The patient may show initial improvement with antibiotic treatment but then stagnates clinically with chronic lid edema, tenderness, and pain. Echographic studies demonstrate thickening of the subperiosteal space and low reflectivity consistent with inflammatory infiltration. This condition often requires surgical drainage to resolve the problem. Echography is a cost effective and safe way to follow-up the effectiveness of treatment.

# Case Study 63
## Subperiosteal Abscess

CDL is a 7-year-old boy who presented to his pediatrician with a history of pain and eyelid swelling around his right eye for several days. The clinical diagnosis of acute sinusitis with early orbital cellulitis was made and he was admitted to the hospital for intravenous (IV) antibiotic therapy. He responded with marked improvement over several days and was discharged on oral antibiotics. He had mild persistent pain and swelling over the next 3 weeks with a low-grade fever.

Plain film x-rays were unremarkable but echography revealed low reflective thickening of the subperiosteal space in the superior nasal orbit (Fig. 147). The diagnosis of a subperiosteal abscess was made and the child was referred to an orbital surgeon for surgical drainage of the abscess.

Expansion of this space by hemorrhage can also result in acute discomfort. This may happen as part of the labor of pregnancy with the increased orbital pressure of the associated valsalva forces. It can also occur spontaneously in pregnancy because of the increased general venous congestion.

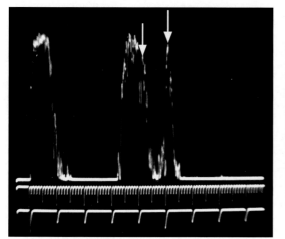 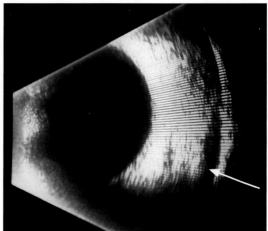

FIG. 147. Left: A-scan of subperiosteal abscess (*vertical arrows*). Right: B-scan of abscess (*arrow*)

# Case Study 64
## Subperiosteal Hemorrhage

MS is a 21-year-old pregnant woman of 34 weeks gestation who noted the sudden onset of severe pain behind her left eye. Examination revealed mild proptosis and upper lid edema. Radiological studies were felt inadvisable because of her pregnancy. Echography demonstrated echolucency of subtenon's space on B-scan and low reflectivity on A-scan (Fig. 148). The diagnosis of subperiosteal

hemorrhage was made and she was treated conservatively with Tylenol and cold compresses with gradual resorption of the blood.

Spontaneous subperiosteal hemorrhage can occasionally occur due to preexisting venous anomalies. The spectrum of orbital varices overlaps with orbital lymphangiomas, either of which can result in spontaneous orbital or subperiosteal hemorrhage.

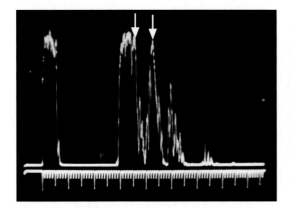 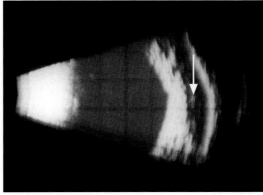

FIG. 148. Left: A-scan of subperiosteal hemorrhage (*vertical arrows*). Right: B-scan of the subperiosteal space (*vertical arrow*)

# Case Study 65
## Bleed into Lymphangioma

LL is a 25-year-old woman who presented with the sudden onset of pain around her right eye and noted a "blood blister" under the upper eyelid with some lid ecchymosis. Echography revealed widening, echolucency, and low reflectivity of the subperiosteal space (Fig. 149). She was treated with cold compresses and the discontinuation of aspirin products. Follow-up ultrasound demonstrated a multicystic lesion consistent with an orbital lymphangioma or orbital varix. She had a history of a similar lesion under her tongue.

Less common causes of pain around the eye and orbit include metastatic tumors from distant sites or secondary invasion from contiguous areas, such as the paranasal sinuses. This pain is especially severe in rapidly expanding lesions that often induce an inflammatory reaction, in cases of perineural invasion, and also in those with bone destruction.

Metastatic invasion of the orbit may give a V pattern of reflectivity on the A-scan. This appearance is due to the manner of infiltration of the orbital tissue by the malignant cells. The area of invasion becomes relatively low reflective because of the dense homogeneity of the neoplastic cell population with a relative paucity of interfaces between different tissue types. Adjacent to the central concentration of cells are areas of higher reflectivity and heterogeneity as malignant cells less densely infiltrate normal orbital tissue. The A-scan spikes in such an area are reflected more strongly by the multiple tissue interfaces. Metastatic tumors in the orbit are generally quite firm to compression when they are imaged on the paraocular examination.

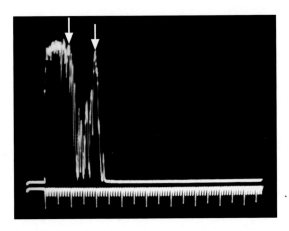

FIG. 149. A-scan of subperiosteal hemorrhage (*vertical arrows*)

161

# Case Study 66
## Orbital Metastasis

LT is a 45-year-old woman with a history of breast carcinoma treated 5 years previously with mastectomy, radiation, and chemotherapy. She had been in remission since that time but presented with painful proptosis of her right eye. She also complained of diplopia and was found to have some restriction of her extraocular motility. Fundus examination did not reveal any choroidal tumors.

The A-scan demonstrated an orbital mass superiorly that was quite hard to compression by the probe on the paraocular examination. Internal reflectivity of this lesion was irregular with a V pattern of higher peripheral spikes that decreased in height towards the center of the lesion and rose again on the opposite side (Fig. 150). The differential diagnosis in this patient included metastatic breast carcinoma of the orbit. This was later confirmed on needle biopsy and she underwent a course of palliative orbital radiation that temporarily relieved her symptoms.

Invasion and destruction of the orbital walls creates high reflective tissue interfaces that are dis-

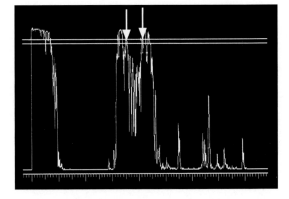

FIG. 150. A-scan of metastatic tumor in the orbit with a V pattern of reflectivity (*vertical arrows*)

played outside the normal boundaries of the orbit. The invasive process erodes the bony walls of the orbit and the ultrasound beam is able to penetrate more deeply than it can normally. The display of signals beyond the usual limits is a clue to the absence of bone.

# Case Study 67
## Sinus Carcinoma

AT was a 54-year-old man who presented with complaints of left orbital pain and persistent tearing for several months. Examination revealed a palpable firmness in the area of the left lacrimal fossa. A-scan demonstrated multiple high reflective spikes from beyond the medial orbital wall consistent with bone destruction (Fig. 151). A CT scan showed a mass that had originated in the left maxillary/ethmoid sinus with obstruction of the nasolacrimal system (Fig. 152). Biopsy was consistent with squamous cell carcinoma.

Orbital lesions that do not invade the bone or periosteum can grow quite large without caus-

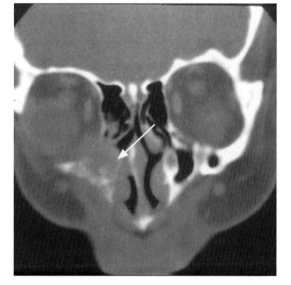

FIG. 152. Computed tomography scan of carcinoma (*arrow*)

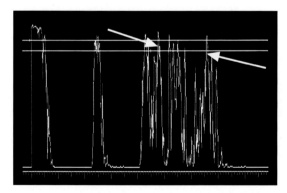

FIG. 151. A-scan of invasion of nasal orbit (*arrows*)

ing any significant degree of orbital pain. Such patients may complain of a low level of discomfort or a vague sense of pressure inconsistent with the size of the tumor. The consistency of the orbital fat and connective tissue is rather elastic. The low resistance anteriorly allows forward proptosis of the globe to an advanced stage before symptoms become apparent.

# Case Study 68
## Cavernous Hemangioma

AL is a 50-year-old man who noted occasional mild sensations of pressure around his right eye that were more apparent when he bent over to pick up something. He lived alone and was not aware of the progressive prominence of his right eye until a friend who had not seen him for several years mentioned it. Examination found 8 mm of axial proptosis with normal visual acuity and full extraocular movements.

Echography demonstrated a high reflective, multiseptate, well-outlined tumor within the muscle cone with a moderately positive angle kappa. It measured 19.13 mm in greatest diameter. The A-scan probe was reapplied with moderate pressure to the globe for 30 seconds, after which the tumor was remeasured and the lesion showed delayed compressibility by reducing in size to 17.53 mm (Fig. 153). Echographic characteristics were quite characteristic of a cavernous hemangioma and the growth was easily removed in total by an orbital surgeon with the subsequent pathological verification of the diagnosis.

The resistance of the orbital tissue is low to forward expansion of tumors even with explosive growth. The degree of discomfort is generally relatively mild even in cases of marked proptosis.

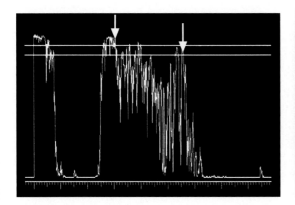 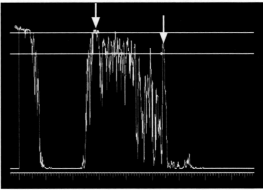

FIG. 153. Left: A-scan of large cavernous hemangioma (*vertical arrows*). Right: A-scan of lesion after compression (*arrows*)

# Case Study 69
## Orbital Rhabdomyosarcoma

AM is a 10-year-old boy who was playing with a wiffle ball when it struck his left eye. There was no apparent injury and he continued playing after a few minutes. The next day his parents noted some mild redness and swelling of his lids on that side, but he had no complaints and went off to school. By that evening the swelling had increased dramatically but he mentioned only a mild pressure feeling. The parents were concerned and took him to the emergency room. An ophthalmologist was called in for a consultation and felt the child had suffered an orbital hemorrhage from the ball. A CT scan showed diffuse orbital opacity with increased tissue volume compatible with the diagnosis of hemorrhage (Fig. 154).

Echography demonstrated a large, firm, very low reflective lesion within the orbit measuring over

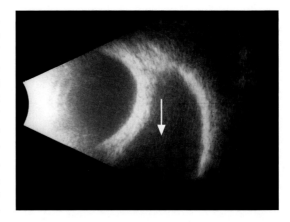

FIG. 155. A-scan of rhabdomyosarcoma (*vertical arrow*)

19.0 mm in greatest dimension (Fig. 155). It was moderately firm to compression. Spontaneous vascularity was noted. The differential included orbital hemorrhage, but a solid mass such as rhabdomyosarcoma could not be ruled out. He was urgently referred for orbital biopsy and frozen sections revealed that it was a rhabdomyosarcoma. The orbit was extenerated, which was standard therapy at that time. Current treatment protocols generally avoid such radical therapy and are based on orbital radiation and chemotherapy.

Echography is a valuable ancillary test in the evaluation of ocular and orbital pain. Its judicious use can often result in the correct diagnosis or aid in the selection of the most effective subsequent testing modality.

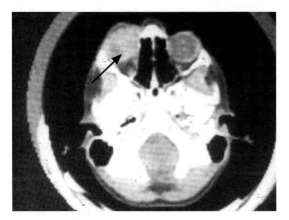

Fig. 154. Computed tomography of rhabdomyosarcoma (*arrow*)

# Part IV
## Blurred Vision

Blurred vision is the *sine quo non* of visual system symptoms. Concern about loss or reduction of the ability to see is a fundamental concern to any normal individual. Rarely, a psychotic patient may mutilate his own eye and suffer permanent damage. This can occur because of distorted feelings of guilt that drive the sufferer to harm himself as punishment for the perceived sin of misuse of his eyes. In the Greek tragedy *Oedipus*, the king puts out his own eyes when he realizes that he has inadvertently killed his father and taken his own mother as wife.

# Case Study 70
## Phthisis Bulbi

TH is a 45-year-old Hispanic woman who was referred for echography to evaluate her eyes regarding any potential for vision. At the age of 25 she had suffered a psychotic episode and stuck a fork into each of her eyes. She had been unable to see light since that time and was mentally stable on medication. Examination found questionable bare light perception in the right eye and no light perception (NLP) in the left. Dense corneal opacities precluded visualization of the fundi.

Echography revealed bilateral phthisis bulbi with total retinal detachments, plaquelike choroidal calcification (Fig. 156), and short globes with axial lengths of 20.34 in the right eye and 21.1 in the left. The referring ophthalmologist was informed that there was no visual potential in either eye.

When the patient presents with the complaint of a reduction in vision, a careful history is essential. Just as with eye pain, historical information must be

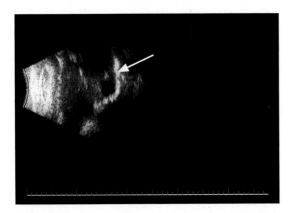

FIG. 156. B-scan of phthisical globe with calcified choroid (*arrow*)

gathered in a systematic way. The benefits of careful attention to the patient's specific complaint are immediate. The subtle nuances that emerge when looking directly at her while she relates the problem in her own words may lead the examiner in a different direction than was initially intended. Really listening, asking pertinent questions, and restating points for clarification are vital history-taking skills that pay important dividends in the final balance sheet of effective, caring medical practice.

The change in vision is analyzed regarding its character. Is it total or partial? Is it persistent or transient? The patient may describe it as a film over the eye or a cloud or a veil. It may be a dark spot in the center or a curtain covering a quadrant of the field of vision. Some patients may find it difficult to articulate the nature of the problem. One elderly lady said, "My vision just doesn't seem right. I can't look at something very long before it goes funny." She had not used the word *double* to describe the problem but on direct questioning she realized that she was seeing two objects. When either eye was covered her symptoms went away.

The location of the visual deficit is important to elicit. The central scotoma of optic neuritis is different than the visual dysfunction of a homonymous hemianopsia. Some patients are not very good at explaining their symptoms and this requires the examiner to ask simple and direct questions to refine exactly where in the field of vision the difficulty lies. It is helpful to ask the patient to look at the examiner's nose at a distance of 1 to 2 feet and first describe what is seen with the normal eye in a case of unilateral visual loss. This eye is then covered and the affected eye is directed at the practitioner's nose. "Now, tell me what you see as you focus on my nose but notice the face around it." This is a valuable technique that can pick up a central or paracentral scotoma, an altitudinal defect, or a general depression in visual perception.

The onset and duration of the decrease in vision is then noted. The sudden catastrophic visual loss of a central retinal artery occlusion occurs over a few minutes to an hour. The slow progressive loss of an optic nerve sheath meningioma can happen over years without the patient being aware of it until it has resulted in substantial depression of vision. *Amaurosis fugax* is Latin for temporary blindness and describes episodes of gray-outs or black-outs of vision that last from seconds to minutes. These fleeting snatches of blindness often have a vascular basis due to transient embolic or vasospastic phenomena. In some cases it is obvious to the clinician that the process resulting in visual loss has occurred over a long time period but the patient has only recently become aware of it. In such cases the patient briefly closed the normal eye and suddenly became aware that the vision was blurred in the opposite eye.

The degree of the reduction in vision is important to note. The evaluation and treatment of profound visual loss is usually urgent. The catastrophic loss of vision of a central retinal artery occlusion is often permanent, but in some cases reversible if heroic measures are taken within the first hour. The vascular occlusion of arteritic optic neuropathy must be emergently treated with high-dose steroids to prevent further visual reduction and to protect the opposite eye. The descending curtain of a detaching retina must be promptly repaired before the macula separates and markedly worsens the prognosis for visual recovery.

The clinician must also pay attention to more subtle degrees of reduction of vision. The patient whose vision is recorded by the technician as 20/20-2 could easily be passed off as normal. However, when that patient is observed while reading the eye chart, it is apparent that it is not a sharp, crisp 20/20, but a slow and hesitating one. This requires the practitioner to deviate from his busy schedule and devote adequate time to more carefully evaluate the problem. Amsler grid testing, pupil evaluation, and possible formal visual field testing may be required.

# Case Study 71
## Optic Nerve Glioma

TM is an 8-year-old boy who had undergone strabismus surgery for esotropia and was also treated with glasses and patching for amblyopia. He had responded over 6 months to treatment with improvement to the 20/30 level of vision in the amblyopic right eye. However, on the next 3-month appointment he had dropped the visual acuity in that eye to 20/40-2. His ophthalmologist felt this was unusual with his parents' careful adherence to the glasses and patching regimen. A careful examination of the optic nerve was performed and early disc pallor was noted that had not been previously observed.

Echography was performed and revealed right optic nerve thickening to 7.45 mm with a negative 30° test, meaning that the nerve thickness stayed the same on abduction of the eye. This suggested a solid enlargement of the nerve versus one due to increased intrasheath fluid (Fig. 157). Magnetic resonance imaging (MRI) scanning was then per-

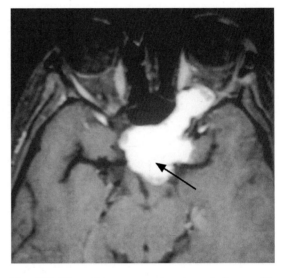

FIG. 158. Magnetic resonance imaging of glioma with involvement of chiasm (*arrow*)

formed and demonstrated fusiform enlargement of the nerve with extension into the optic chiasm (Fig. 158). Neurosurgical exploration later confirmed an optic nerve glioma. The child has been closely followed with repeat scans and thus far the tumor has not grown.

A low threshold of suspicion is very important for the patient in whom "things just don't fit together." The examiner is obligated to explain why a given patient cannot be refracted to 20/20. This is more difficult in someone with existing pathology, such as a cataract or macular degeneration. This can create a trap because the reduced visual acuity can be ascribed to the identifiable problem and the examination stops at this point and a more serious underlying disease process is missed.

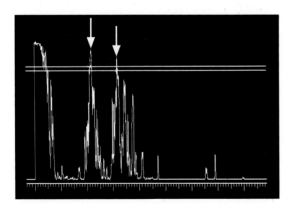

FIG. 157. A-scan of optic nerve glioma (*vertical arrows*)

175

# Case Study 72
## Chiasmal Glioma

TH is a 62-year-old man who saw his ophthalmologist with the complaint that his glasses were not adequately correcting his vision. Examination found visual acuity at the 20/50 level in both eyes and a mild nuclear sclerotic cataract bilaterally. His reduced vision was attributed to the cataracts and he was offered surgery, but the patient stated he functioned adequately in daily life and opted to return in a year. A few months later he experienced severe headaches and sought care at the local emergency room. An MRI scan was performed and a large pituitary tumor was identified with chiasmal compression (Fig. 159). He was sent to a neuro-ophthalmologist for baseline testing before neurosurgery was scheduled to remove the tumor.

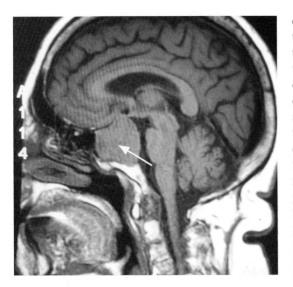

FIG. 159. Pituitary tumor with chiasmal compression (*arrow*)

The consultant recorded bilateral temporal optic disc pallor and a visual field documented a severe bitemporal field defect.

Any associated symptoms can provide helpful clues to the diagnosis of the etiology of the change in vision. A rapid and variable change in refraction in association with increased thirst and urination is suggestive of diabetes. A 35-year-old woman who presents with reduced vision in one eye associated with pain on movement of the eye and paresthesias in her hand over the past year is likely to have a demyelinating disease, such as multiple sclerosis. It is important to ask the patient specific questions about such systemic problems as she may not see the correlation to the visual system and fail to volunteer the information.

Once a thorough history has been taken, the examination should start with a careful refraction to document the best corrected vision. This is the starting point in the evaluation of decreased vision. The eye practitioner speaks in terms of best corrected vision. The patient is usually more concerned about uncorrected vision: "Doctor, I can't see the big E on the chart without my glasses. Does that mean I am legally blind?" The evaluation of early disease processes can only begin in the context of an accurate best corrected visual acuity. The refraction is often relegated to a technician and the patient sees the doctor after this has been done and the pupils dilated. Unfortunately these two critical pieces of information are not available for direct confirmation by the eye professional. If there is any question about their accuracy the patient is asked to return in a day or so to allow the doctor to get a feeling for the refraction and perform a meticulous pupil examination.

Patients often are not aware that there has been a change in the refraction, especially if it mostly involves one eye. They may close one eye for some reason and notice that the vision is blurred in the opposite eye. They then present at the clinician's office with the complaint of a "sudden drop in vision." It is essential that an accurate refraction be performed to initiate the evaluation of the visual system. Echography is sometimes useful in cases of dramatic refractive shift.

# Case Study 73
## Intumescent Lens

TA is a 54-year-old woman who presented with the history of a rapid reduction of vision in her left eye over the past several days. She had only worn glasses for reading up to this time and had no other ocular or systemic problems in the past. Examination found vision OD of 20/25 and OS of 20/100. Slit-lamp examination revealed mild nuclear sclerosis in the right lens and 2+ nuclear sclerosis in the left. The left anterior chamber appeared shallower than the right. Intraocular pressure was 12 mm OD and 19 mm OS

A-scan echography revealed lens thickness OD of 3.41 mm and OS of 5.37 mm (Fig. 160). This was consistent with an intumescent lens. She was referred for cataract surgery because of the shallow anterior chamber and increased pressure.

Echography is also useful in the elimination of certain pathological conditions. Biometry can help to clarify various refractive conditions.

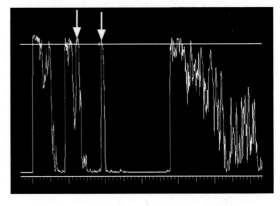

FIG. 160. A-scan of intumescent lens (*vertical arrows*)

# Case Study 74
## Accommodative Spasm

SF is a 15-year-old girl with intractable seizures who had been treated with various antiseizure medications, including a new experimental drug. She had not worn lens correction in the past but presented with complaints of a recent dramatic decrease in vision in both eyes. Examination found uncorrected vision OU of 20/400 and a refraction of −8.00 diopters OD and −7.50 diopters OS. Keratometry measured 44.00 by 43.50 in her right eye and 44.50 by 44.00 in her left. A-scan biometry was performed and the axial length of the right eye measured 23.49 mm and the left measured 23.25 mm (Fig. 161).

These measurements were not consistent with her highly myopic refraction. She underwent atropine cycloplegic retinoscopy with measurements of −0.75 diopters OD and −0.50 OS. These findings were felt to be diagnostic of accommodative spasm. She was treated with cycloplegics and reading glasses for near work. This resolved her

symptoms but over the course of a year she developed −1.50 diopters of myopia as confirmed by cycloplegic retinoscopy and was given appropriate contact lens correction.

If a refraction does not result in a satisfactory level of vision for the patient's age and general ocular status, then the pinhole test should be performed. This test is very useful to separate anterior segment problems, such as corneal irregularities or moderate cataract, from posterior segment abnormalities, such as macular degeneration or optic nerve disease. This is best done after the refraction with the prescription in a trial frame, one eye occluded and a pinhole occluder in front of the eye being tested. The room lights are dimmed and the eye chart is set to a level at which the patient can realistically be expected to see it. He is then told to "move your eye or your head a little until you find the best hole through which to read some letters." He is encouraged to

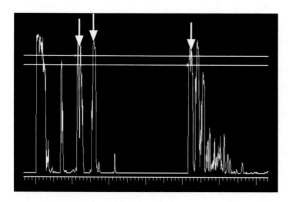 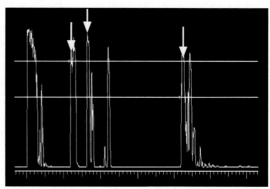

FIG. 161. Left: Axial length of right eye (*arrows*). Right: Left eye (*arrows*) (*First arrow*: cornea, *second arrow*: lens, *third arrow*: retina)

read down the chart as far as possible and given ample time to do this.

The pupils are then examined with attention first drawn to the direct response as the patient looks at a distant target in dim light. A penlight is held about a meter away and a little below eye level and shined directly first at one eye and the briskness and degree of the constriction to light noted. It is then moved to the other side and the process repeated. Then the swinging flashlight or afferent pupil test is performed in which the light is shined directly into one eye with resultant constriction of the pupil. The light is then quickly moved across to the other eye and the response of the pupil is noted. Normally it will just start to dilate as the light is rapidly moved across from the other side and a slight constriction to direct light is noted. However, if there is an abnormality affecting the optic nerve then there is an absence of constriction and an apparent dilation of the pupil to the light as it is moved across. This seemingly paradoxical response is due to the consensual light reflex where the normal eye receives the light stimulus and through nerve pathways via the nucleus of Edinger Westphal constricts the other eye's pupil. When the light is quickly moved across to the abnormal side the direct light response is not sufficient to hold the pupil at the same degree of constriction as the consensual reflex and therefore it seems to relatively dilate. This is not a true dilation to direct light but a relatively lesser degree of constriction.

The role of echography in the evaluation of visual loss is a very important one from the level of daily office practice to specialty referral at the tertiary care center. It complements the clinical examination and provides imaging of the visual system from the anterior segment to the apex of the orbit. It is superior to computed tomography (CT) or MRI in the resolution of intraocular pathology, although immersion techniques may be required to adequately visualize the anterior segment.

Ultrasound is of critical importance in the evaluation of the eye with opaque media of any cause. Sequentially, the anterior most example of media "opacity" starts at the eyelids. A relatively common problem is the squinty patient. Many children and some adults are very photophobic and resist attempts to examine the eye. This can present significant problems when pathology is likely and rarely abnormalities can be missed in a supposedly normal eye.

# Case Study 75
## Retinoblastoma

RM is a 4-year-old child who was brought in by his mother for a routine prekindergarten examination. He was relatively uncooperative for the fundus examination. Indirect ophthalmoscopy was attempted, but only a fleeting view of either fundus could be obtained. The ophthalmologist justifiably felt that the examination was adequate in an otherwise normal child without specific complaints. He told the mother to bring him back in a year unless there were eye problems. A week later he fell off a chair and struck his head and experienced a brief loss of consciousness. A CT scan was obtained at the emergency room with no head trauma noted, but incidentally a calcified mass was detected in the superior temporal periphery of the left eye. He was referred to a pediatric ophthalmologist for fundus examination. This could not be adequately performed in the office so an examination under anesthesia was later performed. A solid mass was noted in the superior temporal fundus of the left eye.

Echography demonstrated a solid mass measuring 8.13 mm in thickness and over 11 mm at the base. A- and B-scan both showed medium-to-high internal reflectivity consistent with calcium deposition (Fig. 162). These findings were highly consistent with retinoblastoma. The child was referred to pediatric oncology for management. His mother was very concerned that the primary ophthalmologist had missed the tumor and asked the pediatric ophthalmologist if she should consider legal action.

Echography performed through closed lids can be easily performed even in the most sensitive patient. It is not uncommon for the practitioner

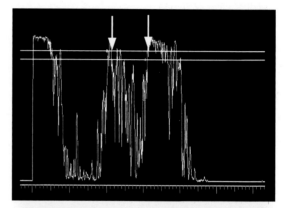

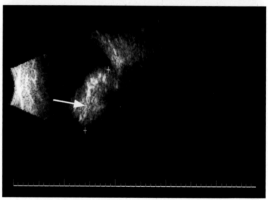

FIG. 162. Top: A-scan of retinoblastoma (*vertical arrows*). Bottom: B-scan of retinoblastoma (*arrow*)

to become frustrated in trying to examine such an individual and fail to adequately visualize the retina. The extra 2 to 3 minutes spent in scanning the globe with the B-scan gives reassurance that significant pathology is not being missed.

183

# Case Study 76
## Posterior Vitreous Detachment with Retinal Tear

AG is a 32-year-old man who was very sensitive to anything around his eyes. He had once tried to wear contact lenses, but gave up when he took over an hour to insert them. He never had successfully completed a glaucoma test because he would not keep his eyes open for tonometry or air-puff testing. He noted the onset of light flashes and floaters in his right eye for several days and presented at the ophthalmologist's office at his wife's insistence. His visual acuity was 20/30-2 OD and 20/20 OS with a myopic correction of −6.00 in each eye. His intraocular pressure could not be measured and the peripheral fundi could not be examined with scleral depression or three-mirror contact lens examination because of the blepharospasm that these procedures precipitated.

Echography was performed through his closed lids and revealed the presence of a total posterior vitreous detachment (PVD) in the right eye with focal vitreoretinal traction with the appearance of an operculum overlying a retinal tear anterior to the 2:00 equator (Fig. 163). He was referred for photocoagulation around the tear with the plan to give him an oral sedative and an injection of lidocaine for a lid block.

Echography can be especially useful in the evaluation of ocular trauma where the eyelids are sometimes edematous precluding adequate visualization of the globe. The ultrasound probe can be gently placed against the closed lids even in a case of suspected globe rupture.

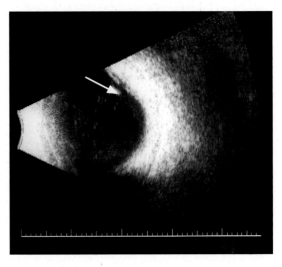

FIG. 163. B-scan of posterior vitreous detachment with traction retinal tear (*arrow*)

# Case Study 77
## Ruptured Globe

MA is a 26-year-old man who ran into a tree while ski racing and suffered multiple facial bone fractures. The eyelids were very edematous and ecchymotic. An attempt to examine the globes in the intensive care unit (ICU) was attempted but was not adequate.

Echography was performed and revealed bilaterally ruptured globes with vitreous incarceration at the site of rupture in the right eye (Fig. 164) and a subretinal hemorrhage in the left eye (Fig. 165). He

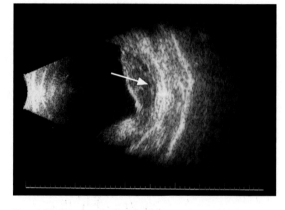

FIG. 165. B-scan of subretinal hemorrhage (*arrow*)

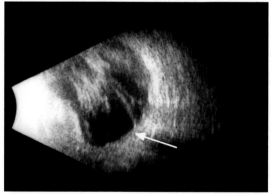

FIG. 164. B-scan of scleral rupture with vitreous incarceration (*arrow*)

was scheduled for surgical repair when his medical condition stabilized.

The eyelids can be weighed down from the edema of mechanical processes. Swelling resulting from trauma, inflammation, or hemorrhage can cause a tense closure of the lid that makes examination of the intraocular structures difficult. Echography is important in evaluation of the globe and orbit in such cases.

# Case Study 78
## Subperiosteal Hemorrhage

TA is an 11-year-old boy who presented with an ecchymotic and ptotic left upper lid. He had awakened 2 days previously with mild aching around the eye and gradually worsening ptosis since that time with a bluish discoloration. He gave a history of a "helmut bump" to the side of his head while playing football 2 days prior to this occurrence but denied any direct injury to his eye. Examination showed almost complete closure of the lid with 2+ tense ecchymosis and mild tenderness. A partial elevation of the eyelid was performed and the globe appeared grossly normal, but the view was inadequate.

Echography was performed and demonstrated a clear vitreous cavity and attached retina. The orbit was imaged by B-scan and an echolucent, well-outlined subperiosteal space was seen in the superior orbit from 10:30 to 12:30 nasally to temporally and back into the mid-orbit posteriorly (Fig. 166). A-scan revealed very low reflectivity (Fig. 167). The differential diagnosis included a subperiosteal hemorrhage or an abscess. The lack of clinical signs

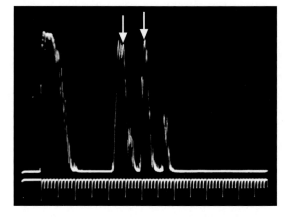

FIG. 167. A-scan of subperiosteal hemorrhage (*vertical arrows*)

of inflammation or infection favored the diagnosis of hemorrhage and the patient was told to return in a few days. He came back with improvement in the ptosis and a normal appearance to the globe.

Congenital eyelid closure includes blepharophimosis that can result in fusion of the eyelids accompanying severe microophthalmos or ultimately anophthalmos. The status of the globe or lack thereof is an important question in infants born with this anomaly.

True anophthalmia in which there is no ocular tissue is extremely rare. It is at the extreme end of the spectrum of microphthalmia, which is defined as an axial length of less than 19.0 mm in a child less than 1 year of age. It may be an isolated occurrence or related to one of several systemic syndromes. If the insult to the embryo occurs before the complete invagination of the optic vesicle, a cyst can form presenting in the newborn as microphthalmos with cyst.

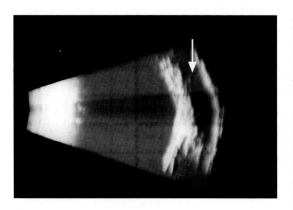

FIG. 166. B-scan of subperiosteal hemorrhage (*vertical arrows*)

# Case Study 79
## Microophthalmos with Cyst

A newborn baby was noted to have a small eye on the right side with partially fused eyelids. There was an impression of the presence of a globe but clinical examination was difficult.

Echography revealed a small vestigial ocular structure with the presence of a rudimentary lens and a large cystic component posteriorly (Fig. 168). The diagnosis of microophthalmos with cyst was made. There was no visual potential in the eye but the child was referred to oculoplastics for appropriate cosmesis of the lids and socket. The cyst became large enough to require intermittent drainage.

The cornea is the window into the eye and anything that clouds this structure can interfere with the patient's view outwards and the examiner's view inwards. Corneal opacification can be due to a number of causes, including edema. Such swelling commonly occurs from failure of the endothelial pump system, but can also result from fluid that has been forced into the epithelium and anterior corneal stroma secondary to increased intraocular pressure.

Immersion echography is helpful in imaging the anatomy of the anterior segment in such cases.

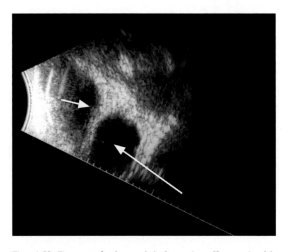

FIG. 168. B-scan of microophthalmos (*small arrow*) with cyst (*large arrow*)

# Case Study 80
## Topamax-Induced Angle Closure

LA is a 50-year-old man who presented with complaints of a rapid reduction in vision and moderate aching pain over the past 24 hours. He denied any previous history of a similar event. His past medical history was positive for a seizure disorder and a recent increase in vascular headaches. He had taken two doses of topamax starting 2 days previously. Clinical examination found visual acuity in both eyes of less than 20/400 but this was improved to 20/70 OD with a −2.50 sphere and 20/80 OS with a −3.50 sphere. He had no history of wearing glasses or contact lenses. There was 2+ corneal edema bilaterally and intraocular pressures of 45 OD and 47 OS. The indirect ophthalmoscope could visualize the optic nerves with a cup to disc ratio of 2/10 OU.

Immersion scanning was performed with a 20-MHz probe and then an ultrasound biomicroscope (UBM; 50 MHz). The angle was very narrow and the ciliary processes were rotated anteriorly (Fig. 169). He was treated conservatively with topical pressure lowering agents and the topamax was discontinued. The pressure returned to normal within 3 days, the corneal edema resolved, and the myopia disappeared.

Inflammatory or hemorrhagic cellular processes may obscure the anterior chamber. Opacification of this compartment by hemorrhage (hyphema) is a relatively common occurrence after ocular trauma. It is vital to evaluate the status of the posterior segment in such a situation. The possibility of a detached retina, choroidal hemorrhage, or ruptured globe demands accurate imaging by echography. Such treatable conditions require immediate attention to provide the best chance of success.

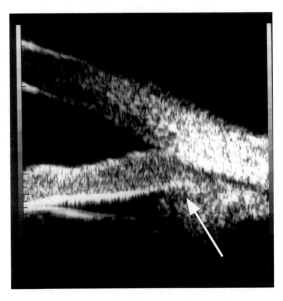

FIG. 169. Ultrasound biomicroscopy of anterior rotation of ciliary body (*arrow*)

# Case Study 81
## Ruptured Globe

TA is a 21-year-old man who was hit in the right eye with a racquetball. He had taken his protective goggles off because they had fogged up and were interfering with his game. He noted the immediate onset of severe pain and rapid reduction in his vision. He presented at the hospital emergency room within an hour and the ophthalmologist was called in for a consultation. He noted vision in that eye of hand motions at 1 m, intraocular pressure of 25 mm, a total eight-ball hyphema in the anterior chamber, and no view of the fundus.

The patient was referred for echography. B-scan revealed a partial posterior vitreous detachment and vitreous incarceration at the superior equator that was suspicious for a choroidal rupture. There was also the appearance of choroidal edema with some degree of hemorrhage (Fig. 170). A-scan detected moderate intravitreal opacities consistent with hemorrhage. It was elected to watch the patient and treat the elevated pressure with topical medications. The posterior segment was followed daily with ultrasound. The vitreous cleared over several days and the fundus could be visualized. The probable rupture site appeared to have self-sealed and the retina was attached. Surgery was not felt to be indicated.

Uveitic conditions can result in media opacities that obscure a view of the posterior segment. Chronic inflammation may lead to anterior chamber reaction, posterior synechiae with a miotic, or, ultimately, an occluded pupil and cataract formation. Such sequelae of uveitis can result in a hazy view of the vitreous cavity and fundus.

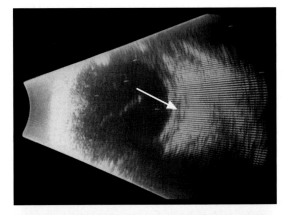

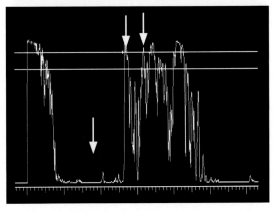

FIG. 170. Top: B-scan of choroidal edema (*arrow*). Bottom: A-scan of vitreous hemorrhage (*first arrow*) and choroidal edema (*second and third arrows*)

Such patients often come to cataract surgery and a preoperative ultrasound is mandatory to evaluate the globe.

# Case Study 82
## Cyclitic Membrane

FA is a 45-year-old woman who presented with complaints of poor vision in her right eye for several months. She had waited for her medical insurance to become effective before seeking medical attention. She initially experienced a red, painful eye, but it had become less irritated over time. Examination found visual acuity in the right eye of 20/80 and in the left eye of 20/20. Intraocular pressure measured 2 mm OD and 15 mm OS. Slit-lamp examination demonstrated 2+ mutton-fat keratic precipitates, 270° of posterior synechiae with a fixed pupil, and a 3+ nuclear sclerotic cataract. The posterior segment could not be visualized.

Echography revealed a partial posterior vitreous detachment with mild intravitreal dotlike opacities. On extreme peripheral view with the B-scan, a high

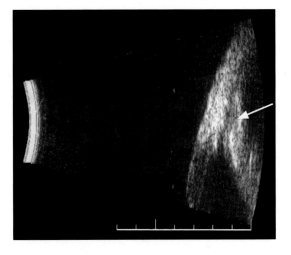

FIG. 172. Twenty-megahertz immersion scan of ciliary body detachment (*arrow*)

reflective membrane was detected retrolentally. An immersion scan was performed and demonstrated a cyclitic membrane bridging the temporal to the nasal ciliary body (Fig. 171). A shallow traction detachment of the ciliary body was present (Fig. 172) that explained the relative hypotony in this eye.

The crystalline lens is remarkable in its ability to focus light on the retina with sufficient plasticity to change shape as the ciliary muscles contract. Lens opacities are ubiquitous as people age and generally require cataract surgery if they interfere with vision. Cataracts that obscure a view of the intraocular contents are an indication for echography. Less dense opacities with an atypical presentation, such as a sector cataract in a younger patient, should also be investigated by ultrasound.

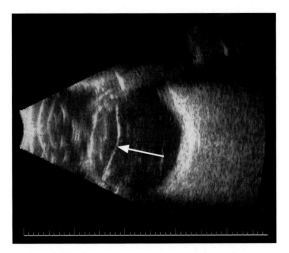

FIG. 171. Immersion scan of cyclitic membrane (*arrow*)

# Case Study 83
## Ciliary Body Melanoma

TB is a 43-year-old man with complaints of a film over part of the vision in his right eye for several months. It had seemed to descend from the lower part of his visual field and grow upwards into the center of his vision. Examination demonstrated best corrected vision in his right eye of 20/60-2 and in his left eye of 20/20. His pupils were equal in size and reactive to light without an afferent defect. Slit-lamp examination discovered a sectorial cortical and posterior capsular lens opacity in the superior part of his lens that was encroaching into the visual axis. Dilated fundus examination was unremarkable with a normal retinal periphery. Because of his relatively young age and the unusual nature of the lens opacity, he was referred for immersion ultrasound examination.

Echography revealed a normal posterior segment. Immersion scanning was done using a scleral shell filled with methylcellulose and the anterior segment was visualized. A solid echodense mass was seen in the ciliary body in contact with the inferior pole of the lens (Fig. 173). The diagnosis was consistent with a malignant melanoma of the ciliary body.

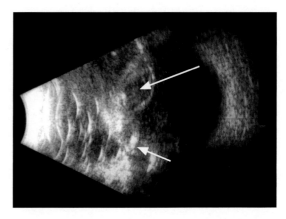

FIG. 173. Immersion scan of melanoma (*small arrow*) touching lens (*large arrow*)

Inadequate visualization of the fundus by the ophthalmoscope should prompt an echographic evaluation of the cataractous eye, especially in a patient who has not been followed over time by his doctor as the cataract progresses. The documentation of a thorough fundus examination within the past couple of years substantially reduces the chances of an unsuspected intraocular melanoma hiding behind media opacity such as a cataract.

# Case Study 84
## Choroidal Melanoma

TS is a 67-year-old woman who had not had an eye examination for several years and complained of progressively decreasing vision in her left eye for over a year. Clinical examination demonstrated a moderately dense nuclear sclerotic and cortical cataract that hindered adequate visualization of the entire fundus. Cataract surgery was scheduled and biometry was performed. There was some difficulty in obtaining a consistent axial length and because the fundus could not be completely examined she was referred for echography.

Ultrasound revealed a solid mushrooming mass near the temporal equator (Fig. 174). A-scan examination demonstrated low-to-medium, regular internal reflectivity with moderate spontaneous internal vascularity (Fig. 175). These findings were highly consistent with a malignant melanoma of the choroid. Cataract surgery was cancelled and the

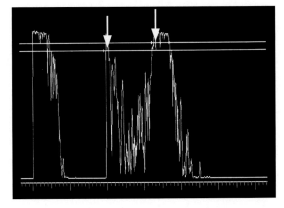

FIG. 175. A-scan of melanoma (*vertical arrows*)

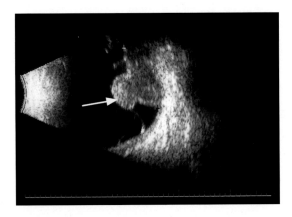

FIG. 174. B-scan of mushrooming melanoma (*arrow*)

patient referred to an ocular oncologist for management of the tumor.

There are a number of reports in the literature of unsuspected intraocular tumors that were not discovered until after cataract surgery. A study by Shields and Augsburger[27] reviewed 21 cases of cataracts that had been removed in the presence of unsuspected choroidal or ciliary body melanomas. They stated, "Since ultrasonography has become readily accessible to most ophthalmologists in countries with advanced medical care, it should be considered as a part of the preoperative evaluation in all patients who have a cataract which is advanced enough to prevent a clear fundus view. It should definitely be performed in patients who have a dense unexplained unilateral cataract." Peter et al. reviewed a series at the Armed Forces Institute of Pathology and found that 5.5% of enucleated eyes (35 of 650) for melanoma were aphakic or pseudophakic. They state, "we believe that most of these tumors were large enough at the time of cataract surgery to have been detected if diagnostic ultrasonography had been performed."[28] Shammas and Blodi[29] state that "a considerable delay in diagnosis and treatment of more than 10% of eyes containing advanced melanomas may result from an inability to visualize the tumor." The possibility of such a potentially life-threatening lesion merits echographic imaging of an eye with a cataract or other media opacity that precludes adequate visualization of the posterior segment.

# Case Study 85
## Choroidal Melanoma

DH is a 72-year-old woman who underwent uncomplicated cataract surgery. The preoperative examination was felt adequate for visualization of all but the superior periphery of the fundus due to a cortical opacity in the upper half of the lens. Postoperative examination with the indirect ophthalmoscope detected a dark elevated lesion at 12:00 near the ora serrata.

Echography confirmed a solid, medium reflective lesion with mild spontaneous internal vascularity (Fig. 176). It was felt to be highly consistent with a malignant melanoma of the choroid and the patient was referred for radioactive plaque treatment. She was informed that there was a small chance that the surgical manipulation during cataract surgery had disseminated some tumor cells into her blood stream. She was referred to her primary care doctor for systemic evaluation.

A subgroup of patients with media opacities masking an unsuspected intraocular tumor is those with longstanding blind or nearly blind eyes with some degree of ocular discomfort. A study from the Armed Forces Institute of Pathology in 1963[29] found that 10% of blind painful eyes harbored malignant melanomas or other tumors. Char states that this percentage of malignancies in such eyes still holds true.[30] Many of these eyes had experienced previous trauma or surgery. It is the standard of care in such an eye to perform diagnostic echography.

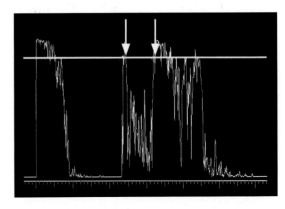

FIG. 176. A-scan of medium melanoma (*vertical arrows*)

# Case Study 86
## Ciliary Body Melanoma

GP is a 56-year-old man who presented with moderate corneal edema, anterior chamber reaction, and a cortical cataract. He gave a history of a lacerated globe by a piece of glass with immediate surgical repair a number of years previously. He had not seen well out of the eye since that time and the vision had gradually deteriorated to bare light perception over the past year. He felt a frequent aching pain in the eye and noticed that it looked red most of the time.

Echography was performed and demonstrated a solid, medium reflective lesion of the temporal ciliary body. It measured 5 mm in thickness and 10.2 mm in basal dimensions. Moderate spontaneous vascularity was noted (Fig. 177). The diagnosis of a ciliary body malignant melanoma was made and the eye was enucleated at the patient's request.

Pathologic examination revealed an epitheloid melanoma of the ciliary body.

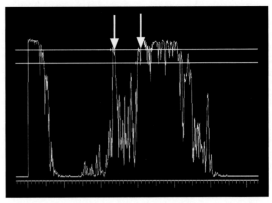

FIG. 177. A-scan of ciliary body melanoma (*vertical arrows*)

# Case Study 87
## Choroidal Melanoma

DW is a 67-year-old man with a 30+-year history of Coat's disease in his right eye. He had undergone laser treatment years ago but had gradually lost the sight in the eye and it had become blind and painful with bullous keratopathy. He was scheduled for evisceration, but the surgeon ordered an ultrasound to eliminate any intraocular tumors.

Echography revealed an inferior dome-shaped mass measuring 3.63 × 6.04 × 8.76mm on B-scan. A-scan demonstrated medium-to-low internal reflectivity (Fig. 178) with a medium angle kappa (sloping internal signals from higher to lower as the sound beam passed through the lesion). Spontaneous vascularity was not seen.

The surgeon was informed that the lesion was suspicious for melanoma and he changed the surgical plan from evisceration to enucleation because of the concern of possible dissemination of a malignant tumor. Pathology confirmed a spindle B melanoma.

A type of media opacity inherent to current cataract surgical techniques is opacification or wrinkling of the posterior lens capsule. After extra-capsular cataract surgery, the posterior capsule may become opacified and wrinkled over time. This occurs in 10% to 50% of cases and is usually treated by YAG laser capsulotomy. One of the potential complications of this procedure is retinal tear and detachment. This is a relatively rare occurrence, but young myopic males are reported to be of higher risk than other groups of patients. It is useful to know if a patient being considered for YAG capsulotomy has a preexisting PVD that would put him at lower risk for a retinal tear because of the absence of vitreoretinal traction.

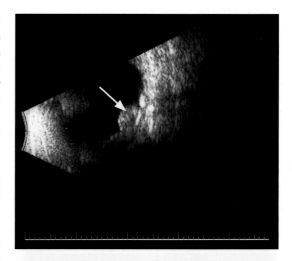

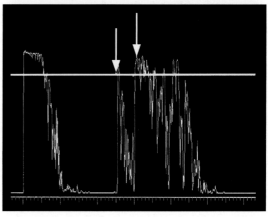

FIG. 178. Top: B-scan of the lesion (*arrow*). Bottom: A-scan of choroidal melanoma (*arrows*)

# Case Study 88
## Posterior Vitreous Detachment

CG is a 52-year-old man who had undergone cataract surgery in both eyes 2 years prior to presentation. Prior to intraocular lens implantation he was highly myopic with a refraction OD of −10.00 and OS of −9.50. He now complained of decreased vision in his right eye and visual acuity was measured at 20/70 in that eye and the left eye at 20/25. Slit-lamp examination showed moderate opacification of the posterior lens capsule in the right eye and slight opacification in the left eye. He was advised to undergo YAG laser capsulotomy on his right eye, but he seemed concerned about potential complications and asked a number of questions concerning the possibility of retinal detachment. His father had gone blind in one eye from a retinal detachment after cataract surgery.

The presence of a posterior vitreous detachment could not be verified on clinical examination because of the opacified posterior capsule. Echography was performed and demonstrated a total PVD (Fig. 179) with no evidence of vitreoretinal traction. He felt reassured that the possibility of a rhegmatogenous retinal detachment was minimal and proceeded with the laser procedure with resultant vision of 20/20 in that eye.

The existence of a PVD is also protective in patients with proliferative diabetic retinopathy. The neovascular scaffold that grows from the retina onto the posterior hyaloid face can undergo traction as the vitreous separates in a PVD and result in vitreous hemorrhage.

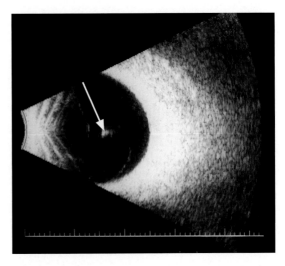

FIG. 179. B-scan of posterior vitreous detachment with Weiss ring (*arrow*)

# Case Study 89
## Vitreous Traction

EI is a 54-year-old woman with a 20-year history of type-1 diabetes. She had undergone panretinal photocoagulation in her right eye for proliferative retinopathy and scatter photocoagulation in her left eye for diabetic macular edema. She presented with a sudden loss of vision in her left eye which started as "seeing dots and streamers in my vision followed by almost total darkness." Examination showed vision in her right eye of 20/30 and left eye finger count at 1 meter. The fundus of the left eye could not be visualized by the ophthalmoscope (direct or indirect).

Echography was performed and revealed a partial PVD with apparent focal traction on a neovascular scaffold on the optic disc (Fig. 180). This finding prompted a recommendation by her ophthalmologist to proceed with vitrectomy within the next several days instead of waiting 6 months for the hemorrhage to clear spontaneously. The concern was that of recurrent hemorrhage with the vitreous-neovascular membrane traction that would reduce the chance of restoration of vision in that eye.

Media opacities, such as vitreous hemorrhage, can hide fundus lesions that are only detectable by echography. The sudden onset of flashes and floaters is often suggestive of a posterior vitreous detachment and this is associated with a retinal tear from 6% to 15% of the time.[31] This is usually detectable on indirect ophthalmoscopy but the presence of vitreous hemorrhage can preclude adequate visualization.

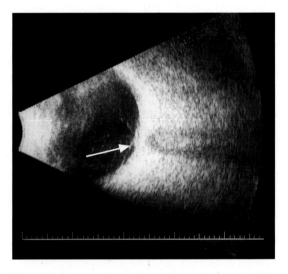

FIG. 180. B-scan of posterior vitreous detachment with traction on neovascular tuft (*arrow*)

# Case Study 90
## Retinal Tear

DJ is a 34-year-old man who noted flashes of light in the right eye for 2 days and then a "lacy cobweb with lots of little black specks" on the day of presentation at his ophthalmologist's office. Examination revealed visual acuity of 20/200 with some variability as he moved his eye around. Ophthalmoscopy found a 2+ vitreous hemorrhage that obscured visualization of the peripheral inferior temporal fundus. Some vitreous membrane formation was noted but retinal detail was hazy.

Echography was performed and demonstrated a total posterior vitreous detachment with moderate intravitreal hemorrhage. An area of vitreoretinal traction was noted at the 5:00 position anterior to the equator. There was the appearance of a flap tear but the adjacent retina was not elevated and no subretinal fluid could be detected (Fig. 181). He was carefully followed by daily echography to verify that the retina was not detaching. When the vitreous hemorrhage had cleared to allow a reasonable view of the fundus, photocoagulation around the tear was performed.

Echography can detect subretinal fluid in the presence of a retinal tear and this provides the retinal surgeon with information to assist in optimizing treatment options from laser to a scleral sponge.

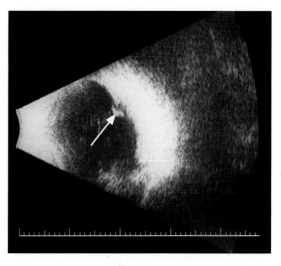

FIG. 181. B-scan of posterior vitreous detachment with vitreous traction on flap tear (*arrows*)

# Case Study 91
## Retinal Tear with Subretinal Fluid

KP is a 32-year-old moderately myopic man who presented with the history of several days of flashing lights and "cobwebs with lots of tiny little dots" in his right eye. His vision was somewhat impaired by the floaters. Examination showed best corrected vision in his right eye of 20/50 by moving his eye back and forth to see through the floaters. The visual acuity in the left eye was 20/20. Fundus examination found a mild vitreous hemorrhage in the right eye with a Weiss ring in the anterior vitreous. There was some clumping of blood inferiorly with obscuration of the view of the retina in the inferotemporal quadrant.

Echography revealed a partial posterior vitreous detachment with moderate intravitreal opacities consistent with hemorrhage. A focal area of vitreoretinal traction was noted at the 7:00 equator consistent with an elevated flap tear with focal subretinal fluid (Fig. 182). This was discussed with the patient and he was advised to reduce physical activity, stop nonsteroidal anti-inflammatory drugs, and return every few days for repeat echography until the vitreous hemorrhage cleared enough to allow treatment of the retinal tear with careful monitoring of the degree of subretinal fluid.

Other causes of vitreous opacification include asteroid hyalosis. This condition is usually idiopathic and often unilateral. It can be dense enough to preclude visualization of the fundus, but yet the patient generally has surprisingly good vision. The reason for this optical paradox is not understood. A patient presenting for the first time to the examiner is best served by an ultrasound evaluation of the eye to rule out fundus pathology.

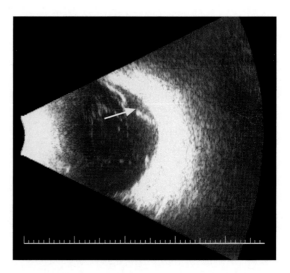

FIG. 182. B-scan of posterior vitreous detachement with vitreous traction and subretinal fluid (*arrow*)

215

# Case Study 92
## Choroidal Melanoma

GP is a 55-year-old woman who presented for a routine eye examination. She stated that for years she had not seen quite as well in her left eye as her right and noticed some floaters against a non-contrast background, such as a blue sky or white wall. Her visual acuity was measured at 20/20 OD and 20/30 OS. Ophthalmoscopy found moderately dense asteroid hyalosis in the left eye and the fundus was poorly seen.

Echography revealed a solid mass lesion near the equator. A-scan demonstrated low-to-medium internal reflectivity with mild spontaneous vascularity. The lesion measured 3.9 mm in height, 6.7 mm in circumferential basal dimension, and 7.2 mm in radial basal dimension (Fig. 183). It was highly consistent with a malignant melanoma of the choroid. A systemic workup was negative for metastases. Options were discussed with the patient and she elected to undergo treatment with a radioactive iodine plaque.

Inflammatory conditions, such as intermediate and posterior uveitis, can opacify the vitreous cavity. This may be idiopathic such as in pars planitis or due to a specific entity, such as toxoplasmosis. Echography is essential in the evaluation of the posterior segment in such conditions. The status of the retina and choroid can best be evaluated by A- and B-scan.

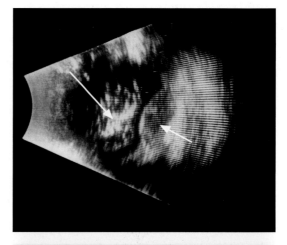

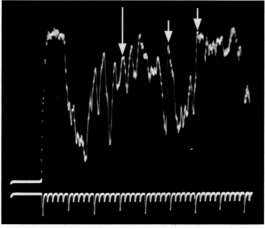

Fig. 183. Top: B-scan of choroidal melanoma (*small arrow*) behind asteroid hyalosis (*large arrow*). Bottom: A-scan of choroidal melanoma (*small arrows*) behind asteroid hyalosis (*large arrow*)

# Case Study 93
## Ocular Toxoplasmosis

MB is a 26-year-old woman who had a history of a "spot" in her left eye since childhood. Her vision had always been good and she was seen by an optical chain store optometrist every few years to update her contact lens prescription. Dilated fundus examination had not been performed during the last several years. She noted the onset of a "film" over her left eye for several days. This progressed to the point where she could only make out vague shapes and forms. She had no complaints of pain or tenderness. Examination by an ophthalmologist found best-corrected vision OD of 20/20 and of hand motions at 1 meter in the left eye. There was a mild anterior chamber reaction with trace flare and cells and dense vitreous cells. Indirect ophthalmoscopy suggested the presence of a lesion just above the macula ("headlight in the fog"). Other fundus details were obscured by the vitreous opacities.

Echography demonstrated 2+ vitreous dot-like opacities and a small solid lesion just above the macula. A- and B-scan of the lesion showed high internal reflectivity and no vascularity (Fig. 184). Calcification wasn't detected. The differential diagnosis included toxoplasmosis and the patient was begun on therapy with triple sulfa and trimethoprim. The vitreous inflammation cleared steadily over several weeks and allowed a view of the fundus with the ophthalmoscope. A yellowish elevated lesion adjacent to an area of chorioretinal scarring was seen which was typical for toxoplasmosis.

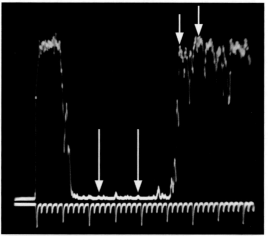

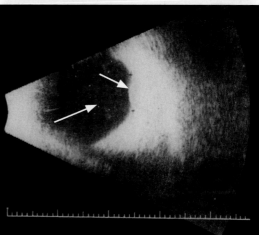

FIG. 184. Top: A-scan of toxoplasmosis lesion (*small arrows*) with vitreous cells (*large arrows*). Bottom: B-scan of toxoplasmosis lesion (*small arrow*) with vitreous cells (*large arrow*)

Neoplastic intraocular lesions can incite vitreous reaction. This is especially true for rapidly growing tumors, such as retinoblastoma. The exophytic type can seed the vitreous with tumor cells and the patient's immune system responds with an outpouring of lymphocytes, polymorphonuclear leukocytes, and other inflammatory mediators. Such vitreous debris can mask the inciting malignancy. Echography is essential in detecting and differentiating such an entity.

# Case Study 94
## Noncalcified Retinoblastoma

DJ is a 2-year-old child who was noted by his parents to have a "wandering eye." He was taken to his ophthalmologist who noted a 30-prism diopter left exotropia. He was unable to see a red reflex in the left eye. The fundus of the right eye was normal. He referred the child for echography.

Dense dotlike vitreous opacities and a solid subretinal mass were imaged but no calcium was detected on B-scan. A-scan demonstrated medium internal reflectivity and mild spontaneous vascularity (Fig. 185). The optic nerve was of normal thickness and no mass lesions were detected in the orbit. The differential diagnosis included a noncalcified retinoblastoma with vitreous seeding. Vitreous aspiration was performed and cytology confirmed the diagnosis of retinoblastoma. The eye was enucleated and chemotherapy was instituted.

Another example of a malignant process with vitreous involvement is central nervous system (CNS) large cell lymphoma. There is a strong correlation between intraocular non-Hodgkin's lymphoma and involvement of the CNS. The vitreous opacities are distinctively larger than other cellular infiltrates that can invade this cavity. This condition is not uncommonly misdiagnosed as chronic uveitis, but a high level of suspicion should exist for lymphoma when a patient over 40 presents with what appears to be intermediate uveitis.

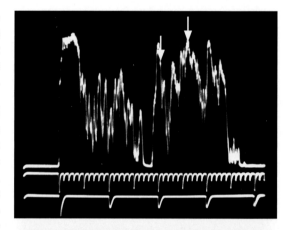

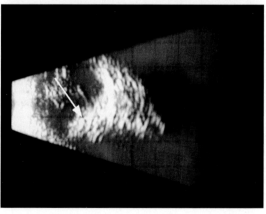

Fig. 185. Top: A-scan of noncalcified retinoblastoma (*vertical arrows*). Bottom: B-scan of the tumor (*arrow*)

# Case Study 95
## Ocular Large Cell Lymphoma

MT is a 52-year-old man who presented with complaints of "spots" in his vision and generalized blurring. His past medical history was unremarkable. Examination of the eye documented visual acuity of 20/20 in the right eye and 20/70 in his left eye. No keratoprecipitates were noted on the corneal endothelial surface and the anterior chamber was clear. The vitreous was hazy with larger yellowish cells floating within it. The diagnosis of pars planitis with intermediate uveitis was made and he was treated with topical and oral steroids. The process was not changed after 2 weeks of treatment so an injection of subtenon's triamcinolone was given. He was seen in another 2 weeks with no improvement.

Echography was performed and 3+ vitreous opacities were noted with focal thickening of the retinochoroid layer (Fig. 186). This finding was felt to be unusual for uveitis so a vitreous biopsy

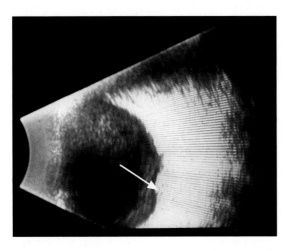

Fig. 186. B-scan of choroidal large cell lymphoma (*arrow*)

was recommended. Cytology demonstrated large cell lymphoma. A spinal tap was performed and showed lymphoma cells in the cerebrospinal fluid. An MRI scan showed enhancement of the brain's meningeal coverings.

A potentially devastating cause of vitreous opacification is endophthalmitis. This can occur via endogenous sources, such as an infection at a distant site in the body. It more commonly is associated with an exogenous seeding of microorganisms, such as penetrating trauma or surgery. The combination of reduced vision, eye pain, and a red angry eye is highly suggestive of infectious endophthalmitis, but the presence of one or more of these findings should raise suspicions for the entity. It is critically important to diagnose endophthalmitis at the earliest stage. This potentially blinding condition can progress over hours, necessitating the institution of appropriate treatment promptly. Mild vitreous opacities may be difficult to detect if the anterior segment is not clear. A patient who has recently undergone intraocular surgery is at risk for endopthalmitis and rapid diagnosis is critical. The classic signs of pain and decreased vision may be subtle especially in the immediate postoperative period when the vision is not expected to be perfectly clear because of mild corneal edema and anterior chamber reaction.

B-scan is useful in demonstrating the formation of membranes and dotlike vitreous opacities, but this is usually a later finding as the process advances to the level of a vitreous abscess. A-scan is helpful in the early stages. The probe is placed against the eye and the gain is increased by 6 decibels above the tissue sensitivity setting ($T + 6$), increases system sensitivity. The vitreous cavity is examined for tiny vertical deflections above the baseline, which can be the first sign of vitreous reaction. As the process advances, the echographic findings become more pronounced. The cellular reaction coalesces into membranes with more prominent opacities on B-scan and higher spikes on A-scan. The retinochoroid layer is thicker as it becomes edematous from the generalized inflammation and in some cases from direct invasion of the tissue by the infectious organisms.

# Case Study 96
## Endophthalmitis

AB is a 72-year-old man who underwent cataract surgery in the right eye and was seen in the office the next day for a postoperative check-up. The cataract was a stage 4 sclerotic nucleus and phacoemulsification had been performed for a prolonged period of time because of the density of the nucleus. He complained of a mild aching pain during the night and blurry vision. Examination found visual acuity of 20/400 in the right eye with a moderate amount of corneal edema and 2 to 3+ cells and flare in the anterior chamber. The vitreous and fundus could not be well seen because of the anterior segment changes of corneal swelling and anterior chamber reaction. He was sent home and instructed to use topical antibiotic and steroid drops. He called later that day and stated that his symptoms were worse and he was concerned. He was brought back to the office and the clinical findings were about the same with possibly a slight increase in the anterior chamber reaction.

The B-scan showed a partial posterior vitreous detachment. However, the A-scan gain was set at $T + 6$ and demonstrated multiple tiny blips in the vitreous cavity (Fig. 187). This was interpreted as early vitreous reaction with a differential diagnosis including hemorrhage or inflammatory cells. In the clinical setting of recent cataract surgery, the diagnosis of endophthalmitis was made and he was referred to a retinal specialist for a vitreous tap and the injection of intraocular antibiotics. As recommended by the collaborative endophthalmitis study, vitrectomy was not performed because the

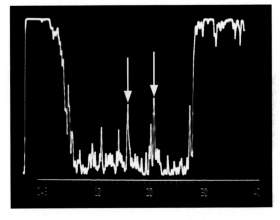

FIG. 187. A-scan of vitreous opacities in aggressive endophthalmitis (*arrows*)

patient had vision at the 20/400 level. If it had been hand motions or worse, then vitrectomy would have been indicated.[32]

He was followed daily over a week with serial A-scans to monitor the vitreous reaction. His clinical symptoms improved concurrently and an adequate view of the fundus could be obtained at this time. He ultimately improved to a visual acuity of 20/40 as the vitreous reaction cleared and the corneal edema resolved. The final culture report was read as "significant *Staphylococcus epidermidis*."

Endophthalmitis can follow an indolent course as a low-grade iritis that does not respond to treatment with anti-inflammatory medications.

# Case Study 97
## Chronic Endophthalmitis

FT is an 80-year-old woman who underwent uncomplicated cataract surgery with intraocular lens implantation and had an unremarkable examination on her first postoperative visit. Her uncorrected visual acuity was measured to be 20/200 in the operative eye. She was noted to have 1+ corneal edema and 1 to 2+ cells and flare. She was seen for follow-up in a week with improvement in her vision to 20/60, but there was a persistent low-grade anterior chamber reaction. The topical steroids were continued and she returned in 2 weeks with vision of 20/70 with 1+ cell and flare in the anterior chamber. A whitish plaque was noted in the periphery of the capsular bag.

Echography was performed and the B-scan was unremarkable. A-scan was done with the gain increased to tissue sensitivity plus 6 decibels. Multiple tiny blips were detected within the vitreous cavity compatible with inflammatory cells (Fig. 188). In the clinical setting of recent intraocular surgery, this finding was most consistent with endophthalmitis. The delayed time course and low degree of inflammatory response suggested an indolent process, such as that caused by propionibacter acnes. An aqueous tap was performed and the diagnosis was confirmed by culture. She failed

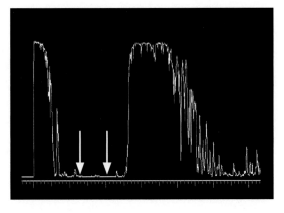

FIG. 188. A-scan of vitreous opacities in indolent endophthalmitis (*arrows*)

to respond to antibiotic treatment and the organism was only eradicated after removal of the intraocular lens and the capsular bag.

The most posterior cause of media opacity is a retrohyaloid or preretinal hemorrhage that obscures the fundus. This can occur spontaneously but is most often due to an underlying vasculopathy, such as diabetes. Echography can be useful in evaluating the retinochoroid layer for abnormalities, such as edema or hemorrhage.

# Case Study 98
## Retinal Macroaneurysm

TM is a 55-year-old woman who had a history of hypertension but stopped her medication because of side effects several years ago. She had not seen her doctor since that time but stated she checked herself on the "blood pressure machine at the grocery store" and it was normal. She presented with a history of an arc of red light in her vision for several days that had not gone away. Examination found visual acuity of 20/50 in the right eye. When she was instructed to look at the examiner's face she stated that there was an "arc of blurring just below the nose." The other eye had a visual acuity of 20/20. Fundus examination found a preretinal

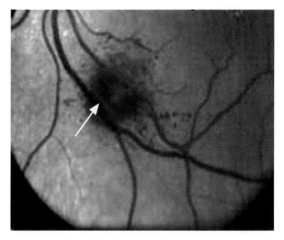

Fig. 190. Fluorescein angiogram of macroaneurysm (*arrow*)

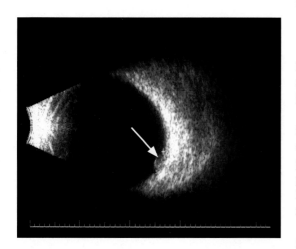

Fig. 189. B-scan of retinal macroaneurysm (*arrow*)

hemorrhage arching along the superior vascular arcades. This area of the retina could not be visualized with the ophthalmoscope.

Echography was performed and demonstrated focal retinal thickening (Fig. 189). The differential diagnosis included a retinal macroaneurysm. The patient was referred for treatment of her blood pressure and the hemorrhage gradually resolved. Fluorescein angiography confirmed a retinal macroaneurysm (Fig. 190).

Blood can condense along the posterior hyaloid face, which increases reflectivity on both A- and B- scan, simulating the high reflectivity of the retina.

# Case Study 99
## Vitreous Hemorrhage

MV is a 55-year-old diabetic who was noted to have early neovascularization of the left optic disc and was advised to return in 4 months to monitor this condition with the possibility of panretinal photocoagulation if it increased. He returned on an emergency basis 3 weeks later with the complaint of loss of central vision in that eye. His visual acuity was 20/25 OD and he could only count fingers in the left eye. The anterior and mid-vitreous were relatively clear but there was preretinal blood obscuring the macular area.

B-scan showed a high reflective membrane attaching at the optic nerve that was very suspicious for retinal detachment. A-scan demonstrated a preretinal vitreous membrane that was about 80% high compared to the initial signal (Fig. 191) and was relatively mobile on eye movements. This was consistent with a partially detached vitreous with blood on the hyaloid face. The patient was told to return in 3 weeks and the blood had mostly resolved. The retina was attached.

Other causes of visual reduction that can be evaluated by echography include astigmatism caused by tilting of the crystalline lens. This may occur from growth of a tumor within the ciliary body pushing on the lens.

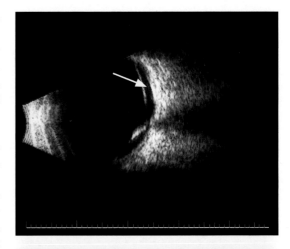

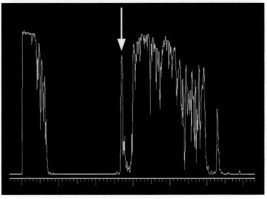

FIG. 191. Top: B-scan of posterior hyaloid face (*arrow*). Bottom: A-scan of the membrane (*arrow*)

# Case Study 100
## Malignant Melanoma of the Ciliary Body with Lens Displacement

TA is a 56-year-old man who complained of a gradual distortion of the vision in his right eye over the past several months. Examination found vision in his right eye of 20/20 and in the left eye of 20/70 with his current glasses. Refraction documented an increased astigmatism of 4 diopters at an axis of 60°. Slit-lamp examination initially appeared unremarkable, but after dilation of the pupils a sectorial cataract at 2:00 was noted. Fundus examination was unremarkable but the cataract blocked an adequate view of the peripheral retina and ciliary body.

B-scan was performed and demonstrated a solid mass lesion in the ciliary body at the 1:00 to 3:00 position. It was difficult to angle the A-scan perpendicular to the tumor, but the impression was that of a medium irregularly reflective lesion with moderate spontaneous vascularity. It was highly consistent with a malignant melanoma of the ciliary body. Immersion B-scan revealed a tumor that appeared to mechanically press on the lens that was felt to explain the irregular astigmatism (Fig. 192).

Another cause of displacement of the crystalline lens is a cyst of the iris and ciliary body that can become large enough to push on the lens. In these cases, a bulge is often noted in the iris on slit-lamp examination. The only way to accurately characterize such a cyst is by immersion echography.

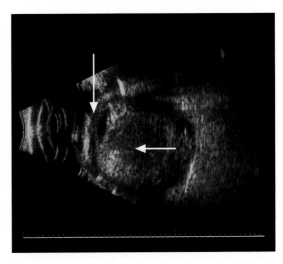

FIG. 192. Immersion B-scan of ciliary body melanoma (*horizontal arrow*) pushing on lens (*vertical arrow*)

# Case Study 101
## Ciliary Body Cyst

DH is a 25-year-old woman who saw her optometrist because of blurred vision in her left eye over several months. Examination was unremarkable except for a 2-diopter increase in astigmatism in that eye and a temporal iris bulge.

An ultrasound biomicroscope (UBM) with a 50-MHz probe visualized the anterior segment and detected multiple iris and ciliary body cysts (Fig. 193). The largest ones was contiguous with the lens. This was felt to be the basis for the increase in astigmatism.

Such cysts have been reported to cause angle closure glaucoma by forward pressure on the iris. Iris and ciliary body cysts are benign lesions but they can rarely be mimicked by cavitary changes in a malignant melanoma of the ciliary body. It is postulated that some melanomas undergo internal necrosis as they outstrip their own blood supply. This necrotic semiliquified tissue has internal reflectivity on echography similar to that of vitreous tissue, and thus appears cystic on A- and B-scan (Fig. 194).

Another category of "lens tilt" astigmatism is zonular dehiscence or laxity. This can be caused by congenital conditions such as Marfan's syndrome, familial ectopia lentis, and homocysteinuria in the phakic patient. The ophthalmologist is often called upon to evaluate patients for such conditions by examining the lens with the slit lamp for the presence of subluxation or displacement.

Pseudoexfoliation of the lens can occur later in life. These patients may have weakening of the zonules that puts them at higher risk for complications in cataract surgery with the implantation of an intraocular lens implant (IOL). In pseudophakic patients with a history of pseudoexfoliation, there are increasing reports of late zonular dehiscence with subluxation of the IOL that was placed in the capsular bag at the time of surgery. In some cases, the IOL may float backward and forwards into the vitreous with one haptec acting as a hinge.

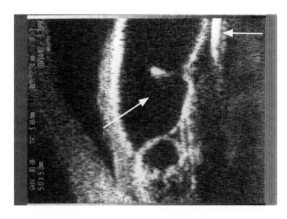

FIG. 193. Immersion scan of large ciliary body cyst (*bottom arrow*) pushing on lens (*top arrow*)

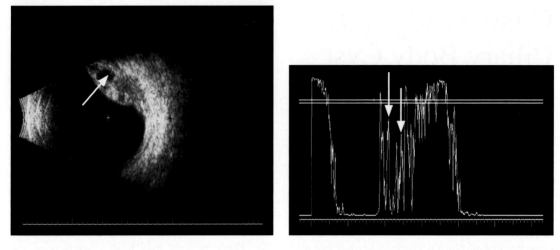

FIG. 194. Left: B-scan of cavitary changes (*arrow*) in ciliary body melanoma. Right: A-scan of cavity in melanoma (*arrows*)

# Case Study 102
## Dislocated Intraocular Lens Implant

SA is a 66-year-old woman with a history of pseudoexfoliation who underwent cataract surgery with the implantation of an intraocular lens implant (IOL) 6 years before presenting to her ophthalmologist with the complaints of fluctuating vision. There was the impression of instability of the IOL on examination but it did not appear to be subluxated.

Immersion B-scan was performed and the IOL was demonstrated to move excessively back and forth into the vitreous with the superior haptec hinged in the ciliary sulcus (Fig. 195). The patient was scheduled for an IOL removal and replacement with an anterior chamber lens.

Difficulty in inserting an IOL at the time of cataract surgery or postoperative malposition of the artificial lens may occasionally be due to a mass in the ciliary body.

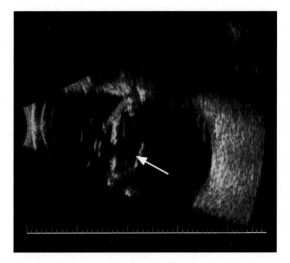

FIG. 195. B-scan of intraocular lens implant dislocated into vitreous (*arrow*)

# Case Study 103
## Ciliary Body Melanoma

EO is a 75-year-old woman who underwent uncomplicated cataract removal with intraocular lens implantation on her left eye followed a month later by surgery on her right eye. On her first postoperative visit, she was told that the lens in the right eye was "a little tilted" but this did not represent a problem. She felt that this eye never saw as well as the opposite eye and she saw distorted images to the right periphery of her vision. One year later, she experienced flashes and floaters in the right eye and was evaluated by her ophthalmologist. He noted the IOL tilt had increased and incidentally diagnosed a posterior vitreous detachment. She dilated poorly and he could not see the temporal peripheral retina well and referred her to a retinal specialist who thought he could just make out a dark shadow in the peripheral temporal fundus. She was referred for echography.

B-scan revealed a nearly spherical mass in the temporal ciliary body in contact with the temporal haptec of the IOL (Fig. 196). The lesion measured almost 12 mm in thickness by 12 mm in basal dimensions. A-scan showed low, regular internal reflectivity with moderate spontaneous vascularity (Fig. 197). These findings were highly consistent with a malignant melanoma of the ciliary body. The tumor was too large for radiation treatment and the patient underwent an enucleation. Pathology confirmed a spindle B melanoma.

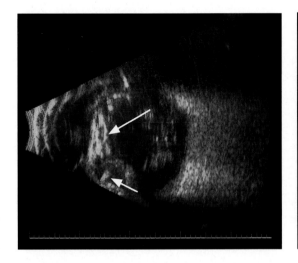 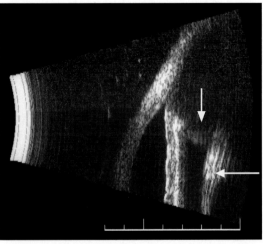

FIG. 196. Left: B-scan of ciliary body tumor (*small arrow*) abutting intraocular lens implant (*large arrow*). Right: 20-MHz A-scan of tumor (*vertical arrow*) and IOL (*horizontal arrow*)

Many types of posterior segment pathology can result in decreased vision. The retina is composed of the rod and cone photoreceptor cells with complex interconnections between them and the bipolar and retinal ganglion cells. This neural tissue is subject to numerous insults from a variety of sources. Many of these are directly visible by means of the direct and indirect ophthalmoscope, but echography is a useful tool when the problem is less apparent.

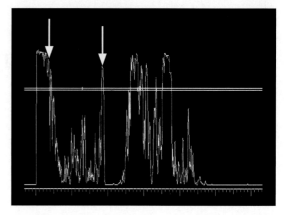

FIG. 197. A-scan directly over ciliary body melanoma (*arrows*)

# Case Study 104
## Shallow Retinal Detachment

TT is a 57-year-old commercial pilot with a history of high myopia. His right eye had suffered penetrating trauma a number of years ago that had been successfully repaired by repair of a corneal laceration and removal of a cataractous lens with implantation of an intraocular lens. He presented to his ophthalmologist with complaints of flickering lights and a shadow in the upper part of his right visual field. Examination found best corrected vision in that eye of 20/20-2. The anterior segment was unremarkable by slit-lamp examination except for an old inferior corneal scar with iris to the cornea. The fundus appeared normal by ophthalmoscopy. He was referred to a neuro-ophthalmologist, who could not find a cause for the symptoms. He returned to his primary ophthalmologist, who performed echography.

B-scan revealed a very shallow detachment of the inferior retina. A-scan confirmed a maximally high and steeply rising spike consistent with retina (Fig. 198). This separation of the retina had been difficult to visualize because of the corneal scar. He was referred to a retinal specialist for surgical repair.

Shallow retinal detachments can be difficult to see because of the subtle degree of elevation above the underlying choroid. An important clue is complaint by the patient of seeing a "shape" or "curving surface" to one side of the field of vision. This history necessitates a very careful fundus examination. Echography is essential if a detachment cannot be visualized on the clinical examination.

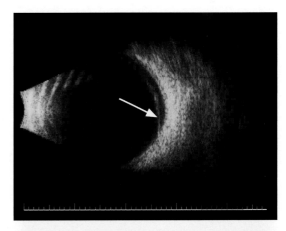

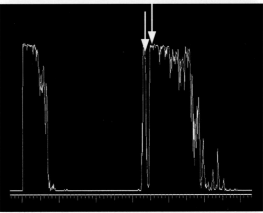

FIG. 198. Top: B-scan of shallow retinal detachment (*arrow*). Bottom: A-scan of the detachment (*arrows*)

# Case Study 105
## Shallow Retinal Detachment

SL is a 43-year-old woman who described seeing an arclike reflection to one side of her left eye. She had a long history of migraine headaches and had often seen scintillating scotomas as part of her visual auras. Her primary care physician increased her migraine medications and told her to see her eye doctor if the symptoms worsened. She noticed the symptom off and on over the next several weeks but learned to ignore it and did not seek medical care because of an extremely busy time at work. She finally called an optometrist when she noticed a smoothly curving surface that was constantly in her temporal field of vision.

Examination found visual acuity in both eyes of 20/20. Her intraocular pressures were 18 in OD and 16 OS. External examination was unremarkable and the fundus was described as normal in appearance. She was instructed to return if her symptoms worsened. She sought a second opinion 2 days later from an ophthalmologist. His initial impression was that of a normal fundus, but her symptoms were distinctive enough that he performed echography.

B-scan revealed a shallow nasal detachment at the equator extending from 1:00 to 4:00 (Fig. 199). She was then referred to a retinal specialist who found a tiny retinal tear at the superior aspect of the detached retina.

Another retinal cause of visual acuity problems is macular hole formation. Donald Gass theorized that horizontal vitreoretinal traction forces at the fovea can initiate hole formation.[33] Such traction can be missed even with contact lens retinal biomicroscopy. The imaging capability of echography can demonstrate partial separation of the posterior hyaloid that is not visible on clinical examination. Optical coherence tomography (OCT) technology is challenging ultrasound in this area and can demonstrate subtle posterior hyaloid separation that is not observable by the standard 10-MHz B-scan. High frequency 15- to 20-MHz B-scan probes focused on the posterior pole are being introduced that will further increase resolution.

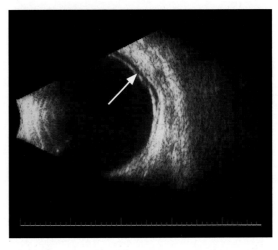

FIG. 199. B-scan of shallow retinal detachment (*arrow*)

# Case Study 106
## Macular Traction

MT is a 70-year-old woman who complained of blurriness of her right eye. She said that sometimes lines appeared wavy. Examination found 2+ nuclear sclerosis bilaterally and mild retinal pigment epithelial changes in both maculae. A fluorescein angiogram was performed and showed a few focal retinal pigment epithelial (RPE) window defects bilaterally but no other abnormalities.

Echography was performed and B-scan demonstrated partial separation of the posterior hyaloid face at the macula (Fig. 200). An impending macular hole was diagnosed and she was carefully followed for further evolution of the process. When she returned in 3 months her symptoms had subsided and repeat echography revealed complete separation of the vitreous. She was reassured that the risk of a macular hole was minimal because of the release of tractional forces.

Several drugs, such as plasmin, are being studied that may induce a PVD. This is postulated to be advantageous in certain high-risk patients, such as those with vitreoretinal traction at the macula, diabetics with high-risk characteristics for proliferative retinopathy, and high myopes with peripheral lattice degeneration. Echography is the ancillary modality in documenting the anatomy of the vitreoretinal interface in one such study.

The choroid contains most of the blood supply to the outer retina. Various disease processes can affect this tissue with resultant decrease in vision. Echography is able to document thickening of the choroid whether due to the edema of an inflammatory process, such as Vogt-Koyangi-Harada syndrome, or the solid thickening of a malignant process, such as en plaque melanoma.

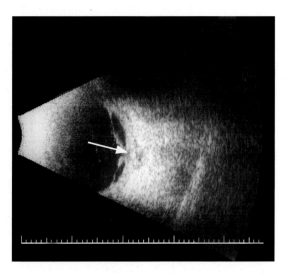

FIG. 200. B-scan of posterior vitreous detachment with macular traction (*arrow*)

# Case Study 107
## Diffuse Choroidal Melanoma

RA is a 52-year-old man who presented with the complaint of a drop in vision in his left eye over several months. Examination found visual acuity in his right eye of 20/25 and his left eye of 20/80-2. Anterior segment examination was normal and the intraocular pressure measured 16 OD and 19 OS. Fundus examination of the left eye found a diffuse grayish thickening of the macula and temporal choroid.

Echography was performed and a medium reflective solid thickening of the choroid was demonstrated with moderate spontaneous vascularity (Fig. 201). The differential diagnosis included lymphoma, metastatic tumor, and en plaque melanoma of the choroid. A needle biopsy later confirmed the diagnosis of melanoma and the eye was enucleated.

Inflammatory cells as part of several diseases can invade the choroid. The adjacent retina and sclera can also be involved.

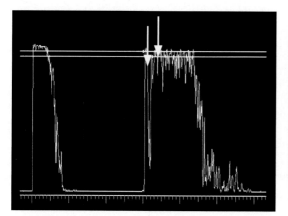 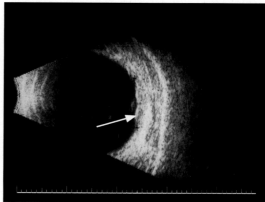

FIG. 201. Top: A-scan of diffuse choroidal melanoma (*arrows*). Bottom: B-scan of tumor (*arrows*)

# Case Study 108
## Sympathetic Ophthalmia

KG is a 43-year-old Hispanic migrant worker who had been struck in the right eye by a piece of metal as he was hammering on a metal rod. He did not seek medical care for several days because of his nonresident status, but finally the pain became intense and he went to the local emergency room. The small hospital in the rural area where he worked did not have an ophthalmologist on staff. The emergency room doctor put the patient on both oral and topical antibiotics and advised the patient to seek out a specialist in a city about 50 miles away. He delayed this for several more days and was finally seen by an ophthalmologist more than a week after the initial injury.

He was found to have a corneal-scleral laceration with iris to the wound. He was taken to surgery, where the laceration was repaired and necrotic uveal tissue was excised. He was noted to have a dense cataract and moderate anterior chamber reaction. The intraocular pressure in that eye was 5 mm and 16 mm in the left eye.

The fundus was imaged with echography and he was found to have diffuse retinochoroidal edema (Fig. 202). It was suggestive of early phthisis bulbi and only palliative treatment with topical anti-inflammatory drugs and cycloplegics was prescribed.

He was lost to follow-up for several months, but then returned to the ophthalmologist with complaints of some aching in his opposite eye with blurry vision. Examination found a phthisical right eye with no light perception and 20/50 in the left eye. Slit-lamp examination of the left eye found a mild flare in the anterior chamber and a slightly hazy vitreous. The retinochoroid layer appeared

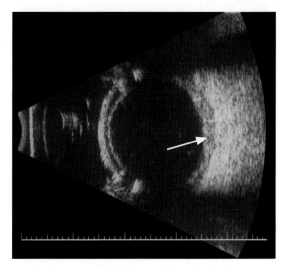

FIG. 202. B-scan of choroidal thickening in pre-phthisis (*arrow*)

edematous and two foci were noted of yellowish infiltrates.

Echography was performed and mild thickening of the choroid was revealed with medium-to-high internal reflectivity (Fig. 203). This differential diagnosis first included sympathetic ophthalmia. The patient was immediately started on high-dose topical and systemic steroids with resolution of the process over several weeks and decreased choroidal thickening.

The optic nerve is derived from the axons of the retinal ganglion cells and is subject to some of the same inflammatory and malignant processes near its exit though the sclera. Its retrobulbar portion can be involved by orbital disease entities that do not involve the intraocular tissues. A common feature

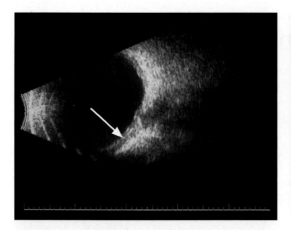 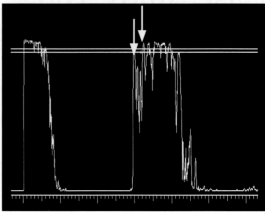

FIG. 203. Left: B-scan of choroid in sympathetic ophthalmia (*arrow*). Right: A-scan of choroid (*arrows*).

of optic nerve pathology is reduced vision and the visual deficit is usually a central scotoma. A helpful test of optic nerve disease is to shine a penlight first in the normal eye and then the abnormal one. The patient is asked to grade the light intensity in each eye on a scale of 1 to 10. Color vision is a very sensitive test in the early phases of optic nerve dysfunction so the same eye-to-eye comparison can be made with a red target such as a mydriatic bottle cap. These findings in association with an afferent pupil defect are highly characteristic of optic nerve involvement by a disease process.

The major processes that can involve the optic nerve are vascular, inflammatory, and neoplastic. Echography is especially helpful with the latter two but specialized ultrasound techniques such as color Doppler are required to evaluate blood flow abnormalities.

# Case Study 109
## Central Retinal Artery Embolus

TH is a 51-year-old man who presented to the emergency room with a history of a sudden loss of vision in his right eye 3 hours previously. He was found to have vision in that eye of light perception with 20/20 in his left eye. An ophthalmology consult was requested and documented a 3+ afferent defect on the right and a cherry red spot in the fovea consistent with marked retinal edema. No emboli were seen.

Orbital color Doppler was performed the next day and the B-scan revealed embolic material posterior to the lamina cribrosa lodged in the central retinal artery (Fig. 204). This observation prompted a workup for a source. Carotid duplex scanning showed only a focal atherosclerotic plaque that was considered nonsignificant. Transesophageal echocardiography was performed and a calcific plaque was noted on the aortic valve. He was scheduled for open heart surgery with valve replacement.

The most common solid tumors of the optic nerve include gliomas in children and meningiomas in adults.

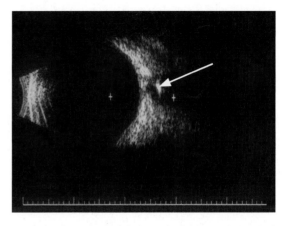

FIG. 204. B-scan of embolic material in central retinal artery (*arrow*)

# Case Study 110
## Optic Nerve Sheath Meningioma

JB is a 37-year-old woman with complaints of gradually decreasing vision over the past 9 months in her right eye. It seemed to fluctuate and at first she ascribed the symptom to overuse of her eyes on the computer. However, it continued when the stress of work had decreased and she became concerned enough to seek attention.

Examination found vision in the right eye of 20/30-1 and the left eye of 20/20. Exophthalmometry measured 2 mm of proptosis of the right eye. Intraocular pressures and the anterior segment were normal in both eyes. A 1+ afferent pupil defect was noted in the right eye. Fundus examination revealed engorged vessels on the surface of the right optic disc. A visual field examination demonstrated a central scotoma on the right and a normal field on the left.

An A-scan revealed thickening of the right nerve that measured 9.4 mm compared to 3.8 mm on the left. The nerve sheaths were abnormally thickened relative to the optic nerve (Fig. 205). A 30° test was negative on the right, which suggested a solid thickening of the nerve and was evidence against excess optic nerve sheath fluid as the cause.

An MRI scan demonstrated thickening of the optic nerve sheath consistent with optic nerve sheath meningioma (Fig. 206). The echographic and MRI findings were felt to be diagnostic and obviated the need for a nerve sheath biopsy. She was observed and as the vision declined she was referred for radiation therapy.

The optic nerve is subject to mechanical compression by processes other than neoplasms. Orbital hemorrhage subsequent to trauma can compress the nerve and result in visual loss.

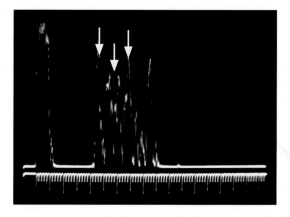

FIG. 205. A-scan of optic nerve sheath meningioma (*vertical arrows* contacting nerve sheath and *small middle arrow* touching nerve parenchyma)

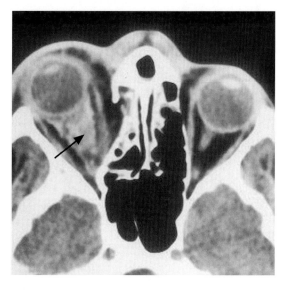

FIG. 206. Magnetic resoance imaging of optic nerve sheath meningioma (*arrow*)

# Study 111
## Optic Nerve Sheath Hemorrhage

HA is a 25-year-old man who was struck by a car while riding his bike. He was thrown onto the pavement and suffered head injury with a concussion. He was evaluated in the emergency room with CT scanning and no skull fracture was noted. He was admitted for overnight observation in the hospital. The next morning he complained of hazy vision in his right eye. An ophthalmology consult was obtained and the examination found vision OD of 20/80 and OS of 20/20. A 2+ afferent pupil defect was noted in the right eye. Slit-lamp and fundus examination were unremarkable. The CT scan was reviewed and showed widening of the right optic nerve sheaths (Fig. 207).

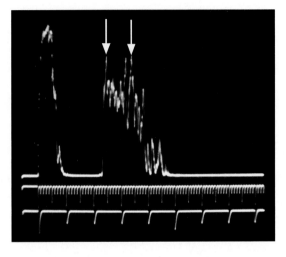

FIG. 208. A-scan of optic nerve sheath hemorrhage (*small vertical arrows* point to optic sheath)

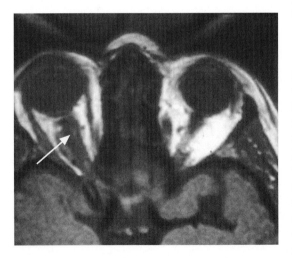

FIG. 207. Computed tomography scan of widened optic nerve sheath (*arrow*)

Echography showed thickening of the right nerve that was measured at 5.4 mm versus 3.2 mm on the left (Fig. 208). The nerve sheath appeared to be thickened. There was a mildly positive 30° test with reduction of the right nerve sheath-to-sheath diameter to 4.1 as he looked to the right. In the clinical setting of trauma, these findings were felt to be most consistent with optic nerve sheath hemorrhage. The patient was carefully observed for 24 hours with frequent monitoring of his visual acuity. The plan was to perform optic nerve sheath decompression if his vision did not improve. The vision recovered to 20/25 over the next several days and was 20/20 by 2 weeks. Ultrasound was repeated several times during this period and the optic nerve sheath reduced to a diameter of 3.5 mm.

Computed tomography and MRI are exquisite methods to image the optic nerve in its course as it exits the globe until it reaches the chiasm. However, subtle degrees of thickening can be missed. Echography has the advantage of quantifying the nerve thickness and, by means of the 30° test, it is possible to differentiate excess nerve sheath fluid from solid thickening of the sheaths and nerve parenchyma.

Pseudotumor cerebri is defined as increased intracranial pressure in the absence of mechanical obstruction to cerebrospinal fluid outflow. These patients are commonly women in the 20-to-mid-40 age group who are obese with a history of headaches. Radiologic imaging studies show normal to undersized ventricles. They are found to have papilledema on clinical examination and may give a history of visual gray-outs or black-outs.[34]

# Case Study 112
## Optic Nerves in Pseudotumor Cerebri

BA is a 34-year-old moderately obese woman with a 6-month history of increasingly severe headaches and intermittent obscurations of vision in the right eye. Her primary care physician noted bilateral papilledema and referred her to an ophthalmologist.

Ophthalmologic examination documented vision in both eyes of 20/25 and moderate papilledema on fundus evaluation. Visual field studies revealed bilateral blind spot enlargement worse on the right and moderate peripheral constriction. An MRI scan was obtained and no mass lesion was detected. The ventricles were of normal size and the optic nerve diameters were interpreted as qualitatively normal.

Echography was performed and A-scan revealed optic nerve thickness of 4.5 mm OD and 4.98 mm OS (Fig. 209). A 30° test was performed and was positive for excess sheath fluid bilaterally with reduction OD to 3.48 mm and OS to 3.72 mm (Fig. 210). The diagnosis was felt to be consistent with pseudotumor cerebri and she was referred for optic nerve sheath fenestration because of the visual field defects and increasing amaurotic symptoms.

A change in vision is the most common presenting complaint of patients seeking attention for ocular problems. A good clinical history and examination can clarify most of these, but echography provides a rapid and cost-effective ancillary technique to assist in the workup of less obvious pathology in the globe and orbit.

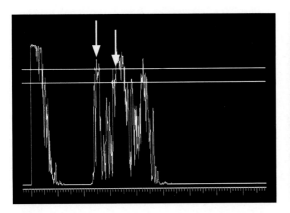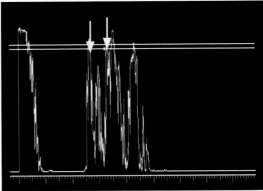

FIG. 209. Left: A-scan of increased optic nerve sheath fluid in pseudotumor cerebri right eye. Right: Left eye (*vertical arrows*)

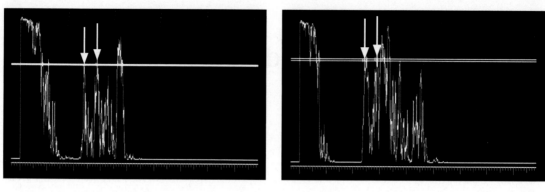

FIG. 210. Left: A-scan of right optic nerve after 30 degree test. Right: A-scan of left optic nerve after 30 degree test.

# Part V
## Bulgy Eyes

Echography is a valuable diagnostic technique for the evaluation of orbital pathology. The incredible advances in computerized imaging capability with computed tomography (CT), magnetic resonance imaging (MRI), and positron emission tomography (PET) scanning have seemingly supplanted the role of ultrasound in orbital diagnosis, but this modality has much to offer. B-scan still occupies an important niche especially in the anterior half of the orbit, but A-scan brings a unique capability to the orbit by providing quantitative data for the evaluation of orbital lesions. The ability to accurately measure structures, such as the optic nerves, extraocular muscles, and lacrimal glands, in conjunction with tissue pattern analysis of tumors and other lesions complements the morphological analysis provided by the other imaging modalities.

Orbital diagnosis requires a systematic and methodical approach including a careful history, physical examination, and the judicious and cost-effective use of imaging technology. A common presentation of many kinds of orbital pathology is proptosis. This term is usually applied to space-occupying lesions, whereas exophthalmos generally applies to the protrusion of the eyes seen in Graves' orbitopathy.

Patients with prominent eyes are encountered commonly in general ophthalmic practice. The patient herself or a family member may have noticed the change in eye position or the practitioner may be the first to bring it to the attention of the patient.

# Case Study 113
## Optic Nerve Glioma

TR was a 6-year-old child who had been treated with glasses and patching for anisometropic amblyopia and accommodative esotropia over several years. His vision in the right eye was 20/25 on the most recent examination and the left had improved with therapy to 20/50. His family had changed their health insurance and because their ophthalmologist was not on the plan they elected to seek consultation with a different doctor. He noted that the patient's left eye appeared prominent under amplification by the high plus spectacle lenses the child was wearing. Hertel exophthalmometry was performed and showed a measurement of the right eye of 15 mm and the left of 18. He also documented the presence of a subtle afferent pupil defect on the left side.

Echography was performed and revealed thickening of the left optic nerve of 6.98 mm compared to 3.4 mm on the right. The nerve substance was thickened and the optic nerve sheaths appeared normal (Fig. 211). The 30° test was negative,

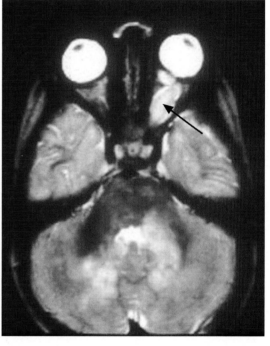

FIG. 212. Magnetic resonance imaging of optic nerve glioma (*arrow*)

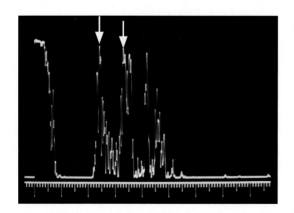

FIG. 211. A-scan of optic nerve glioma (*arrows*)

which supported a solid process of the left optic nerve as opposed to excess optic nerve sheath fluid. The echographic findings were consistent with an optic nerve glioma.

This diagnosis was supported by MRI scanning that demonstrated fusiform optic nerve enlargement on the left back towards the optic chiasm (Fig. 212). The chiasm appeared uninvolved by the tumor. It was elected to follow the child without treatment with serial MRI scans to ensure that the neoplasm was not growing posteriorly. The treatment of the amblyopia with glasses and patching was continued.

Exophthalmos can be simulated by retraction of the upper lids. Their normal position is just above the superior limbus and elevation above this level can give the appearance of prominence of the globe. The most common cause of retraction is thyroid-related eye disease. The causes of this finding are multifactorial and according to Doxanas and Anderson[35] include sympathetically innervated muscle contraction, infiltration of the levator muscle by glycopro-teins and mucopolysaccharides, and overaction of the levator palpabrae/superior rectus muscle complex in response to a fibrotic inferior rectus muscle that tethers the globe with resultant hypotropia.

The spectrum of Graves' disease ranges from simple hyperkinetic lid retraction to congestive ophthalmology with conjunctival chemosis and edema of orbital tissues. It is possible to image the levator/superior rectus complex by echography and thickening of these structures may be an early echographic sign of Graves' orbitopathy.

# Case Study 114
## Levator/Superior Rectus Complex in Graves' Disease

SB is a 43-year-old woman with a history of radioactive iodine treatment of hyperthyroidism 10 years before she presented to her ophthalmologist with the complaint that "my eyes seem bigger." She stated that her thyroid hormone levels had recently been checked and were normal. Examination revealed vision in both eyes of 20/20 and normal slit-lamp examination. There was 1 mm of scleral show bilaterally and mild lid lag. Hertel exophthalmometry was performed and measured 18 mm OD and 19 mm OS.

A-scan demonstrated normal to upper limits of extraocular muscle quantitative measurements bilaterally. However B-scan qualitatively showed thickening of the levator/superior rectus complex (Fig. 213). She was diagnosed with early congestive Graves' ophthalmopathy and was advised to be followed up in 6 months or to return sooner if she noted symptoms, such as reduced vision or diplopia.

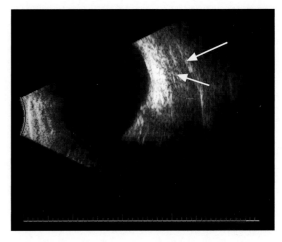

FIG. 213. B-scan of superior rectus (*small arrow*)/levator (*large arrow*) complex in Graves' disease

# Case Study 115
## Noncongestive Graves' Disease

CJ is a 53-year-old woman with a history of hyperthyroidism who noted prominence of her eyes over several months. She was referred to an endocrinologist who diagnosed Graves' orbitopathy and referred her for echographic confirmation. This showed several thickened extraocular muscles bilaterally, which was consistent with her diagnosis. She was lost to follow-up for several years and then presented to her endocrinologist with the concern that her left eye was "bulging out more." Exophthalmometry measurements were basically unchanged from the previous ones (OD 20 mm and OS 22mm). An MRI scan showed borderline enlargement of several muscles, but no mass lesion was detected. An orbital surgeon was consulted and recommended orbital decompression.

She sought a second opinion and was referred for echography, which showed that the muscle measurements had actually decreased from the ones taken 3 years ago (Fig. 214). Her increasing

eye prominence was felt due to increased lid retraction and not from extraocular muscle thickening. She was given the option for a relatively simple levator recession operation to lower the left upper lid and advised not to undergo orbital decompression with its greater risk of complications.

If the examiner suspects proptosis, it is recommended that he stand behind the seated patient without leaning forward and look down at the top of her head. Then her head is gently tilted back and normally her supraorbital ridges should first be seen followed by the malar prominences. The corneas are not normally seen unless proptosis is present. This is especially apparent if the eyes are asymmetric in their protrusion forward. Another technique is to place a card so it simultaneously touches the supraorbital ridge and malar prominence. The eyeball should not be in contact with the card unless it is proptotic. The impression of proptosis should be confirmed by exophthalmometry measurements.

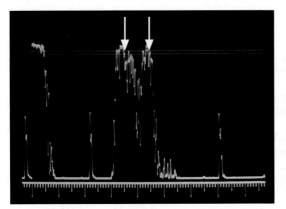 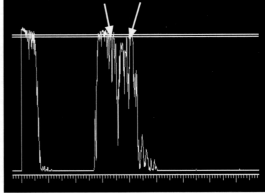

FIG. 214. Left: A-scan of superior rectus muscle (*arrows*). Right: Same muscle 4 years later (*arrows*)

In some cases of orbital pathology the globe is not proptosed, but is displaced in the horizontal plane. Inferior displacement suggests a lesion in the lacrimal gland or superior orbit such as lymphoma, lateral displacement is suspicious for a lesion in the ethmoid or sphenoid sinus, medial displacement suggests lacrimal gland enlargement, and superior displacement suggests a lesion in the maxillary sinus.

The 30cc space comprising the orbit is subject to a wide variety of pathological states. An accurate differential diagnosis is dependent upon a combination of clinical history and examination in conjunction with appropriate imaging studies. In spite of such careful analysis the clinician is not uncommonly surprised at the final pathological diagnosis.

A systematic approach is essential to clinical diagnosis in the orbit. Ben Simon et al.[36] propose a system of orbital tumor diagnosis primarily based on CT and MRI findings. Utilizing the combination of location, content (e.g., density and contrast enhancement on CT and intensity on MRI), soft tissue characteristics, bone characteristics, and associated features a systematic approach to orbital lesions is outlined.

An example of such an integrated diagnostic scheme with the incorporation of echographic findings is shown as applied to a cavernous hemangioma, the most common orbital tumor in adults (Table 1).

Such a scheme can be generated for almost all of the orbital pathology encountered in clinical practice with high diagnostic accuracy for many lesions. An expanded table is illustrated in Part VIII. The ultimate objective of the practitioner is to make a correct diagnosis without the need to surgically invade the orbit for diagnostic biopsy. This goal is realistic for a number of conditions but uncommon entities, such as orbital myxoma or orbital fibroma, require biopsy to make the final diagnosis.

The general categories of disease processes that can affect the orbit include neoplastic, inflammatory/infectious, vascular, and traumatic. There are many different entities that can involve the orbit and relatively few ways in which they can interact with the tissues in the crowded bony orbital space. The history is the first step in placing orbital pathological processes into one of these categories. The patient's perception of a change in appearance is often the basis for presentation to the clinician. Her concern about an eye that appears larger on one side or an eyelid abnormality noted when applying her makeup may be the reason she has sought medical consultation.

Orbital tumors often present with some type of displacement of the globe in either the anterior/posterior direction or in the coronal plane with horizontal or vertical misalignment. Benign lesions tend to grow slowly and a considerable amount of time may pass before the patient becomes aware of the abnormal eye position.

This is especially true with axial proptosis, which often is not evident unless someone besides the patient views the eyes off angle. The globe can be pushed forward to a considerable degree before it is recognized. Exophthalmometry is an important tool to quantitate the amount of proptosis. Migliori[37] studied normal subjects and found that Caucasian males had average exophthalmometry measurements of 16.5mm to 21.5mm and females averaged 15.5mm to 20mm. Black adults averaged about 2mm more than whites for both men and women.

TABLE 1. Example from Table 3 in Part VIII.

| History | Physical examination | Imaging | Echography | Computed tomography | Magnetic resonance imaging |
|---|---|---|---|---|---|
| Slow painless proptosis | Axial proptosis | Location | Muscle cone | Muscle cone | Muscle cone |
| | | Contents | "Sawtooth" (high, regular reflectivity) | Homogeneous | T1 hypointense |
| | | | | | T2 hyperintense |
| | | | Medium angle kappa | | |
| | | Soft tissue characteristics | Round, encapsulated | Round, circumscribed | Round |
| | | Bone | Normal | Normal | Normal |
| | | Associated features | Global flattening | Optic nerve and muscle displacement | Optic nerve and muscle displacement |

# Case Study 116
## Cavernous Hemangioma

TP is a 43-year-old woman who presented with the complaint that her eyelashes were brushing against her glasses for the past several weeks. Examination found vision in the right eye of 20/25 and the left of 20/20. She had full range of extraocular movements and no horizontal or vertical displacement of the eye. Hertel exophthalmometry was performed and OD measured 24 mm with OS at 17 mm. Her driver's license photo had been taken 5 years previously and there was no apparent proptosis of the right eye when the picture was inspected with a magnifying lens. Fundus examination was remarkable for the presence of choroidal folds in the right eye.

Echography was performed and an intraconal well-outlined mass was noted on B-scan. A-scan revealed medium internal reflectivity and angle kappa with a "saw-tooth" pattern consistent with a cavernous hemangioma (Fig. 215). The lesion decreased from 15 mm to 13 mm upon compression by the probe through the closed lid for over a minute. No spontaneous vascularity was noted.

The patient underwent an excision of the tumor, which was easily removed *in toto* with the aid of a cyroprobe. The pathological diagnosis was a cavernous hemangioma (Fig. 216) with characteristic large blood-filled cystic spaces.

Another tumor that may be found in the retrobulbar space with resultant axial proptosis is the hemangiopericytoma. This potentially malignant lesion has been confused with cavernous hemangioma on imaging studies, but A-scan characteristics are usually quite helpful in distinguishing between these two entities.

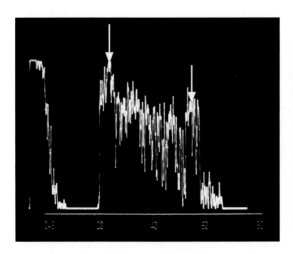 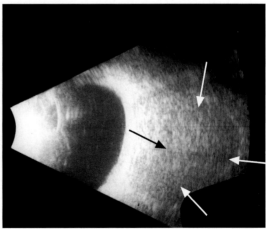

FIG. 215. Left A-scan of cavernous hemangioma (*vertical arrows*). Right: B-scan of the lesion (*arrows*)

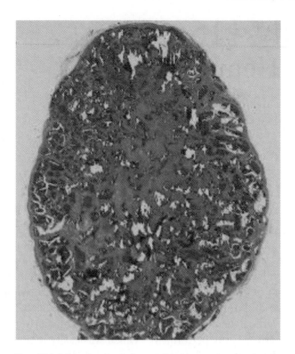

FIG. 216. Microscopic structure of cavernous hemangioma

# Case Study 117
## Hemangiopericytoma

HO is a 42-year-old woman who presented with the complaint that her left eye appeared larger than her right. She was not exactly certain when the problem started but felt it was probably over several months. Examination found vision in both eyes of 20/20 and 5 mm of left proptosis on Hertel exophthalmometry. Fundus examination was normal and no choroidal folds were noted. CT scanning revealed a rounded isodense lesion behind the globe that mildly enhanced after the injection of a contrast agent. The differential diagnosis included a cavernous hemangioma.

Echography showed an encapsulated moderately echolucent tumor on B-scan with irregular low-to-medium reflectivity and moderate vascularity on A-scan (Fig. 217). The regular "sawtooth" pattern typical of cavernous hemangioma was not appreciated so the ultrasound findings were inconsistent with this diagnosis and more typical for other well-circumscribed lesions, such as hemangiopericytoma, neurilemoma (Antoli A type Schwannoma), neurofibroma, or histiocytoma.

Because of the malignant potential of this tumor, a total excision of the lesion was performed and pathology confirmed a hemangiopericytoma. The patient was followed up every 3 months with clinical examination and echography for the first year with plans to increase the time interval to every 6 months the second year and then annually.

Lesions in the medial orbit such as frontal ethmoidal mucoceles tend to displace the globe laterally as they grow. A mass effect is created as it pushes into the orbit behind a very thin layer of bone on the surface. Internally a mucous membrane-lined cavity filled with mucinous material is found.

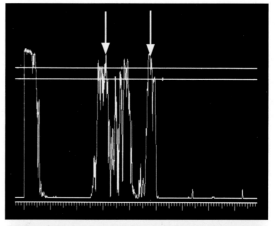

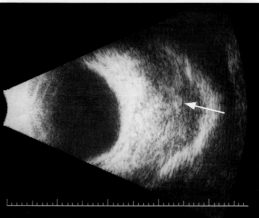

FIG. 217. Top: A-scan of hemangiopericytoma (*vertical arrows*). Bottom: B-scan of the lesion (*arrow*)

# Case Study 118
## Mucocele

GB is a 52-year-old woman with a history of chronic sinus disease who visited her daughter whom she had not seen for almost a year and was noted to have a left eye that "was pushed way off to the left." The patient had not been aware of this but did notice it after her daughter's comments. She presented to an ophthalmologist who measured lateral displacement of the left eye of 5 mm compared to the right. This measurement was performed by placing one end of a millimeter ruler on the middle of the nose on the same horizontal level as the center of the pupil. This measurement was then repeated for the opposite eye. The patient had a full range of motility and had experienced no diplopia.

Echography was performed and revealed an encapsulated lesion in the left superior nasal orbit. B-scan demonstrated a high reflective surface suggestive of calcification. A-scan showed low internal reflectivity. The probe was placed on the inferotemporal globe and directed to the 11:00 orbit. As it was angled over the lesion, a high spike "jumped up" and then disappeared as the probe was angled a little further. This phenomenon was consistent with a bone defect in the lateral wall of the frontal ethmoid sinus. The first spike was reflected from the normal medial orbital wall but this disappeared when the defect was encountered. The second spike then arose as a reflection of the sound beam from the medial wall of the sinus because the beam passed into the sinus without hindrance. As the probe was angled further the sound beam once again was reflected by the orbital bone that bounded the sinus cavity (Fig. 218). These findings were very consistent with a mucocele causing a bone defect. Echo spikes were also detected from the right ethmoid sinus cavity and both maxillary sinuses, consistent with chronic sinusitis.

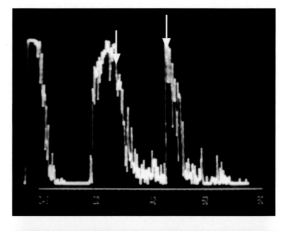

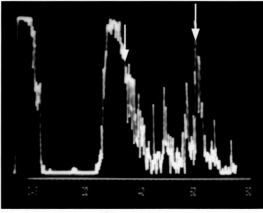

FIG. 218. Top: A-scan of orbital portion of mucocele (*vertical arrows*). Bottom: A-scan of extension of mucocele into sinus (*vertical arrows*)

A CT scan confirmed the presence of a large cystic lesion with a thin bony rim as it extended into the orbit (Fig. 219). The patient was referred to an otolaryngologist for sinus surgery and removal of the mucocele. Surgery was performed in conjunction with an orbital surgeon and the eye soon returned to its normal position.

Lid swelling and displacement of the globe may include symptoms such as the pain of acute sinusitis or a more indolent pressure pain as occurs in chronic sinus disease. The paranasal sinuses are a common source of discomfort around the eyes. Patients often describe a pressure sensation that is made worse on bending over. There is frequently a history of previous sinus disease but paraocular pain may be the first sign of sinus infection.

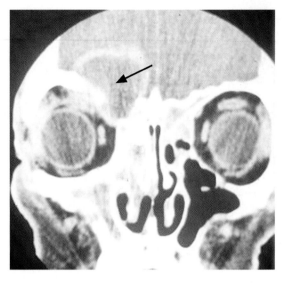

FIG. 219. Computed tomography scan of mucocele (*arrow*)

# Case Study 119
## Dacryoadenitis to Acute Sinusitis

QH was a 13-year-old child who presented to her pediatrician with complaints of eye pain. He did not appreciate any abnormalities of her eyes but there was mild swelling of the eyelids. An x-ray was obtained and was interpreted as normal. She was referred to an ophthalmologist for a consultation that day. The globes were normal, but A-scan revealed marked signals from both ethmoid sinuses consistent with sinusitis (Fig. 220). She was started on antibiotics and decongestants with resolution of her symptoms over several days.

Downward displacement of the globe is seen with lesions such as lacrimal gland tumors. Traditional teaching has been that 50% of lacrimal gland lesions are nonepithelial, such as lymphomas and inflammatory infiltrations. The other 50% are epithelial tumors, such as pleomorphic adenomas (benign mixed tumors) and adenocystic carcinomas. This concept has been challenged by Shields,[38] who found that inflammatory and lymphoid lesions are two to three times mores common than epithelial tumors.

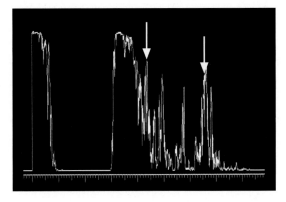

FIG. 220. A-scan of ethmoid sinus signals (*vertical arrows*)

The pleomorphic adenoma is the most common "benign" neoplasm of the lacrimal gland, although this lesion has malignant potential if it is not completely excised. These tumors usually grow slowly and painlessly with proptosis and downward displacement of the eye.

# Case Study 120
## Pleomorphic Adenoma of Lacrimal Gland

HH is 42-year-old man who presented with the complaint of some swelling of the right upper eyelid over several months. Examination by an ophthalmologist found vision in both eyes of 20/20 and mild temporal edema of the right upper lid. Exophthalmometry was performed with the OD measuring 21 mm and OS 19 mm. There was also found to be 4 mm of inferior displacement of the right eye. Palpation of the orbit found a firm mass in the area of the right lacrimal gland.

Echography demonstrated an encapsulated tumor of the right lacrimal gland on B-scan and medium reflectivity with a moderate angle kappa on A-scan (Fig. 221). Minimal spontaneous vascularity was noted. The differential diagnosis included a pleo-morphic adenoma and a cavernous hemangioma, but the superotemporal location outside of the muscle cone was most consistent with a tumor of the lacrimal gland with the echographic features of a benign mixed tumor. CT scan demonstrated a mass in the superotemporal orbit with mild molding of the bone, but no bone destruction.

The patient was referred to an orbital surgeon for an en bloc excision of the tumor. Biopsy was not recommended because of the danger of violating the capsule with potential malignant recurrence of the lesion.

The lacrimal glands can be a source of globe displacement and lid swelling due to infection or nonspecific inflammation.

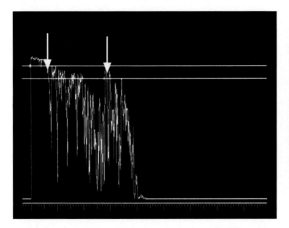 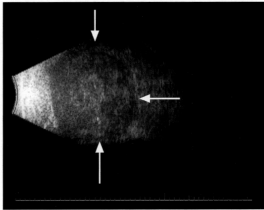

FIG. 221. Left: A-scan of pleomorphic adenoma (*vertical arrows*). Right: B-scan of lesion (*arrows*)

# Case Study 121
## Dacryoadenitis

BS is a 23-year-old woman who complained of moderately severe pain around her left eye for 2 days. She had gone to a local emergency room and a CT scan was performed with no apparent abnormalities. She was sent home on pain pills and told to follow up with her eye doctor. She presented the next day to an ophthalmologist with worsening of the pain. Examination found vision in both eyes of 20/25 and a normal anterior segment by slit-lamp examination. Subtle s-shaped swelling of the left upper lid was noted and there was some tenderness to palpation in the superotemporal orbit.

Echography was performed and the right lacrimal gland measured 11.47 mm and the left measured 13.4 mm (Fig. 222). A-scan showed medium-to-high reflectivity bilaterally but there was a relatively low area centrally in the left gland. The diagnosis of a probable dacryoadenitis was made and she was started on a course of oral antibiotics with resolution of her symptoms in a few days. Repeat echography in 3 weeks demonstrated left lacrimal gland thickness of 12 mm.

Orbital pseudotumor, including that involving the lacrimal gland, is rare in children. Infectious or idiopathic dacryoadenitis is more common and is usually self-limited with mild symptoms of temporal upper lid swelling and tenderness. Echography provides a rapid and cost-effective method to evaluate the lacrimal gland in an office setting.

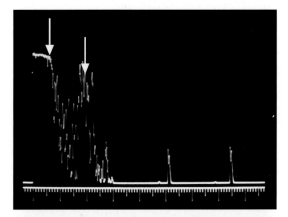
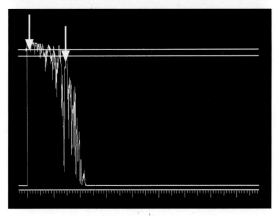

Fig. 222. Top: A-scan of lacrimal pseudotumor (*vertical arrows*). Bottom: Normal opposite gland (*vertical arrows*)

# Case Study 122
## Chronic Dacryoadenitis

MS is a 4-year-old child with a history of progressive left upper lid swelling over several weeks. Examination of the eyes was unremarkable except for moderate nontender edema of the lid. The parents stated that the child had not complained of pain in that area at any time. A CT scan showed enlargement of the left lacrimal gland without apparent involvement of the orbital bone. The differential diagnosis included a solid tumor such as a pleomorphic adenoma, lymphoma, and pseudotumor. An oculoplastic surgeon was consulted and was concerned that the lack of pain and tenderness supported a solid tumor of the gland as compared to an inflammatory process.

Echography revealed an enlarged left lacrimal gland with low-to-medium and relatively regular internal reflectivity (Figs. 223 and 224). The findings were most consistent with an inflammatory process, such as pseudotumor, with malignant conditions, such as lymphoma, included in the differential.

The surgeon was very reluctant to perform an excisional biopsy of a possible pleomorphic

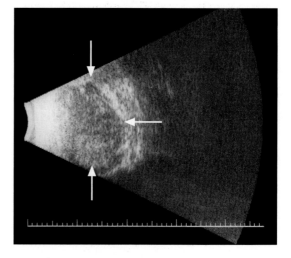

FIG. 224. B-scan of gland (*arrows*)

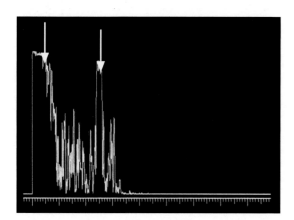

FIG. 223. A-scan of lacrimal gland (*arrows*)

adenoma because of the risk of converting the lesion to a more aggressive malignancy, but largely on the basis of the echographic findings the biopsy was performed. The pathology report stated that the final diagnosis was "chronic or smoldering pseudotumor of the lacrimal gland (dacryoadenitis)."

Another cause of globe malposition and lid swelling with orbital pain is orbital pseudotumor. Various series report the incidence of this inflammation to occur in 5% to 7% of orbital disease processes.[39] Modern imaging techniques have allowed the subcategorization of orbital pseudotumor into the inflammation of specific orbital structures, such as the extraocular muscles. Acute pain made worse by moving the eye is suggestive of inflammatory myositis.

# Case Study 123
## Orbital Myositis

AC was a 21-year-old woman who lived in the Amana colonies in Iowa. She presented to the emergency room with the complaint of severe pain in her left eye starting the previous day. She stated that it was made worse on looking to the left and she also experienced double vision when she did this. Examination showed normal vision in both eyes with some swelling of the left eyelids with mild proptosis. The nasal conjunctiva showed moderate injection, especially over the insertion of the medial rectus muscle.

Only first-generation CT scans were available at that time and the patient was scanned with that modality. The radiologist reported "nonspecific left orbital fullness." She was referred to the eye department for echographic evaluation. The right orbit was normal and the left orbit revealed thickening of the medial rectus muscle and tendon on B-scan and low internal reflectivity on A-scan (Fig. 225).

The diagnosis of medial rectus myositis was made and she was started on high-dose prednisone with rapid improvement in her symptoms over several days. A complete systemic workup was performed to rule out an inflammatory process, such as collagen vascular disease, but all of the tests were normal.

Globe displacement with pain secondary to a neoplastic process is generally an ominous symptom suggestive of perineural infiltration by a malignancy. Such symptoms may be associated with adenocystic carcinoma. It is the most common malignant tumor of the lacrimal gland and pain occurs in up to 80% of these patients.

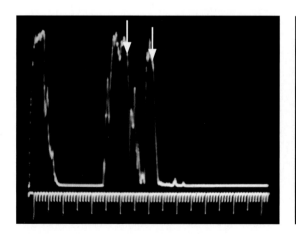
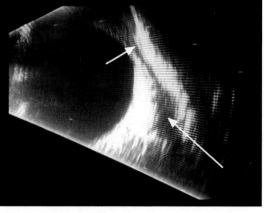

FIG. 225. Left: A-scan of thickened extraocular muscle (*vertical arrows*). Right: B-scan of muscle tendon (*small arrow*) and muscle belly (*large arrow*)

# Case Study 124
## Adenocystic Carcinoma of the Lacrimal Gland

SC is a 27-year-old man who presented with complaints of an intermittent boring pain for several months around his left eye. Examination revealed fullness in the superotemporal orbit and some tenderness to palpation. Otherwise, the examination was unremarkable. A plain film x-ray was obtained and showed some evidence of erosion of the bone on that side. CT was performed and demonstrated a lacrimal mass with bone invasion.

Echography was performed and A-scan showed irregular internal reflectivity with a central low area (Fig. 226). Mild spontaneous vascularity was detected. The findings were consistent with a lacrimal gland malignancy with the differential diagnosis including adenocystic carcinoma. This was later confirmed on biopsy and orbital exenteration was advised.

Subtle displacement of the globe can be missed in the early stages even by experienced observers.

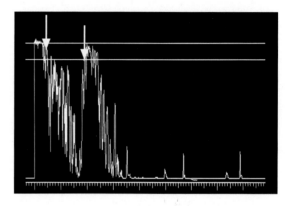

FIG. 226. A-scan of adenocystic carcinoma of lacrimal gland (*vertical arrows*)

# Case Study 125
## Sinus Squamous Cell Carcinoma

EW was a 62-year-old engineer who noted difficulty in closing his left eye starting 4 months prior to presentation. Numerous specialists, including a neurologist, for the evaluation of an atypical Bell's palsy, had seen him. He had undergone three MRI scans, two CT scans, two lumbar punctures, and numerous blood tests, including serology, to rule-out Lyme disease. He had recently noted a further reduction of vision in his left eye and had consulted with his local ophthalmologist, who diagnosed an inferior retinal detachment and referred him to a retinal specialist for surgery. The retinologist did not feel the retina was detached but suspected a choroidal detachment and referred him for echography.

Examination prior to the ultrasound found moderate lagophthalmos of the left eye and 2 mm of superior displacement of the globe. B-scan showed a 24-mm orbital mass indenting the eye inferiorly. A-scan revealed a very low reflective orbital lesion with a bone defect in the orbital floor with a maxillary sinus component to the lesion (Fig. 227). Because of these findings, the patient was asked about any skin lesions and he pointed out a lesion under his moustache that had lately been growing.

The echographic findings were suspicious for either a primary sinus carcinoma invading the orbit or perineural spread of a squamous cell carcinoma of the skin. The diagnosis of squamous cell was confirmed on orbital biopsy.

Another symptom of orbital disease associated with globe displacement is diplopia. The workup of this symptom starts with evaluation of the extraocular musculature and proceeds intracranially if a more proximate cause is not found.

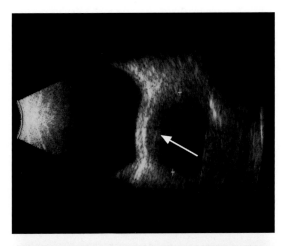

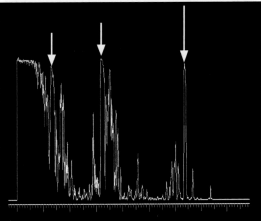

FIG. 227. Top: B-scan of orbital lesion compressing globe (*arrow*). Bottom: A-scan of orbital component (*small arrows*) and sinus component (between *second* and *third arrow*)

Most causes of diplopia originating in the orbit result from mechanical difficulties with the extraocular muscles, such as infiltration, compression, or entrapment. The most common entity causing muscle dysfunction in the orbit is Graves' disease. Initially the muscles may show inflammatory changes and later can become fibrotic and noncontractile. They may not appear enlarged on imaging studies at this stage.

According to Gorman,[40] the pathophysiology of Graves' disease involves muscle swelling caused by the accumulation of inflammatory cells and water binding glycosaminoglycans (GAGs) followed by subsequent muscle fibrosis. It is believed be an autoimmune disease where CD4 T lymphocytes become sensitized to an antigen common to thyroid and orbital tissue.[41] The most common antibody in Graves' patients binds with the thyrotropin receptor (TSH-R). There are two distinct subtypes of thyroid orbitopathy: congestive with retrobulbar deposits of GAGs and myopathic with impaired extraocular muscle function.

# Case Study 126
## Graves' Disease

JN is a 16-year-old boy who presented with double vision on looking to the right for several weeks. Examination found vision in both eyes of 20/20 and mild proptosis of the left eye compared to the right. There was mild lid lag of the left eyelid. He was found to have 15 prism diopters of exotropia on right gaze. Forced duction testing was positive for restriction of adduction on the right. He had no history of diabetes or thyroid abnormalities.

Echography was performed and demonstrated thickening of the left lateral rectus muscle, which measured 5.2 mm compared to 3.8 mm for the right lateral rectus. A-scan demonstrated irregular internal reflectivity (Fig. 228). Thyroid function testing was normal and the clinical findings were atypical for Graves' disease with abnormality of only the lateral rectus muscle.

Because he was orthotropic in primary gaze, it was elected to observe him and repeat an examination in 3 months. At that time his clinical findings were unchanged but repeat echography showed thickening of several other extraocular

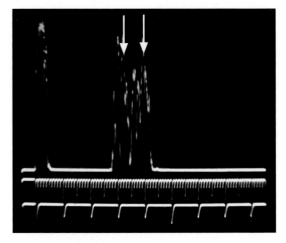

FIG. 228. A-scan of lateral rectus muscle in Graves' disease (*vertical arrows*)

muscles bilaterally, which supported the diagnosis of Graves' disease.

Other infiltrative processes of the extraocular muscles include malignant processes such as lymphoma and metastatic tumor.

# Case Study 127
## Metastasis to Extraocular Muscle

KB was a 54-year-old woman who presented to her ophthalmologist with a history of increasing diplopia over several months. Examination found proptosis of her right eye of 4 mm compared to her left. She had 2 mm of left upper lid ptosis. Her driver's license photo taken 3 years previously did not show these changes. CT scan showed marked enlargement of several extraocular muscles.

Echography was performed and demonstrated thickening of the right superior rectus (9.3 mm), the right medial rectus (8.4 mm), and borderline thickening of the left superior rectus (5.8 mm) and the left lateral rectus (4.5 mm). However, reflectivity on A-scan was low-to-medium and regular in the right superior and medial recti (Fig. 229).

The finding of low internal reflectivity in a markedly thickened extraocular muscle in conjunction with minimal pain was not typical for Graves' disease, so a biopsy of the right superior rectus was performed. The pathological diagnosis was consistent with malignancy probably due to metastasis. Systemic evaluation found an infiltrative ductal carcinoma of the left breast.

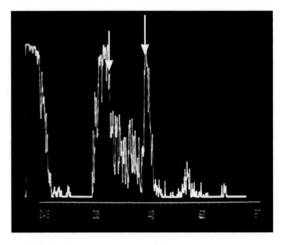

FIG. 229. A-scan of markedly thickened muscle in metastatic cancer (*vertical arrows*)

Other malignant processes, such as lymphoma, can sometimes invade the extraocular muscles as part of systemic disease, but in some cases it acts as a local process confined to the orbit.

# Case Study 128
## Lymphoma of Extraocular Muscle

AG is an 81-year-old woman with a 3-month history of double vision on looking to the left. She reported minimal discomfort when she moved the eye horizontally. Examination found mildly reduced abduction of the left eye and focal injection at the insertion of the left lateral rectus tendon. The remainder of the ocular examination was unremarkable except for cataract formation consistent with her age.

Echography was performed and demonstrated thickening of the left lateral rectus muscle measuring 5.4 mm with low reflectivity on A-scan (Fig. 230). The tendon was not abnormally thickened. The differential diagnosis included an infiltrative process by inflammatory or malignant cells.

A systemic evaluation by her primary care physician was unremarkable. A conjunctival biopsy performed at the lateral rectus tendon was positive for B-cell lymphoma. She was treated with local radiation to the orbit and followed closely by an oncologist for the development of any systemic signs of lymphoma.

The incidence of relapse at a distant site in the body is 20% to 25% for low-grade lymphoma of the ocular adnexae and 40% to 60% for higher grades.[42] The probability of systemic lymphoma is relatively low when it is confined to the conjunctiva and increases when the eyelids are involved. According to Coupland et al., lymphomas of the ocular adnexa represent about 8% of all extranodal lymphomas.[43] The incidence of systemic involvement summarized from several series is 35% for lymphoma of the orbit, 20% for that of the conjunctiva, and 67% for lymphoma of the eyelid. Lymphoma occurs systemically in 35% of cases where there is bilateral orbital involvement.

Orbital biopsy of lymphoid lesions may be read by the pathologist as "lymphoid hyperplasia" or "atypical lymphoid hyperplasia," which is categorized as a benign process. This low-grade lesion is at one end of a spectrum with highly aggressive monoclonal lymphoma at the other end. However, the incidence of eventual systemic involvement is reported to be 25% to 30% for these "benign" lesions.[44] The probability of systemic occurrence by lesions classified as reactive lymphoid hyperplasia is a function of the monoclonality of the B-cells.

Diplopia and proptosis can be due to vascular congestion that can cause extraocular muscle thickening and dysfunction simulating Graves' disease. A high-flow arteriovenous fistula is usually readily diagnosable by its rapid onset with pulsating exophthalmos, an audible bruit, and a red eye with arterialization of the conjunctival and episcleral veins. They are often related to traumatic head injury and are responsible for about 75% of high-flow carotid cavernous fistulas.

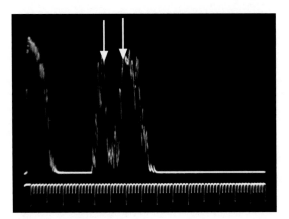

FIG. 230. A-scan of lymphoma of extraocular muscle (*vertical arrows*)

# Case Study 129
## Superior Ophthalmic Vein in Carotid Cavernous Fistula

AM is a 52-year-old man who was knocked to the ground by falling canisters and bumped the back of his head on the cement floor. He did not recall losing consciousness and was cleared by the emergency room to return to work the next day. He was asymptomatic for a few months but then began to experience severe headaches. He was diagnosed with migraines and treated with beta blockers with partial relief. In the following year he began to see double and was seen by an ophthalmologist, who prescribed prisms in his glasses that allowed him to see without diplopia in primary gaze. During this time he also noted that his right eye was red much of the time. He did not appreciate any unusual noises in his head.

He returned to his ophthalmologist, who suspected the patient had Graves' disease and ordered a thyroid workup and referred him for echography. A-scan revealed diffuse thickening of most of his

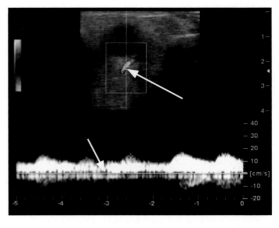

FIG. 232. Doppler frequency analysis (*small arrow*) of arterialized superior opthalmic vein (*large arrow*)

extraocular muscles with heterogeneous reflectivity consistent with Graves' orbitopathy. However, B-scan demonstrated a markedly dilated right superior ophthalmic vein with spontaneous vascularity (Fig. 231). This finding was confirmed with orbital color Doppler that demonstrated reversal of flow with arterialization of the vein with a flow velocity of 13.68 cm/s on the pulse tracing (Fig. 232). The other orbit appeared normal.

A stethoscope was applied to the eye through closed lids and a faint bruit could be heard. Blood was noted in Schlem's canal on gonioscopy and the intraocular pressure was 20 mm OD and 15 mm OS. He was referred for angiography with the plan to close the fistula by the injection of embolic material through the catheter.

Dural sinus fistulas are generally subtler and may occur spontaneously in middle-aged women.

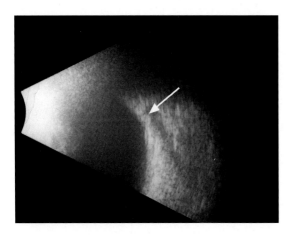

FIG. 231. B-scan of dilated superior opthalmic vein in carotid cavernous fistula (*arrow*)

# Case Study 130
## Superior Ophthalmic Vein in Dural Sinus Fistula

SJ is a 58-year-old woman who presented with intermittent diplopia over several months. She also mentioned that her eyes were always red with a mild aching sensation. She denied hearing her "pulse" at night while lying in bed. There was no history of trauma to her head. She had undergone radioactive iodine therapy for hyperthyroidism 10 years previously and her thyroid levels were maintained at normal levels by medication. Examination found vision in both eyes of 20/25 and intraocular pressures of 23 mm OD and 24 mm OS. Slit-lamp examination showed tortuous dilation of conjunctival vessels bilaterally. A stethoscope was applied to both globes through closed eyelids and no bruit was appreciated.

Echography revealed diffuse thickening of her extraocular muscles bilaterally with irregular reflectivity on A-scan (Fig. 233). Dilation of the superior

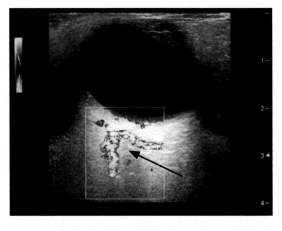

FIG. 234. Color doppler of dilated superior ophthalmic vein in low-flow fistula (*arrow*)

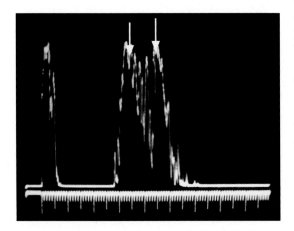

FIG. 233. A-scan of extraocular muscle in cartotid cavernous fistula (*vertical arrows*)

ophthalmic veins bilaterally was detected. Orbital color Doppler imaging substantiated venous dilation and showed reversal of flow with low-flow arterial pulse waves of 3 cm/s in the superior ophthalmic veins (Fig. 234).

Because of the elevated intraocular pressure and diplopia, the patient was advised not to wait for spontaneous closure of the fistula but to proceed with angiography. The diagnosis of a dural sinus fistula was confirmed and embolic material was injected through the catheter to close the fistula with resolution of her diplopia and reduction of her intraocular pressure to under 20 in both eyes.

Another symptom of orbital pathology in association with proptosis is reduction of visual acuity due to lesions that directly involve the optic nerve, such as glioma, or invade the optic nerve sheaths, as with meningioma.

# Case Study 131
## Optic Nerve Sheath Meningioma

SB is a 40-year-old woman who noted some reduction in vision in her left eye during pregnancy. Examination was performed and found visual acuity OD of 20/20 and OS of 20/40-1. A 1+ afferent pupil defect was present in the left eye and Hertel exophthalmometry showed 2 mm of proptosis on that side. Fundus examination on the left found slight pallor of the optic disc with a possible retinochoroidal "shunt" vessel at the inferior margin. It was considered inadvisable to do CT scanning, with its attendant radiation exposure, during her pregnancy. She was given the option for an MRI scan but did not want to risk the unknown effects of a strong magnetic field on her developing fetus and was referred for echography.

B-scan showed a possible widening of the optic nerve shadow but this was not definitive. Calcification of the left nerve sheath could not be detected. A-scan measured optic nerve thickness on the right of 2.51 mm and on the left of 7.40 mm with widening of the optic nerve sheaths and a normal optic nerve parenchyma width (Fig. 235). The 30° test was negative for increased optic nerve sheath fluid so the differential diagnosis included a solid lesion of the nerve, such as meningioma, glioma, lymphoma, and metastatic tumor.

Her age at presentation and the appearance of the optic disc were most consistent with meningioma. It was elected to observe her without treatment and reevaluate after she delivered the baby. A CT scan was performed at that point and showed calcification of the optic nerve sheath that was highly consistent with nerve sheath meningioma.

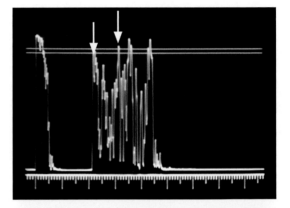
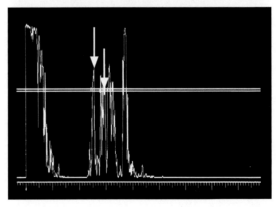

FIG. 235. Top: A-scan of optic nerve sheath meningioma (*vertical arrows*). Bottom: Normal contralateral optic nerve (*vertical arrows*)

Her vision was stable at 20/40 and there was no evidence of posterior extension intracranially so no treatment was offered, but radiation was planned in the future if the vision decreased.

Optic nerve sheath meninigiomas are generally slow-growing tumors and can be observed unless the vision progressively deteriorates. Nerve sheath biopsy to confirm the diagnosis is hazardous and often results in profound loss of vision. Echography provides a cost-effective and safe technique to correlate the clinical findings with growth of the tumor.

# Case Study 132
## Optic Nerve Sheath Meningioma

VA is a 75-year-old woman who noted some blurring of her right eye over several months. Examination found vision OD of 20/50 and OS of 20/25. She had a 2+ afferent pupil defect in her right eye and 2 mm of proptosis. Fundus exam found slight pallor of the right optic disc.

Echography showed thickening of the right optic nerve sheath with a sheath-to-sheath diameter of 8.7 mm (Fig. 236) compared to 3.2 mm for her left nerve. The findings were consistent with an optic nerve sheath meningioma and were confirmed on CT scan with calcification of the nerve sheath (Fig. 237).

She was followed up with every 3 months without treatment, but was noted after 12 months to have reduction of vision to 20/70 on the right. Echography demonstrated further thickening of the sheath to 7.6 mm. She was referred for stereotactic radiation therapy with improvement in visual acuity to 20/30.

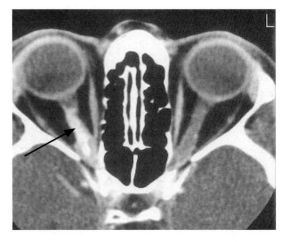

FIG. 237. Computed tomography scan of optic nerve sheath meningioma (*arrow*)

A- or B-scan is not reliable in demonstrating calcification of the optic nerve sheaths in the orbit because of the high reflectivity of adjacent orbital tissue. This is not the case in the globe, where the high reflectivity of calcified lesions stands out in distinct relief against the low reflective vitreous gel. MRI scans are also not helpful in detecting sheath calcification. The imaging technique of choice to display orbital calcification is CT scanning.

An uncommon process that involves the nerve sheaths is an idiopathic process referred to in the literature by various names, such as perioptic hygroma, optic hydrops, or meningocele.[45] In this condition, there is increased cerebrospinal fluid in the intrasheath space of unknown etiology. These patients may present with symptoms of reduced vision and can have fundus findings including atrophy of the optic disc, disc swelling, and choroidal folds.

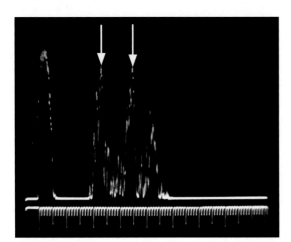

FIG. 236. A-scan of optic nerve sheath meningioma (*vertical arrows*)

# Case Study 133
## Optic Nerve Sheath Hygroma

HH is a 9-year-old child who failed his vision test in school. He had first noted problems the previous summer that he characterized as difficulty in seeing in dim light. His parents took him to an optometrist who documented vision in the right eye of 20/25 and the left of 20/20. Cycloplegic refraction was +1.00 OD and +0.50 OS. The fundus exam showed mild choroidal folds on the right while the optic discs had a normal appearance. Exophthalmometry measured 18 mm bilaterally.

Echography showed bilateral increased optic nerve sheath diameter with a slightly widened sub-arachnoid space on A-scan. B-scan demonstrated patulous retrobulbar optic nerve sheaths (Fig. 238).

A CT scan was performed and showed dilatation of the optic nerve sheaths. A spinal tap was performed and showed normal opening pressure. The diagnosis of optic nerve sheath meningocele was made and it was elected to follow the child with biannual eye exams and echography. His vision and optic nerve sheath diameter were unchanged over 5 years.

Choroidal folds are a variable finding in this condition. They are possibly due to a masslike effect of the increased nerve sheath fluid pushing on the posterior globe. However, choroidal folds are not generally found in other cases of excess sheath fluid, such as the papilledema associated with pseudotumor cerebri. Their presence on fundus examination should always prompt an investigation of the orbit to eliminate a mass lesion. This can easily be accomplished in the office as part of the initial examination.

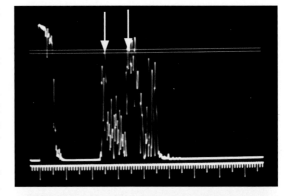

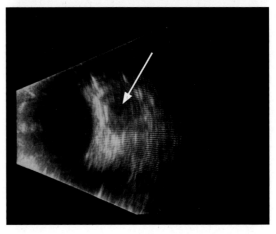

FIG. 238. Top: A-scan of optic nerve sheath hygroma (*vertical arrows*). Bottom: B-scan of dilated optic nerve (*arrow*)

# Case Study 134
## Orbital Hematic Cyst

JJ is a 26-year-old man who complained of reduced vision in his left eye over several weeks. Examination by his ophthalmologist found uncorrected vision OD of 20/20 and OS of 20/60, but this eye could be refracted to 20/20 with a +2.50 lens. Hertel exophthalmometry showed 2 mm of proptosis OS. Fundus examination found choroidal folds in this eye.

Echography was performed at this time and showed a low reflective well-outlined lesion in the retrobulbar space (Fig. 239). The differential diagnosis included cystic lesions, such as a hematic cyst, dermoid, or lymphangioma. The patient gave no history of trauma. He opted for surgical removal of the lesion and a cystic structure was found with blood breakdown products consistent with a hematic cyst. The patient experienced a complete resolution of his symptoms after surgery.

Hematic cysts are rare orbital lesions that are most often subperiosteal and may or may not be related to trauma.[46] A fibrous capsule surrounds an area of inflammatory reaction to blood or blood breakdown products, such as hemosiderin.

Mass lesions in the orbit that are separate from the optic nerve can cause reduced vision by direct compression of the optic nerve. This is more common with slowly growing tumors that enlarge over time to the degree that they can press on the nerve with varying degrees of proptosis.

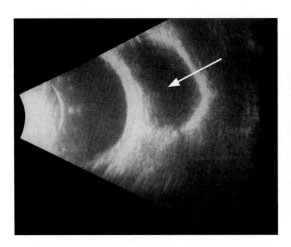 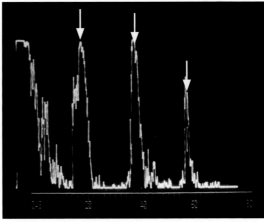

FIG. 239. Left: B-scan of hematic cyst (*arrow*). Right: A-scan of lesion (*first two arrows*). Multiple signal (*third arrow*)

# Case Study 135
## Cavernous Hemangioma

BC is a 10-year-old boy who failed his vision test in school and was referred to an optical shop to be fitted for glasses. The optometrist found visual acuity OD of 20/20 and OS of 20/40+2. Fundus examination revealed some swelling of the left optic disc so he was then referred to an ophthalmologist. Optic disc edema was confirmed and the presence of choroidal folds was also noted. Exophthalmometry measured 15 mm OD and 18 mm OS.

Echography was performed and B-scan revealed a round, well-outlined lesion in the muscle cone with some indentation of the posterior sclera. A-scan measured the lesion to be 9.92 mm in greatest diameter with medium internal reflectivity with a cavernous pattern. There was a moderate angle kappa (Fig. 240). Spontaneous vascularity was not detected. The lesion decreased in diameter by 2 mm with mild sustained pressure of the probe against the globe for 2 minutes through closed lids. These findings were highly characteristic of a cavernous hemangioma.

Computed tomography scan confirmed a round, well-outlined lesion in the muscle cone consistent with a hemangioma. He was referred to an orbital surgeon who completely removed the lesion with the aid of a cryoprobe. Follow-up examination found a reduction in the optic disc edema and improvement in visual acuity to 20/25+2.

The A-scan reflectivity of a cavernous hemangioma is based on the tissue architecture. The relatively large blood-filled cystic spaces provide a homogenous medium for the sound beam to traverse so the height of the echo spikes begins to drop towards baseline. However, the sound beam then encounters a septa and becomes high due to the

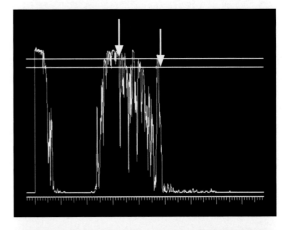

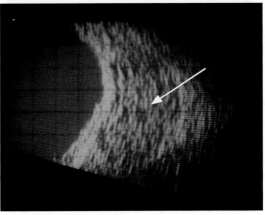

FIG. 240. Top: A-scan of cavernous hemangioma with angle kappa (*arrows*) (I). Bottom: B-scan of lesion (*arrow*)

interface reflection. This pattern is repeated as it travels through the lesion and gives a characteristic "saw-tooth" or "honeycomb" pattern sometimes referred

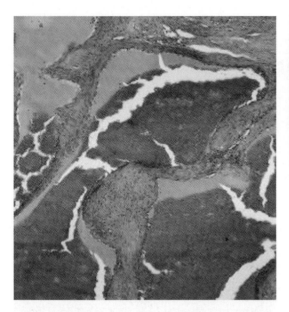

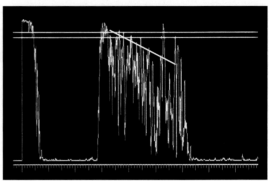

FIG. 242. Diagram of angle kappa

FIG. 241. Microscopic anatomy of cavernous hemangioma

to as "cavernous,"' as correlated to the microscopic structure of the tissue (Fig. 241). The angle kappa, as described by Ossoinig, refers to the slope of a line drawn along the tops of the vertical spikes within the lesion (Fig. 242). These tumors have a significant angle kappa because sound energy is absorbed and scattered as the beam travels through the tumor.

Another vascular lesion that can put pressure on the optic nerve is a lymphangioma. This lesion can entwine itself around orbital structures and will sometimes undergo spontaneous hemorrhage into its cystic spaces with marked expansion of the cyst with resultant pressure on orbital tissue.

# Case Study 136
## Orbital Lymphangioma

CM is a 7-year-old girl who presented to her pediatrician with sudden proptosis of her left eye over the course of one day. Examination found marked proptosis and numerous tiny serous-filled cysts of the conjunctiva in the inferior fornix. She was urgently referred to an ophthalmologist for evaluation. He found vision in her right eye of 20/20 and her left eye of 20/50-2 with a 2+ afferent pupil defect. Hertel exophthalmometry measured the anterior position of the right eye at 11 mm and the left at 17 mm.

Echography was performed with B-scan showing a large, low reflective lesion adjacent to the optic nerve with multiple smaller cysts adjacent to it. A-scan revealed an 11-mm encapsulated cystic structure with very low internal reflectivity (Fig. 243). Spontaneous vascularity was not detected. The optic nerve thickness was thicker on the left, measuring 4.2 mm compared to the right, which measured 3.4 mm. There was a mildly positive 30° test with the left nerve reducing to 3.6 mm when she looked to the left. The diagnosis of an orbital lymphangioma with spontaneous hemorrhage was made. A multicystic lesion was confirmed on MRI scan (Fig. 244).

Because of the concern about optic nerve compression, an orbital surgeon was contacted and needle aspiration of the cyst was performed under ultrasound guidance. Ten cubic centimeters of blood was extracted and the eye immediately became less proptotic on the operating table. Examination in the office the next day showed an exophthalmometry measurement of 14 mm and improvement in visual acuity to 20/25. It was elected to not attempt surgical removal of the tumor because of its extensive entanglement

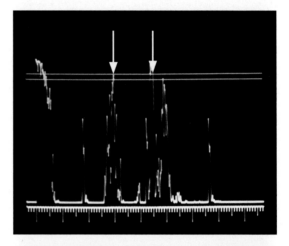

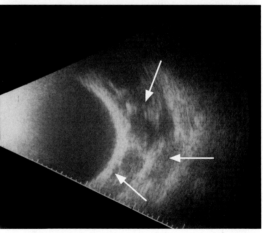

FIG. 243. Top: A-scan of orbital lymphangioma (*vertical arrows*). Bottom: B-scan of lymphangioma with large cyst and several smaller cysts (*arrows*)

with the optic nerve and extraocular muscles, but to manage the patient conservatively by aspiration of cyst fluid contents as needed to protect

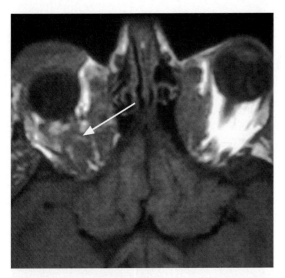

F<sub>IG</sub>. 244. Magnetic resonance imaging scan of lymphangioma (*arrow*)

the optic nerve and to help maintain facial comesis.

Another cause of optic nerve compression is "malignant" Graves' disease with pressure on the nerve in the orbital apex from massively enlarged extraocular muscles. About 1/3 of patients with Graves' orbitopathy experience a more aggressive disease course, with signs of inflammation, progressively reduced ocular motility, and possible optic nerve compression.[47] This fulminant course occurs more commonly in elderly patients who smoke. Some studies have suggested a male predominance but this finding is not consistent.

# Case Study 137
## Graves' Orbitopathy

HN is an 80-year-old male who presented with rapidly progressive proptosis and reduced vision over the period of a month. He gave a long history of smoking and no past history of thyroid disease. Examination found visual acuity OD of 20/100 and OS of 20/200. Intraocular pressures were 23 mm in the right eye and 24 mm in the left. Hertel exophthalmometry measured 22 OD and 23 mm OS. He had moderate lid edema and conjunctival chemosis. Slit-lamp examination showed mild corneal epithelial stippling bilaterally with poor tear film coverage. Fundus examination was unremarkable except for age-related macular drusen and retinal pigment epithelial changes. Visual field testing showed moderate peripheral depression.

Echography was performed with B-scan showing diffuse enlargement of the extraocular muscles. A-scan found significant enlargement of both superior recti with the right measuring 7.75 mm and the left 7.5 mm. The other muscles were diffusely enlarged. Internal reflectivity was generally heterogeneous but the superior recti were relatively medium reflective (Fig. 245). The optic nerves measured 4.5 mm OD and 4.3 mm OS with an equivocal 30° test on the right and a negative test on the left. CT scan demonstrated obvious thickening of the extraocular muscles at the orbital apex with apparent compression of the optic nerve.

He was urgently referred to an orbital surgeon, started on high-dose intravenous (IV) steroids and scheduled for surgery the next day. Orbital decompression was performed and the patient noted improvement in his vision later that evening. The IV steroids were continued for several days and he was discharged on oral prednisone after his visual acuity had been documented to substantially improve in both eyes.

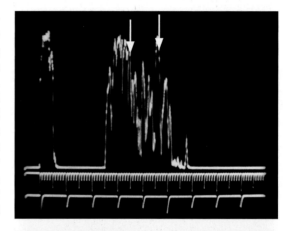

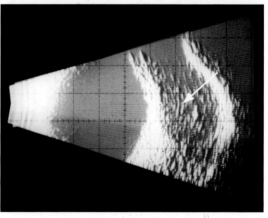

Fig. 245. Top: A-scan of markedly enlarged extraocular muscle (*vertical arrows*). Bottom: B-scan of muscle (*arrow*)

Optic nerve dysfunction can occur in the setting of Graves' disease by other mechanisms than compression by enlarged extraocular muscles.

# Case Study 138
## Increased Orbital Fat in Graves' Disease

GB is a 26-year-old woman who presented with complaints of reduced vision in her right eye over several weeks. Examination showed moderate lid lag and stare bilaterally with mild exophthalmos of 19 mm OD and 18 mm OS. Visual acuity was 20/50 OD and 20/25 OS with a 1 to 2+ afferent pupil defect on the right.

Echography was performed and demonstrated essentially normal extraocular muscle and optic nerve measurements bilaterally. There was an increase in the orbital fat volume on A-scan examination (Fig. 246), more on the right than on the left. CT scan confirmed an increase in orbital fat volume and showed straightening of the optic nerve (Fig. 247).

It was concluded that she had an optic nerve "on stretch" due to relative exophthalmos from increased orbital fat and connective tissue volume without significant extraocular muscle involvement. An orbital decompression was performed to reduce orbital volume and reduce the tension on the optic nerve. Her visual acuity was noted to improve.

Orbital inflammatory processes can involve the optic nerve directly, as in optic neuritis, or secondary to the involvement of other ocular tissues. Echography is most helpful in imaging the retrobulbar portion of the nerve with the appearance of the T sign where the nerve sheaths merge with inflamed sclera. Otherwise, ultrasound is less useful in demonstrating inflammatory changes of the orbital portion of the nerve, which is better shown on MRI scanning after injection of enhancing agents (Fig. 248).

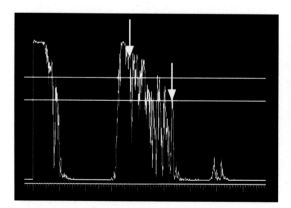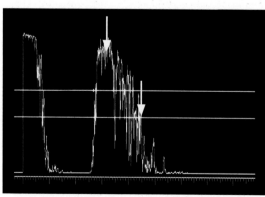

FIG. 246. Left: A-scan of increased orbital fat in the right eye (*vertical arrows*). Right: A-scan of orbital fat in the left eye (*arrows*)

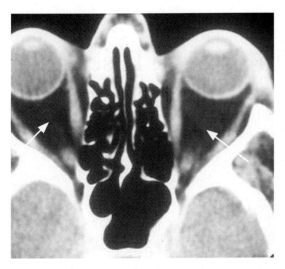 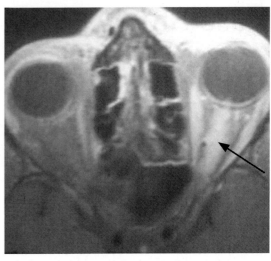

FIG. 247. Computed tomography scan of increased orbital fat (*arrow*).

FIG. 248. Magnetic resonance imaging scan of optic neuritis (*arrows*).

# Case Study 139
## T Sign in Retrobular Neuritis

CW is a 25-year-old woman who presented with complaints of pain and reduced vision in her left eye for about a week. Examination found visual acuity of 20/20 OD and of 20/60-2 OS with a 3+ afferent pupil defect. The left eye was mildly proptotic. Fundus examination showed a normal right optic disc and moderate edema of the left disc with several focal hemorrhages. Some perivascular sheathing was noted peripherally.

Echography of the left orbit revealed increased lucency of subtenon's space and the optic nerve sheaths with the appearance of a T sign (Fig. 249). A-scan measured the right optic nerve to be 3.5 mm and the left 3.7 mm, which was within normal limits for optic nerve thickness.

Magnetic resonance imaging scan showed optic nerve sheath enhancement after contrast injection, but no white plaques were noted in the brain as would be expected in demyelinating disease, such as multiple sclerosis. Systemic evaluation found a significantly positive antinuclear antibodies (ANA), which supported the diagnosis of systemic lupus erythematosis. She was treated with high-dose IV steroids with improvement in her vision in the left eye to 20/25. She subsequently experienced recurrences of her optic neuritis with response to steroids, but she began to have similar episodes in the right optic nerve. She eventually

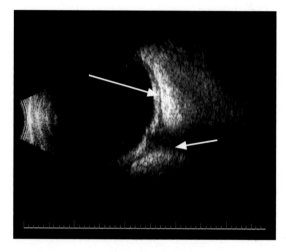

FIG. 249. T sign–scleral thickening (*large arrow*) and adjacent optic nerve thickening (*small arrow*)

suffered some atrophy of both nerves but maintained functional vision.

Idiopathic inflammation at the orbital apex, such as in the Tolosa-Hunt syndrome, can result in reduction of vision in conjunction with motility disturbances. This syndrome usually presents with the abrupt onset of painful ophthalmoplegia involving the third, fourth, and sixth nerves. There is often associated hypesthesia of the skin in the distribution of the first division of the fifth trigeminal nerve.

# Case Study 140
## Tolosa-Hunt Syndrome

JC is a 71-year-old woman who presented with the complaints of pain and reduced vision in her left eye for several days. Examination found visual acuity of 20/70 OD with a 3+ afferent pupil defect and acuity of 20/25 OS. Two millimeters of proptosis of the right eye was measured. She was also noted to have almost total ophthalmoplegia and reduced sensitivity of the periorbital skin. The remainder of the examination was normal except for mild nuclear sclerotic cataracts in both eyes.

Echography with B-scan was normal, but A-scan revealed thickening in the orbital apex in the area of the superior orbital fissure (Fig. 250). The extraocular muscles and optic nerve in the mid- and anterior orbit were of normal thickness. MRI scan was performed and showed enhancement of the cavernous sinus and superior orbital fissure (Fig. 251). A systemic workup was negative except for mild elevation of her sedimentation rate.

She was diagnosed with the Tolosa-Hunt syndrome and treated with high doses of oral prednisone. Her painful ophthalmoplegia rapidly improved, as did her visual acuity. She had only slight residual sixth nerve palsy after 2 weeks and the steroids were slowly tapered over another 3 weeks.

Pathology of the anterior orbit can cause visible abnormalities of the eyelids or periorbital tissue. A change in appearance of these areas even in the absence of other symptoms, such as pain, visual loss, or diplopia, can be the basis for presentation to the ophthalmologist.

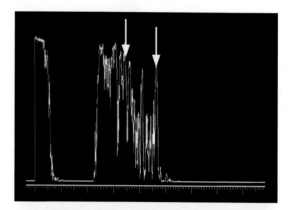

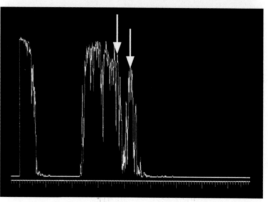

FIG. 250. Top: A-scan of thickened orbital apex in the right eye (*arrows*). Bottom: A-scan of normal apex in the left eye (*arrows*)

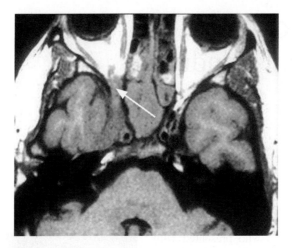

FIG. 251. Magnetic resonance imaging scan of orbital apex
(*arrow*)

# Case Study 141
## Orbital Infantile Hemangioma

CB is a 1-year-old boy who was noted by his parents to have some bluish swelling of the left upper eyelid shortly after birth. They attributed it to birth trauma but became alarmed when the swelling increased dramatically over 2 weeks. They observed that the lid became more swollen and reddish when the baby cried vigorously. The pediatrician, who obtained a CT scan that same day that was interpreted as showing diffuse orbital swelling, saw the child. A mass such as rhabdomyosarcoma could not be ruled out. The patient was referred to a pediatric ophthalmologist with the operating room on call for a possible emergency biopsy that evening.

A-scan revealed an orbital lesion that occupied the mid- and anterior orbit. A-scan showed heterogeneous internal reflectivity with areas of medium-to-high reflectivity interspersed with a relatively low area (Fig. 252). Rapid spike movements were detected consistent with arterial blood flow. This was confirmed when a hand-held obstetrical Doppler unit with a special probe adapted for the orbit was held against the lid. There was a moderately loud sound of arterial blood flow that persisted when the probe was angled in different directions. This was consistent with a highly vascular lesion. The combination of irregular internal reflectivity and arterial blood flow was most consistent with a hemangioma of the infantile type, or capillary hemangioma (benign hemangioendothelioma).

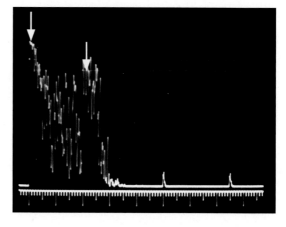

FIG. 252. A-scan of infantile hemangioma (*vertical arrows*)

Biopsy was cancelled and the child was treated with high-dose oral steroids with reduction in size of the tumor over several weeks. The parents were advised that the lesion would spontaneously involute over the next year or two and treatment should only be considered if the vision was threatened by amblyogenic factors, such as a ptotic lid occluding the visual axis or asymmetric astigmatism caused by pressure of the lesion on the globe.

Treatment of capillary hemangiomas often involves the use of the intralesional injection of steroids that reduces the systemic side effects versus a higher risk with the oral route.

# Case Study 142
## Orbital Infantile Hemangioma

RC is a 2-year-old girl with a history of a vascular lesion involving the left upper lid and anterior orbit. It was diagnosed as a capillary hemangioma and intralesional injection of steroids was recommended to the parents because the tumor was enlarging rapidly and threatening to obstruct the visual axis. The child was referred for echography to substantiate the diagnosis and direct the steroid injection.

Echography by A-scan showed a 17-mm lesion with irregular internal reflectivity and marked vascularity on examination with an obstetrical Doppler unit. A low reflective area with marked spontaneous vascularity was noted (Fig. 253) and a marking pen was used to outline this highly vascular area. A triamcinolone injection of 1 cc was performed with avoidance of the area with the highest blood flow to reduce the possibility of retrograde injection of steroid into the retinal arterial vasculature. The injection was accomplished without difficulty

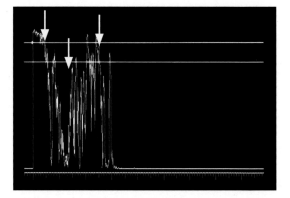

FIG. 253. A-scan of low reflective high flow area (*middle arrow*) in infantile hemangioma (*small vertical arrows*)

and the lesion regressed significantly over the next several weeks.

Varices can occur in the orbit but sometimes present as more visible lesions in the paraocular area.

# Case Study 143
## Orbital Varix

PC is a 72-year-old man whose wife noted a lump in the corner of his left eye that extended onto the nose. His ophthalmologist noted a serpiginous lesion under the skin that collapsed under gentle pressure. The conjunctiva was moderately injected nasally, but not temporally. Echography was performed and showed a low reflective soft lesion (Fig. 254). An obstetrical Doppler unit was applied and transmitted sounds from the nasal artery were heard but not from the vascular lesion. This was consistent with a varix without arterialization of blood flow.

Orbital varices can also occur in the mid- and anterior orbit as either primary vessel wall anomalies or secondary to vascular malformations. They may present with intermittent proptosis as they dilate secondarily to valsalva-induced increased venous pressure. They may remain undetected for years.

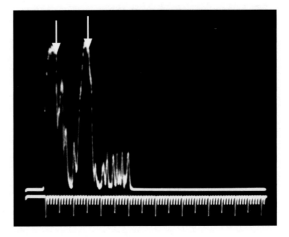

FIG. 254. A-scan of orbital varix (*vertical arrows*)

# Case Study 144
## Orbital Arteriovenous Malformation

RG is a 25-year-old man who presented with the history of bulging of his right eye when he felt increased pressure in his head when lifting weights or bending over and picking up heavy objects. Examination found vision in both eyes of 20/20 and normal intraocular pressures. Proptosis of his right eye was measured at 23 mm when he performed a valsalva maneuver and his left eye exophthalmometry measurement was normal at 18 mm.

Echography showed a normal right orbit before valsalva and a low reflective encapsulated lesion in the mid-orbit after he increased venous pressure by bending over and bearing down (Fig. 255).

The most common marginal lid lesion encountered in clinical practice is the chalazion (stye). This often starts as a focal tender bump at the lid margin that may come to a head and involute spontaneously or with the application of warm compresses. However, it may evolve into a more chronic form called a chalazion. Generally, echography has little or no role in these lesions except in atypical presentations.

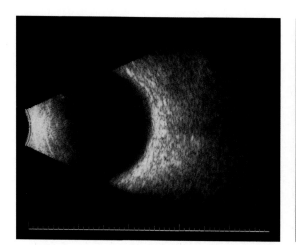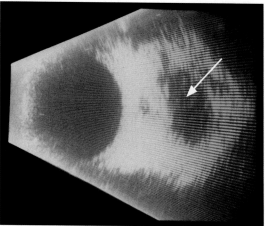

Fig. 255. Left: B-scan of orbital arteriovenous malformation before Valsalva. Right: B-scan after Valsalva (*arrow*)

# Case Study 145
## Lymphoma of Eyelid

CT is a 35-year-old man with a reddish focal swelling in his right lower lid that fluctuated in size over several months. He was seen by his primary care doctor and diagnosed with a chalazion. He had tried hot packs, oral antibiotics, and was seen by an ophthalmologist who injected steroids into the lesion, but it persisted.

Echography was performed and showed a 1-cm encapsulated lesion with medium internal reflectivity on A-scan (Fig. 256). The differential diagnosis included an inflammatory infiltrate but a lymphoid lesion could not be ruled out. Because of this possibility and the persistence of the tumor, a biopsy was performed.

The pathological diagnosis was a B-cell lymphoma and a systemic workup was initiated with no evidence of lymphoma at other sites. Nevertheless, the patient was informed that the probability of a distant focus of lymphoma was 60% to 70% because of the involvement of the ocular adenexae.

Bulges in the nasal canthus are often related to pathology of the nasolacrimal system. Obstruction of the nasolacrimal duct is quite common in newborns and is generally a self-correcting problem but can be treated by probing. Rarely, an infant is born with a tense cystic bulge in the area of the nasolacrimal fossa. This is called a dacriocystocele or lacrimal sac mucocele. It may be of the regurgitating type when mucous and fluid can be expressed

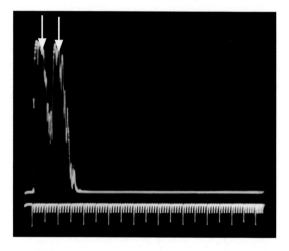

FIG. 256. A-scan of atypical chalazion (*vertical arrows*)

through the punctum when the examiner presses on the sac. If secretions cannot be expressed due to obstruction or kinking of the common canaliculus, then it is of the nonregurgitating type and can result in marked distention of the lacrimal sac.

Echography is useful in such cases by demonstrating a well-outlined and low reflective structure without vascularity. The A-scan can be placed inside the nose. If the mucocele descends into the nasal cavity it is best treated by a myringotomy blade from the nasal end because it may not respond to probing of the system performed through the punctum.

# Case Study 146
## Dacriocystocele

TE is a 3-day-old infant who was noted to have a moderately firm swelling in the corner of the left eye. This increased over the next 2 days so the parents sought ophthalmic consultation. The doctor was relatively certain the lesion was a lacrimal sac mucocele. The differential diagnosis included a meningoencephalocele, but the lack of pulsations made this unlikely.

Echography demonstrated a well-outlined echolucent lesion on B-scan with regular low reflectivity on A-scan. The A-scan probe was placed inside the nose and a high reflective membrane was encountered that was consistent with a mucocele of the sac (Fig. 257). An otolaryngologist performed an incision with a myringotomy blade and under the same anesthesia an ophthalmologist performed nasolacrimal probing. Mucinous fluid gushed out and the distended lacrimal sac was decompressed.

Rarely, tumors can originate from the lacrimal sac. When a patient presents with the complaint

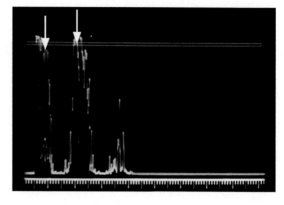

FIG. 257. A-scan inside nose of dacriocystocele (*vertical arrows*)

of tearing, the sac on the involved side should be palpated. Bloody tears are especially suggestive of a neoplasm. Firmness may indicate dacrioliths in the sac that may require surgical removal, but also may indicate a neoplasm.

# Case Study 147
## Hemangiopericytoma of Lacrimal Sac

JR is a 34-year-old man who presented with complaints of epiphora on the left side for several months. He had been given antibiotics and decongestant nasal sprays by his primary care physician without relief of the tearing. He was referred to an ophthalmologist, who noted some fullness in the nasolacrimal fossa and found a firm lesion on palpation.

Echography revealed a moderately echodense encapsulated lesion on B-scan and a regular medium reflective growth with moderate spontaneous vascularity on A-scan (Fig. 258). CT scan showed an isodense process in the lacrimal sac without bone destruction or invasion. The patient was referred for a dacriocystorhinostomy with the plan to perform a concurrent excisional biopsy of the lesion. A reddish firm tumor was found at surgery.

Pathology demonstrated a cellular lesion with vascular elements consistent with a hemangiopericytoma of the lacrimal sac. The patient was followed serially with ultrasound to eliminate recurrence of the tumor.

Other tumors can also rarely involve the lacrimal sac and include epithelial tumors, such as squamous cell carcinoma, adenocarcinoma, and oncocytoma. Nonepithelial tumors, such as rhabdomyosarcoma, lymphoma, plasmocytoma, and leukemia can also be found.

Epiphora can be the first sign of an extensive process invading the medial orbital bony wall and may even extend intracranially.

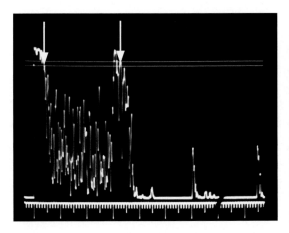
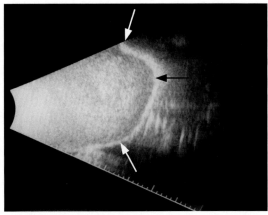

FIG. 258. Left: A-scan of hemangiopericytoma of lacrimal sac (*vertical arrows*). Right: B-scan of lesion in lacrimal sac (*arrows*)

# Case Study 148
## Orbital Meningioma

CW is a 43-year-old woman who gave a history of tearing and "sinus pressure"' on her left side for several months. Examination found firmness in the entire medial bony orbit. The left eye was displaced medially about 3 mm compared to the right eye.

Echography showed numerous A-scan spikes emanating from the area of the lacrimal sac and deep ethmoid/sphenoid sinus complex (Fig. 259). CT scan revealed an extensive bony intracranial lesion that involved the greater wing of the sphenoid that was very suspicious for a meningi-

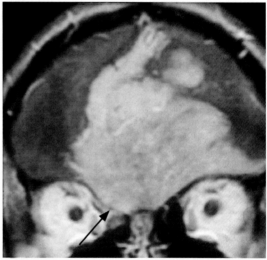

FIG. 260. Computed tomography of meningioma invading nasal orbit (*arrow*)

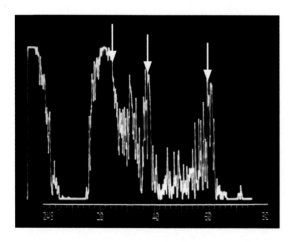

FIG. 259. A-scan of meningioma invading lacrimal sac (*first two vertical arrows*) and paranasal sinuses (between *second* and *third arrows*)

oma (Fig. 260). This diagnosis was confirmed on biopsy.

Occasionally, a foreign body that strikes the periocular area will lodge in the eyelids. Any history of high-speed projectiles hitting the eye or adnexae, especially without safety goggles being worn, should prompt a careful examination for a tiny self-sealing entry wound in the lids or globe. The threat to the eye is greatly increased by the entry of a foreign body into the ocular contents.

# Case Study 149
## Eyelid Thickness

CP is a 23-year-old man who was involved in a motor vehicle accident with shattered glass from the windshield striking his eye. He went to an emergency room where the doctor "picked out many pieces of glass from the eye." He later felt focal tenderness in the lid and was convinced that he could palpate a small firm object under the eyelid skin. He was seen by an ophthalmologist who was not able to palpate any foreign object in the lid. The patient demanded that some sort of "x-ray" be performed to find the object. The doctor felt radiographic studies including CT would not show a piece of glass so the patient was referred for echography.

Standard contact B-scan did not show any foreign body signals in the globe or anterior orbital tissue but the image of the eyelid was hidden in the probe's 5-mm dead zone. An immersion scan with a 20 MHz probe was performed utilizing a soft silicone immersion shell filled with methylcellulose to back the probe away from the lid to display its full thickness (Fig. 261). No foreign body signal was detected and the patient was reassured that there was nothing to worry about.

The differential diagnosis of proptosis and other malpositions of the eye is a long one. Echography provides a rapid and inexpensive method to quickly diagnose many of these entities in an office setting. The quantitative ability of the A-scan can provide a focused differential diagnosis in most cases and can correctly characterize the lesion in many cases.

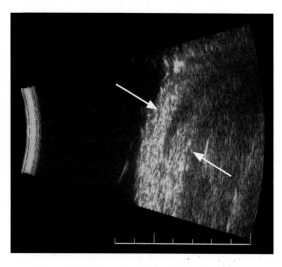

FIG. 261. Immersion scan of normal eyelid (*arrows*)

# Part VI
## Lumps and Bumps

Echography is extremely valuable in the evaluation of lumps and bumps in and around the eye. It is the most valuable of the various imaging techniques in the evaluation of intraocular lesions. The approach to intraocular tumors has changed dramatically in the last 25 years. Prior to that time, eyes were often enucleated because of the suspicion of intraocular melanoma. Ferry published a major intraocular tumor pathology study from the Armed Forces Institute of Pathology (AFIP) in the 1960s and found that 20% of eyes enucleated with the diagnosis of malignant melanoma harbored other mostly nonmalignant lesions. This study was criticized because it was performed before indirect ophthalmoscopy and fluorescein angiography were widely used in the evaluation of intraocular tumors. Ferry repeated the study in the 1970s when these modalities were part of routine practice and the same 20% misdiagnosis rate was found.[48]

The list of lesions misdiagnosed as choroidal melanomas with their incidence in the pathology series includes:

| | |
|---|---|
| Choroidal nevi | 20% |
| Retinal pigment epithelial hypertrophy | 10% |
| Metastatic tumor | 8% |
| Subretinal hemorrhage | 7% |
| Disciform scar | 7% |
| Choroidal detachment | 6% |
| Retinal detachment | 5% |
| Choroidal hemangioma | 4% |
| Retinal hamartoma | 3% |
| Vortex veins | 1% |
| Posterior scleritis | 1% |
| Reactive lymphoid hyperplasia | 1% |

Many of these lesions can be readily diagnosed by careful ophthalmoscopy but this becomes more difficult as a direct function of the opacity of the ocular media. Such obscurations to the passage of the light from the ophthalmoscope are not inhibitory to the sound beam of the echographer. This modality is essential in the accurate characterization of a number of intraocular lesions. The most difficult clinical differentiation is among solid tumors of the fundus, such as metastatic tumors, hemangiomas, and large nevi, even when they are not obscured by media opacification. A-scan allows tissue differentiation that is especially valuable in separating choroidal melanomas from the various mimickers.

Since the second AFIP study, echography has dramatically impacted the accuracy of the evaluation of intraocular tumors. This technique began to be used more extensively in the 1980s and the rate of specificity for the diagnosis of choroidal melanoma increased significantly. The latest data from the Collaborative Ocular Melanoma Study (COMS) documents a diagnostic accuracy of 99.7%, although atypical lesions were not included.[49] Standardized echography was the primary ancillary tool used in this study. Ultrasound has become the standard in detecting and diagnosing intraocular tumors. According to Trubo, "the gold standard in evaluating ocular tumors remains ocular ultrasound, including both A- and B-scan ultrasound." He quotes Timothy Murray who states, "it is clearly better than the best MRI scan, the best CT scan or the best PET scan that we have."[50] This level of reliability approaches that of microscopic tissue sections as studied by the pathologist. Echography is unable to differentiate cell types, but the tissue architecture created by collections of cells has a direct correlation to the reflectivity patterns on A-scan. This is especially important in an organ, such as the eye, in which biopsy may be hazardous.

Current radiologic techniques, such as magnetic resonance imaging (MRI) and computed tomography (CT) rely mostly on gross morphology and are not able to differentiate tissue at the resolution of ultrasound. Positron emission tomography (PET)/CT technology does its imaging in the biochemical realm. It displays the concentration of radioactively tagged glucose and other molecules as they are metabolized in different tissues. Finger et al. reviewed two cases of intraocular melanoma in which the first evidence of liver metastases was focal hot spots on PET/CT scanning.[51] This finding was noted before liver function tests became abnormal. However, this technology is not widely available and is relatively expensive. The usefulness of PET scans for the characterization intraocular tumors has not been established.

B-scan echography is similar to MRI and CT scanning as it provides valuable morphologic information about the size and shape of ocular and orbital lesions. Lesions such as ocular melanomas often have an almost pathognomonic mushroom shape on B-scan (Fig. 262). This shape is due to the constriction of the "neck" of the tumor as it erodes and breaks through Bruch's membrane into the subretinal space.

Rarely, a rapidly growing metastatic tumor breaks through Bruch's membrane. B-scan also allows an overview of the local surround of a lesion. It can demonstrate subretinal fluid and the extent of any retinal detachment (Fig. 263). It provides a picture of tumor proximity to the optic nerve, which is an important prognostic factor (Fig. 264). B-scan is essential in measuring the basal dimensions of a lesion, which enables the calculation of total tumor volume when combined with the very precise thickness measurements attainable by A-scan.

The use of A-scan enables a peek inside the tissue being studied. Histological characteristics are directly correlated to the characteristics of the spikes. The major A-scan criteria for the diagno-

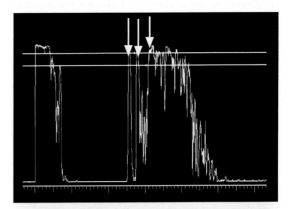

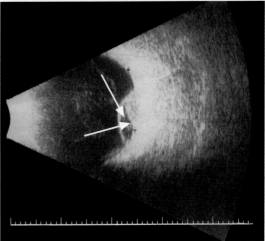

FIG. 263. Top: A-scan of subretinal fluid (*first two arrows*) over choroidal melanoma (*second* and *third arrows*). Bottom: B-scan of subretinal fluid (*vertical arrow*) over melanoma (*horizontal arrow*)

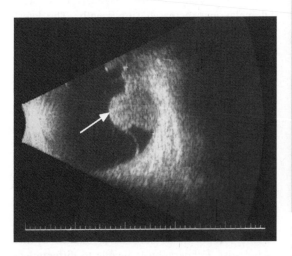

FIG. 262. B-scan of choroidal melanoma with mushrooming shape (*arrow*)

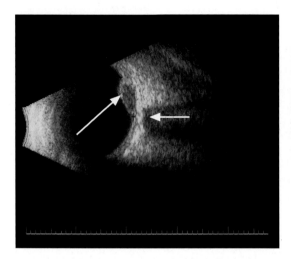

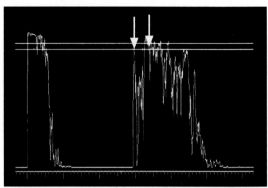

FIG. 266. A-scan reflectivity of choroidal melanoma of 50% (*first arrow*) surface of melanoma and (*second arrow*) on sclera

FIG. 264. B-scan of proximity of choroidal melanoma (*large arrow*) to optic nerve (*small arrow*)

sis of choroidal melanoma include a solid tumor surface spike, low-to-medium and regular internal reflectivity, and spontaneous vascularity. The internal features of reflectivity are determined by the cellular architecture of the lesion. Melanomas are densely cellular in a relatively homogenous pattern of distribution. There are some interfaces largely due to the presence of blood vessels, especially arterioles (Fig. 265). This rather uniform structure with few interfaces results in the sound wave traveling through the tissue with relatively minor

reflection of sound back to the probe. The average height of the spikes range from almost baseline up to about 60% compared to the lesion surface spike (Fig. 266). The spikes do not vary significantly in vertical extension with rare exceptions (Fig. 267). Ciliary body melanomas tend to be medium reflective with more irregularity of the spikes as compared to more posterior lesions. This is due to the bumpier shape of this area of the uveal tract. Also, some melanomas have necrotic or cystic areas and this does affect the regularity of the echo signals as the sound beam traverses these regions (Fig. 268).

Vascularity with arterial blood flow is generally present in choroidal melanomas and is a major differential feature in the echographic criteria. The detection of spontaneous vascularity is difficult in lesions under 2.5 mm in thickness because of the limitations upon

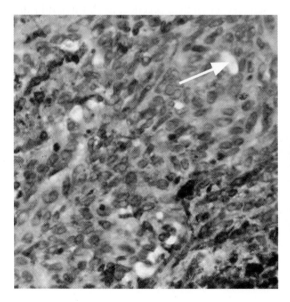

FIG. 265. Path slide of vessel in a melanoma (*arrow*)

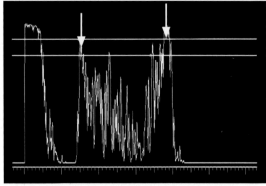

FIG. 267. A-scan of irregular choroidal melanoma reflectivity (*first arrow*) surface of melanoma and (*second arrow*) on sclera

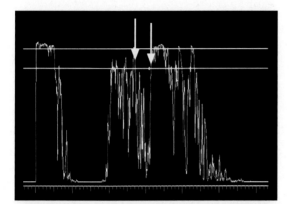

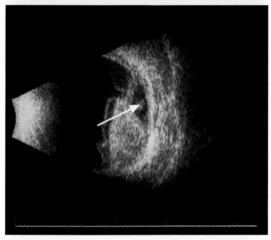

FIG. 268. Top: A-scan of ciliary body melanoma with cavitary changes (*vertical arrows*). Bottom: B-scan cavity (*arrow*)

the examiner in resolving subtle movements in such a relatively small space. An increase in thickness with

the appearance of spontaneous vascularity usually indicates a more aggressive nature of the tumor, with conversion from a choroidal nevus to a melanoma. This characteristic is also useful in determining the response of a melanoma to radiation treatment by either plaque therapy or proton beam irradiation. The disappearance of vascularity on echography in conjunction with a change to more irregular internal reflectivity is evidence that there has been response to therapy. The rapid flickering movements of the spikes on A-scan have their counterpart in the dancing pixels on the B-scan. The resolution of vascularity is directly dependent on the sensitivity of the A- and B-scan unit. It is difficult or even impossible to evaluate in vector A-scans and some B-scans. The examiner should first look for spontaneous vascularity on B-scan by increasing the size of the image on the screen. During this time, the tumor is centered in the middle of the display and the probe is held steady while the examiner moves forward to carefully study it. These movements can also be seen on the A-scan as rapid vertical movements independent from microsaccadic eye movements. They should be graded in intensity on a scale of 1 to 4.

The presence of all of these characteristics (low-to-medium reflectivity, spontaneous vascularity, and mushroom shape) results in diagnostic accuracy of 99.7% for choroidal melanoma. Such capability approaches histology and is exceptional among the various disciplines of imaging technology. The advantages of such sensitivity and specificity are invaluable in clinical practice, as illustrated in the following case study.

# Case Study 150
## Choroidal Melanoma Treated with Radioactive Plaque

WP is a 52-year-old man who complained of a shadow in his right eye for several months. He went initially to an optometrist, who could not improve his vision with refraction and documented a depression on automated perimetry in his temporal field of vision. Ophthalmoscopy revealed a darkly pigmented nasal tumor. The patient was referred for echography.

Ultrasound demonstrated a solid, low reflective and regular lesion with marked spontaneous vascularity that measured 6.53 mm in thickness (Fig. 269). B-scan revealed a mushroom-shaped tumor that measured 11.9 by 12.1 mm in basal dimensions. Subretinal fluid extending inferiorly was noted (Fig. 270). The patient was evaluated systemically with liver function tests, a chest x-ray, and a thorough skin examination. No evidence of metastatic disease was found. Therapeutic options were discussed with the patient and he elected to have a radioactive iodine 131 plaque applied to the tumor.

He was seen for follow-up echography in 6 months and the tumor volume was slightly reduced from the pretreatment measurements. However, on A-scan the internal reflectivity was higher and more irregular than before radiation (Fig. 271). Only slight spontaneous vascularity was noted. On B-scan an echolucent area was noted in subtenon's space corresponding to the location of the plaque (Fig. 272).

It is not uncommon after radiation treatment for melanomas to be the same size or larger than before treatment. This usually does not indicate growth, but is probably due to necrosis and edema caused by the radiation damage to the malignant cells. Such changes may persist for up to 6 months. After this time there is generally some reduction in the volume of the tumor but it rarely disappears completely. The patient should be reassured that

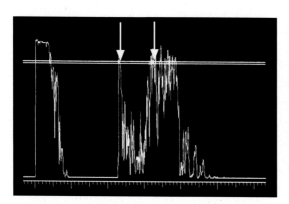

FIG. 269. A-scan of typical choroidal melanoma (*vertical arrows*)

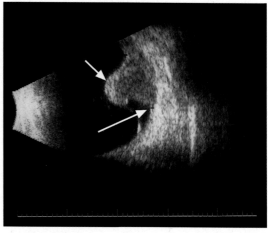

FIG. 270. B-scan of melanoma (*small arrow*). Subretinal fluid (*large arrow*)

persistence of a lesion is not evidence of failure of the treatment to destroy the tumor, but is simply a scar that has little chance of growing.

The echographic criteria that support the diagnosis of choroidal melanoma are equally valuable in eliminating this malignant tumor from the other differential considerations of fundus lesions. Internal reflectivity that is higher than 60% of

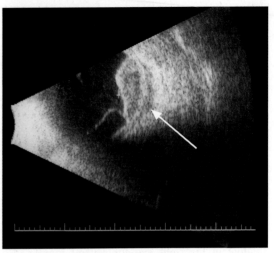

Fig. 272. B-scan of subtenon's echolucency post-radiation treatment of choroidal melanoma (*arrow*)

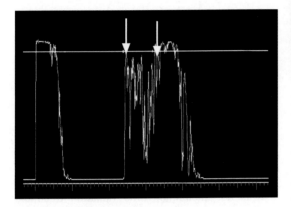

Fig. 271. A-scan of postradiation changes in choroidal melanoma (*vertical arrows*)

the initial spike height is inconsistent with the diagnosis of melanoma. Occasionally an interface within the tumor resulting from an area of cavitation or necrosis may result in a spike or two that is at this 60% level, but the average spike height will remain below this threshold.

# Case Study 151
## Pseudomelanoma

TD is a 52-year-old man who was seen for a routine eye exam by his optometrist and found to have a lightly pigmented fundus lesion near the nasal equator of his left eye. It was assumed to be a melanoma and the patient was so informed. He was referred to a retinal specialist for the initiation of therapy. The retinologist agreed that it was most likely a choroidal melanoma, but before treatment was begun a fluorescein angiogram was performed and the man was sent for echographic examination.

Ultrasound was performed and A-scan demonstrated medium-to-high internal reflectivity with mild irregularity (Fig. 273). Spontaneous vascularity was not detected. The differential diagnosis was most consistent with a choroidal hemangioma, but a metastatic tumor could not be ruled out. Melanoma was considered to be unlikely. The retinologist proceeded on the assumption it was a melanoma in spite of the echographic findings and scheduled the patient for radioactive plaque therapy, but first performed a fine needle biopsy of the lesion. The initial pathology report was suspicious for melanoma so the plaque placement proceeded. The final cytology report ruled out melanoma but a specific tissue diagnosis could not be given. Echography was repeated and showed no change in the volume of the lesion. The patient was followed over several years with serial ultrasound exams and no change in size or internal reflectivity characteristics was noted.

Many suspected nevi and small melanomas are followed over time without treatment. The conversion of choroidal nevi to malignant melanomas is projected to be relatively rare.[52] About 7% of individuals are estimated to harbor nevi and with an incidence in the United States of about 3000 new cases a year, the conversion rate would be about 1/8000 to 1/9000. However, some clinicians argue that most melanomas arise de novo and do not originate from preexisting nevi. It is reasonable to obtain fundus photos and baseline echography for a nevus documented for the first time by the examiner in a given patient. This is especially true if it meets one or more of the criteria for suspicious nevi as outlined by Shields et al.[53]

These criteria include subretinal fluid, orange pigment, thickness greater than 2 mm, symptoms of a shadow or surface in the patient's field of vision, and proximity to the optic nerve. The probability of growth by a suspicious choroidal lesion (under 2 mm in thickness) is about 4% if none of these risk factors are present. There is a 34% chance if one risk factor is present, and 63% chance if 3 or more are present. COMS found that about 31% of the entire group of small ocular melanomas had grown to medium or large size after 5 years.

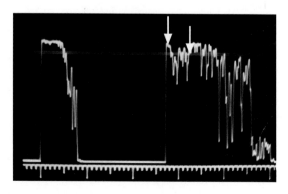

FIG. 273. A-scan of pseudomelanoma (*vertical arrows*)

Besides its value in following suspected nevi over time for an increase in thickness, A-scan is particularly useful for characterizing changes in the internal structure of a specific lesion. A change in the height and regularity of the A-scan reflectivity pattern typical for a nevus to one more consistent with a melanoma is very suggestive of the transition to a more aggressive type of tumor. The patient should be informed of this change and given the option to continue following the lesion or the choice of different treatment modalities.

# Case Study 152
## Conversion of Nevus to Melanoma

BP is a 56-year-old woman who was incidentally noted to have a pigmented temporal choroidal lesion in her right eye on a routine examination by her ophthalmologist. It was moderately pigmented and estimated to be just over 2 mm in thickness and about 5 mm in basal diameter. Baseline echography was performed and documented a lesion measuring 1.55 mm in thickness by 5.2 mm by 5.8 mm in basal dimensions. It was medium-to-high reflective on A-scan with slight irregularity of the echo spikes (Fig. 274). These findings were felt to be consistent with a nevus and the patient was instructed to return in 6 months for follow-up. The lesion appeared unchanged clinically at that time.

Echography was repeated and demonstrated a mild increase in overall volume of the lesion to 1.98 mm by 5.5 mm by 5.8 mm. However, internal reflectivity on A-scan was now more medium reflec-

tive than noted on the initial examination (Fig. 275). This change in reflectivity was suspicious for an increase in cellular infiltration of the choroid consistent with conversion from a nevus to a melanoma. The situation was discussed with the patient and she elected to return in 3 months for repeat echography. That examination revealed a further small increase in tumor volume and the appearance of spontaneous vascularity. She elected to undergo radioactive plaque treatment after a systemic workup, including liver function tests, chest x-ray, and dermatologic survey, found no evidence of metastases.

Benign nevi can grow over time and a slight increase in thickness alone would not necessarily be a reason to initiate therapy. However, the value of A-scan is to demonstrate changes in internal reflectivity suggestive of a change in the mitotic activity of the cells.

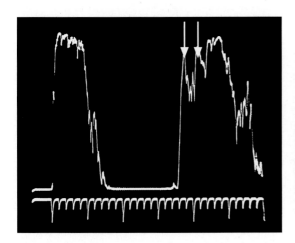

FIG. 274. A-scan of large nevus (*vertical arrows*)

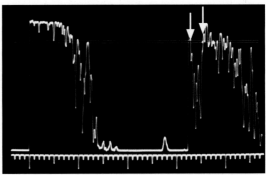

FIG. 275. A-scan of the nevus in Figure 254 with lower reflectivity over time (*vertical arrows*)

# Case Study 153
## Nevus Transforming to Melanoma

DF is a 56-year-old man who complained of slight visual distortion in his right eye on presentation to his optometrist. Examination showed visual acuity of 20/20-2 in that eye and 20/20 in his left eye. The anterior segment examination was normal but fundus examination showed a lightly pigmented submacular lesion. Fluorescein angiography was ordered and the lesion demonstrated initial hypofluorescence with delayed spotty leakage and staining. Echography was performed and displayed a high reflective lesion measuring 1.11 mm in thickness and just under 5 mm in basal diameter. The patient was seen a year later with no change in symptoms or echographic findings.

He presented a year from that examination with complaints of further distortion and reduction of vision in the right eye. Clinical examination showed a reduction in vision to 20/60-2 with distortion of the central lines on amsler grid testing. Fundus examination was not definitive for an increase in size of the lesion, but there was some question of subretinal fluid overlying the growth. The patient was told that his visual symptoms were possibly due to "leakage of fluid" from the growth.

Echography was performed and demonstrated an increase in thickness to 2.5 mm and basal dimensions of 6.1 mm. A scan now showed medium and slightly irregular internal reflectivity (Fig. 276). It was concluded the lesion was transforming from a nevus to a melanoma. The options were presented to the patient with further observation of an enlarging melanoma or radioactive plaque treatment with loss of his central vision. After a negative systemic workup he elected to proceed with radiation treatment.

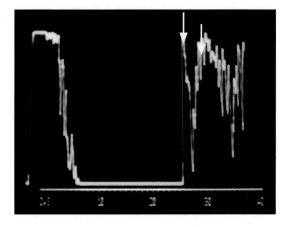

FIG. 276. A-scan of nevus (*vertical arrows*) enlarging with lower internal reflectivity

Melanomas will sometimes invade the sclera without significant anterior growth over time. The incidence of scleral infiltration is higher in larger tumors. Shammas and Blodi reported a 12.6% incidence in tumors with basal diameters less than 10 mm and 32.3% in lesions with diameters greater than 10 mm.[54] Rarely, a relatively small lesion with borderline thickness of around 2 mm is actually a malignant melanoma growing posteriorly with extrascleral extension. There is no way to detect such posterior growth other than by imaging studies. Echography is the most sensitive and least expensive of these diagnostic techniques, although it cannot reliably detect microscopic invasion of the sclera. However, Ossoinig feels that a "ragged" posterior tumor spike is suggestive of scleral invasion (Fig. 277). An echolucency in the retroscleral

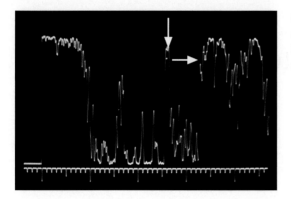

space on B-scan and low reflectivity on A-scan are suggestive of posterior extension. Ultrasound can be more sensitive than CT or MRI in detecting this occurrence.

FIG. 277. A-scan of choroidal melanoma (*vertical arrow*) with scleral irregularity suggestive of tumor invasion (*horizontal arrow*)

# Case Study 154
## Choroidal Melanoma with Extrascleral Extension

ON is a 73-year-old man who was noted to have a lightly pigmented choroidal lesion in the right eye on a routine examination by his ophthalmologist. Fundus photographs were taken and the patient was instructed to return in a year. He came back almost 2 years later with no new symptoms. Fundus examination and photographs were consistent with no change in the choroidal lesion and he was told to return in another year. The patient was in another state on vacation several months later and was advised to see his son's ophthalmologist when he complained about some loss of vision in the opposite eye. Examination revealed a branch vein occlusion in the left eye with mild macular edema and visual acuity of 20/50. The right eye had visual acuity of 20/30 and the original choroidal lesion was noted. Because the previous records were not available, echography was performed.

B-scan demonstrated an elevated choroidal lesion with basal dimensions of 5.3 mm by 6.1 mm. There was an echolucency in subtenon's space directly posterior to the growth (Fig. 278). A-scan revealed a thickness of 5.27 mm and medium, regular internal reflectivity. Moderate spontaneous vascularity was detected. These findings were very suspicious for a malignant melanoma with extraocular extension. The patient was referred for enucleation with possible exenteration that was to be determined by the presence or absence of an intact subtenon's capsule at the time of surgery. A tumor with extension through the sclera but encapsulated by an intact subtenon's capsule was identified. It was elected to only enucleate and not exenterate the orbit. The patient showed no evidence of recurrence after 2 years of follow-up.

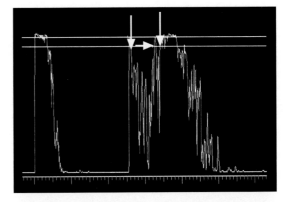

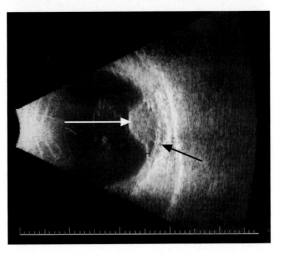

FIG. 278. Top: A-scan of choroidal melanoma (*first vertical arrow*) with extrascleral extension (between *horizontal* and *second vertical arrow*). Bottom: B-scan of extrascleral extension (*small arrow*)

Choroidal melanoma will rarely invade the optic nerve, as reported in 0.6% to 3.7% of cases.

Shields states, "most uveal melanomas have little tendency to invade the optic disc. Even tumors that are adjacent to the disc tend to stop abruptly at the optic disc margins." He adds that some melanomas with a diffuse growth pattern have a tendency to grow into the substance of the nerve and can be confused with papilledema. Such tumors have an extremely poor prognosis.[55] This frequency of nerve invasion is in contrast to retinoblastoma, in which an incidence of 29% is reported.[56]

# Case Study 155
## Choroidal Melanoma with Optic Nerve Invasion

NA is a 67-year-old woman who noted a drop in the vision in her right eye, but delayed seeking medical attention for several months. She was finally seen by an ophthalmologist who documented vision in that eye of 20/70-2 and 20/30 in the left eye. A 2+ afferent defect was noted. Fundus examination showed a darkly pigmented lesion adjacent superiorly to the optic nerve. Echography was performed and revealed a low-to-medium reflective tumor measuring 4.2 mm in thickness and 13.8 mm in basal diameter (Fig. 279). The optic nerve was measured by A-scan to be 2.66 mm, which is within normal limits.

Because of the poor visual acuity and the presence of an afferent defect, the patient was referred for an MRI scan of the optic nerve. It demonstrated slight nonspecific enhancement after the administration of a contrast agent. The patient chose to have the eye enucleated as opposed to exenteration. Every effort was made to obtain a long segment of the retrobulbar optic nerve. The pathological report showed that the surgical margin at the distal end of the optic nerve segment was clear and only the anterior part was invaded by melanoma cells.

Choroidal melanomas will uncommonly present as a diffuse process and not a solid tumor. This is reported to occur in 4% to 5% of cases and has a metastatic risk of 24% at 5 years. According to Shields et al., the risk of metastasis is higher in a lesion with a large basal diameter and poorly defined margins.[57] Such lesions are misdiagnosed about half of the time.

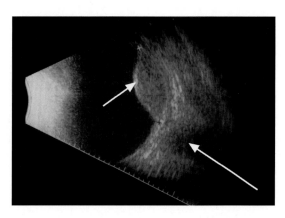

FIG. 279. B-scan of choroidal melanoma (*small arrows*) adjacent to optic nerve (*large arrow*)

# Case Study 156
## Diffuse Choroidal Melanoma

TY is a 25-year-old man who was noted on routine examination to have a dark choroidal lesion with poorly defined margins. Echography revealed low reflective choroidal thickening in the area of the lesion on A-scan and an irregular surface on B-scan (Fig. 280). The differential diagnosis included an infiltrative process either by inflammatory or neoplastic cells. A systemic workup for malignancy was negative. He returned for follow-up in 3 months and the lesion had increased in size. Because of the high probability of diffuse melanoma, the eye was enucleated and pathology confirmed the diagnosis of epitheloid melanoma.

The low-to-medium and regular internal reflectivity of melanomas as imaged by the A-scan is the result of a dense, homogenous cell population with relatively few tissue interfaces to reflect the sound waves. On the other hand, choroidal nevi have a less dense population of melanocytes that are loosely interspersed within the normal choroid. This results in multiple interfaces from which the sound beam is reflected resulting in higher reflectivity than is seen in melanomas on the A-scan (Fig. 281).

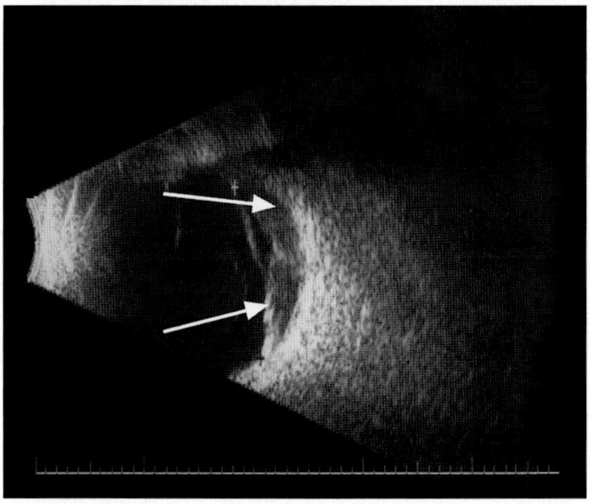

Another pigmented choroidal tumor with high internal reflectivity on A-scan is the melanocytoma (Fig. 282). This lesion is generally dome shaped on B-scan, but a case of a "mushrooming" melanocytoma has been reported.[58] These lesions most often originate from pigmented cells within the optic disc, although they can occur anywhere in the uveal tract. They generally are heavily pigmented, with a jet-black appearance with a feathered edge that extends into the adjacent retina. Their clinical appearance allows an accurate diagnosis in most cases. Their malignant potential is very low, but there have been reports of transformation to a melanoma. They do not replace the choroid with a dense homogenous population of cells as the case

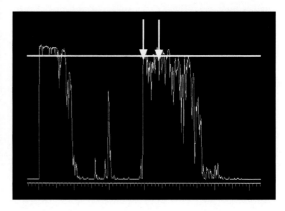

FIG. 280. B-scan of bumpy choroidal melanoma (*arrows*)

FIG. 281. A-scan of choroidal nevus (*arrows*)

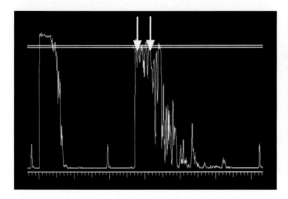

FIG. 282. A-scan of melanocytoma (*arrows*)

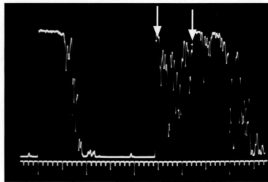

FIG. 283. A-scan of metastatic tumor to the choroid (*arrows*)

with melanomas, but infiltrate the choroidal tissue in a less compact distribution.

An analogous situation on the cellular level occurs as metastatic tumors invade the choroid. These lesions invade the uveal tract in a sporadic pattern with areas of dense tumor cells and "fingers" of partial choroidal infiltration by the malignant cells. A-scan performed on these tumors will be irregular, with low spikes corresponding to the more homogenous areas of malignant infiltration and higher spikes corresponding to the more heterogeneous areas (Fig. 283). The lower reflective and regular areas can be confused with a choroidal melanoma if only that part of the lesion is imaged. The entire tumor must be scanned with particular attention to more irregular portions. The overall echographic picture of metastatic tumors usually includes irregular internal reflectivity with high and low echo spikes on A-scan.

An important differential point is the rarity of echographically detectable spontaneous vascularity in metastatic tumors. These lesions are relatively flat compared to choroidal melanomas, which causes difficulty in visualizing the rapidly moving vertical spikes on A-scan. In addition, these tumors often lack the larger arterioles that are seen in melanomas. The examiner must carefully analyze the ultrasound screen for the rapid flickering movements visible on standardized A-scan and many B-scan units. It is helpful to enlarge the image with the zoom control and to look at the screen at a distance of a few inches. The degree of vascularity can be graded on a scale of 1 to 4+. The higher degrees of spontaneous movement are generally seen in larger melanomas. Their absence in a choroidal tumor over 3 mm in thickness should bring the diagnosis of melanoma into question.

# Case Study 157
## Metastasis to Choroid

HA is a 57-year-old woman with a history of breast cancer 5 years prior to her presentation. The tumor was first detected as a small nodule and was resected via a lumpectomy. She received a short course of chemotherapy and no radiation. She had been followed with annual exams by her oncologist and no evidence of recurrence or systemic spread of the tumor was noted.

She saw her ophthalmologist complaining of some distortion in vision in the right eye for the previous 3 weeks. His examination documented vision 20/30-2 OD and 20/20 OS. A paramacular yellow-orange lesion was noted and she was referred for echography. B-scan revealed a dome-shaped high reflective lesion near the macula. A-scan demonstrated a thickness of 2.17 mm and medium-to-high reflectivity (Fig. 284). Spontaneous vascularity was not observed. The differential diagnosis first included metastatic tumor, but a subretinal disciform lesion could not be ruled out. Fluorescein angiography did not demonstrate choroidal new vessels. Her primary ophthalmologist informed the patient that there was a possibility that she had a metastatic breast lesion in her eye. Echography was repeated in a month and no change in the size or internal structure of the lesion was noted. This fact was more consistent with a neoplasm than subretinal blood.

Since her initial diagnosis of breast cancer, the patient had been actively participating in healthy lifestyle choices, including good nutrition with an emphasis on antioxidants, exercise, and stress reduction. She was involved in the American Cancer Society and ran a support group for cancer survivors. She had a very difficult time accepting the diagnosis of metastatic disease. She sought other opinions nationally and was seen by several prominent ocular oncologists.

She finally underwent a fine needle biopsy of the ocular lesion that substantiated the diagnosis of metastatic breast cancer. A systemic workup had failed to reveal any other lesions so she underwent

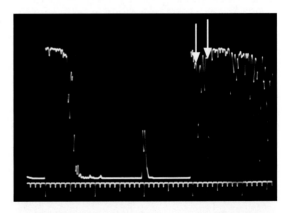

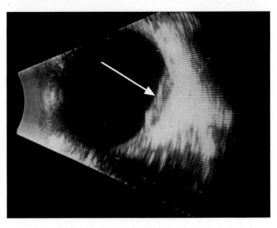

FIG. 284. Top: A-scan of choroidal metastatic tumor (*arrows*). Bottom: B-scan of tumor (*arrow*)

chemotherapy and focal radiation treatment to the choroidal lesion with a partial loss of central vision. There was no evidence of recurrent metastatic lesions to the eye or elsewhere over a 2-year follow-up.

Metastatic lesions to the globe and orbit commonly occur in systemically ill cancer patients with a known primary tumor that has already metastasized elsewhere in the body. They are often undetected in this location because such patients are usually preoccupied with the cancer treatment and its side effects and do not seek ophthalmologic care unless there are significant problems with vision. They frequently die from the cancer before the ocular metastasis is diagnosed. Several studies of autopsy series of patients who succumbed to metastatic cancer of various types found a 4% to 8% incidence of metastatic lesions in the eye and orbit.[59] Most of these had been undiagnosed while the patients were alive. It was concluded that metastatic tumors to the globe and orbit are the most common malignancies that invade these structures. The rich vascular supply of the choroid predisposes it to invasion by metastatic cells. According to Madhavi and Finger,[60] this tissue has a metastatic efficiency index that is the highest for any site in the body that has been investigated.

According to Shields et al., the most common metastatic tumors to the choroid are breast carcinomas in women.[61] These lesions are bilateral in about 33% of cases and tend to be multifocal. They are relatively flat on the average, measuring about 2 mm. The next most common cancers that invade the eye are from the lung and are more often found in men. These tumors not infrequently present in the eye before the primary in the lung is diagnosed. Other less common primary cancers that metastasize to the eye are from the gastrointestinal tract, kidney, thyroid gland, and skin. Shields found no primary site in 51% of the cases in his series.

The diagnostic accuracy of metastatic tumors to the choroid by echography is less than that of malignant melanoma. This is mainly due to the relative lack of thickness when these lesions are first detected because internal structure cannot be adequately analyzed in a lesion in the range of 2 mm or less. Usually only a differential diagnosis can be given by the echographer, with a specificity of about 80%. In fact, some metastatic tumors will behave like melanomas by aggressively invading the choroid with a densely homogenous cell population. Such lesions can be misdiagnosed on A-scan. Examples include metastatic lung carcinomas, testicular carcinomas, and carcinoid tumors.

# Case Study 158
## Metastasis to Choroid

TS is a 56-year-old man with a long history of smoking. His medical history was positive for mild hypertension and borderline cholesterol. He presented to his optometrist with complaints of a shadow in the nasal field of vision in his right eye. His visual acuity measured 20/20 in both eyes and the external segment examination was normal. Fundus examination found a cream colored, dome-shaped lesion near the temporal equator. He was referred for fluorescein angiography, which revealed an area of choroidal hypofluorescence in the area of the lesion with adjacent pinpoint hyperfluorescence.

The patient was referred for echography and a solid lesion measuring 5.6 mm in thickness by 9.83 mm by 7.6 mm in basal dimensions was detected. A-scan revealed medium and regular internal reflectivity without evidence of spontaneous vascularity (Fig. 285). The differential diagnosis first included choroidal melanoma. His primary care physician performed a systemic evaluation and a chest x-ray detected a suspicious nodule in the apex of the left upper lobe of the lung. Bronchoscopy was performed and biopsy of an apical lesion was determined to be poorly differentiated lung carcinoma. He was treated with a lobectomy of the left upper lobe and followed-up by his ophthalmologist several months later. A second choroidal lesion was detected in the right eye supernasally. This strongly supported the diagnosis of metastatic lung carcinoma in spite of the initial echographic findings.

The most common entities in the differential diagnosis of metastatic choroidal tumors are subretinal disciform lesions and choroidal hemangiomas. Fluorescein angiography is essential in the

diagnosis of active subretinal neovascularization (Fig. 286), but is less secure in burned out disciform lesions with gliotic scarring. Echography in such lesions usually demonstrates one or more

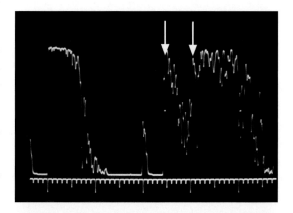

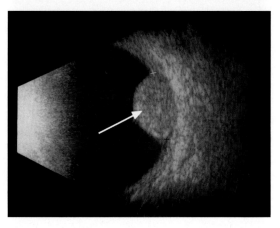

FIG. 285. Top: A-scan of metastatic tumor to the choroid (*arrows*) simulating a choroidal melanoma. Bottom: B-scan of the tumor (*arrow*)

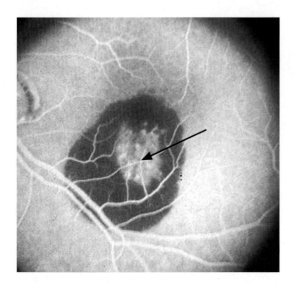

FIG. 286. Fluorescein angiogram of a subretinal disciform lesion (*arrow*)

medium-to-high spikes probably reflected from a scarred Bruch's membrane, and this irregularity of internal structure cannot be distinguished from metastatic tumor. It is important to repeat the ultrasound in a few weeks. Generally, recent subretinal hemorrhage will organize as the blood reabsorbs and the thickness of the lesion will decrease. A malignant process will tend to increase in dimension over time.

# Case Study 159
## Subretinal Hemorrhage

WA is a 72-year-old man who presented with the complaint of a rapid decrease in vision of his left eye. Examination found visual acuity of 20/30–2 OD and 20/80+1 OS. Fundus examination of the right eye showed only mild macular pigmentary changes. The left macula was seen to have a bulging dark lesion with adjacent subretinal

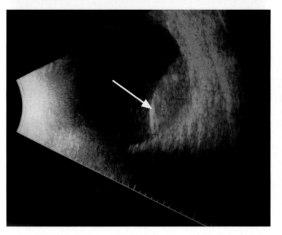

hemorrhage. A neoplasm could not be ruled out. Fluorescein angiography showed mostly hypofluorescence throughout the macular area.

B-scan revealed a dome-shaped lesion with moderate spontaneous internal vascularity. A-scan demonstrated thickness of 4.9 mm and regular internal reflectivity (Fig. 287). The pattern was suspicious for subretinal hemorrhage, but a malignant lesion could not be ruled out. The patient was asked to return for repeat ultrasound in 3 weeks. On the return visit, A-scan measured the thickness at 1.50 mm with a high internal spike (Fig. 288). This was interpreted as a resolving subretinal hemorrhage with formation of a disciform scar.

Disciform lesions are easier to diagnose when they are submacular than when they are more peripheral. Age-related macular degeneration is the most frequent cause of irreversible visual loss in the elderly. Statistically it is much more likely

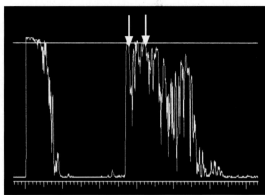

FIG. 287. Top: A-scan of acute subretinal hemorrhage (*arrows*). Bottom: B-scan of the process (*arrow*)

FIG. 288. A-scan of resolving subretinal neovascularization (*arrows*)

that a macular lesion in this age group is due to subretinal neovascularization than to a metastatic lesion or melanoma. However, peripheral disciform lesions are much less common than the submacular process, which makes the distinction less certain in this location. Fluorescein angiography is helpful if active subretinal neovascularization with leakage of vessels is present.

The echographic findings can be equivocal, which necessitates follow-up ultrasound in a few weeks to see if the lesion is increasing or decreasing in size. A subretinal hemorrhage will generally partially resolve with a reduction in thickness. A-scan will often concurrently demonstrate increased irregularity of the internal structure. If such changes do not occur, then a tumor should be suspected.

# Case Study 160
## Subretinal Disciform Scar

SG is a 78-year-old woman who had a history of mild dry macular degeneration bilaterally. Her medical history included a history of breast cancer 8 years prior to presentation that had been in remission after a mastectomy, radiation therapy, and a course of chemotherapy. She was seen for a routine annual examination by her ophthalmologist, who noted a raised grayish lesion in the right temporal fundus near the equator. She had no subjective symptoms due to this process but the clinician referred her for echography to rule out a neoplasm.

A-scan revealed a 3.1-mm lesion near the temporal equator with moderately irregular internal reflectivity, including a high internal spike (Fig. 289). The differential included an eccentric subretinal disciform lesion, metastatic tumor to the choroid, and a choroidal hemangioma.

The patient was reevaluated by her primary care physician with a systemic workup, including a bone scan that did not show evidence of metastatic tumor. She was scheduled for repeat ophthalmic examination and echography 2 months after the initial exam. Clinical evaluation showed no apparent change in the lesion and ultrasound measured the same thickness and demonstrated no change in internal reflectivity. She was scheduled for another follow-up exam 3 months later, and again no change in thickness or reflectivity was noted. The dormancy of this lesion was most consistent with a gliotic subretinal disciform scar and it was planned to follow her on a biannual basis.

The other major differential considerations in the evaluation of possible choroidal metastatic disease include hemangiomas and atypical melanomas. Choroidal hemangiomas have a microscopic structure that is honeycomb-like with multiple blood-filled cystic spaces (Fig. 290). As the sound beam travels through this tissue, it is reflected by the septae between the blood-containing cavities. If the cystic spaces were larger, the reflectivity of the A-scan spikes would become lower as the sound wave was propagated through the homogenous blood. This does occur in orbital cavernous hemangiomas. However, the spaces in hemangiomas of the choroid are small enough relative to the sound beam that there is not enough time for the reflectivity to become very low before it strikes another septum and results in a high reflective spike. Therefore, the A-scan characteristics of a choroidal hemangioma are relatively high spikes with a regular structure (Fig. 291).

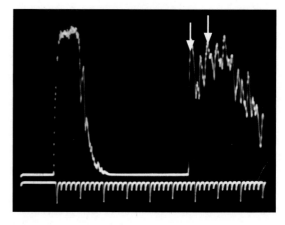

Fig. 289. A-scan of an eccentric disciform lesion (*arrows*)

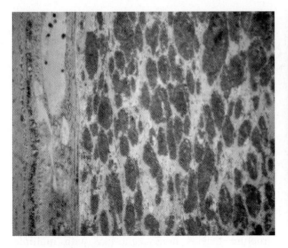

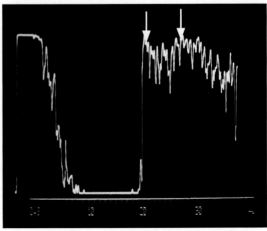

FIG. 290. Microscopic anatomy of a choroidal hemangioma

FIG. 291. A-scan of a choroidal hemangioma (*arrows*)

# Case Study 161
## Choroidal Hemangioma

TA is a 52-year-old man who complained of some visual distortion in his right field of vision for several weeks. He was seen by an ophthalmologist who documented visual acuity of 20/30-2 OD and 20/20 OS. Ophthalmoscopic examination found a yellow-orange elevated lesion just below the macula. Fluorescein angiography was performed and demonstrated mottled leakage of dye within the lesion that increased over several minutes. These findings were consistent with a choroidal hemangioma but an amelanotic melanoma or metastatic tumor could not be eliminated completely.

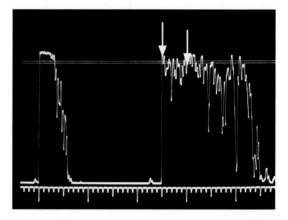

FIG. 293. A-scan of a choroidal hemangioma (*arrows*)

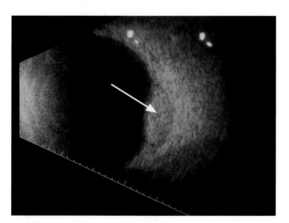

FIG. 292. B-scan of a choroidal hemangioma (*arrow*)

B-scan showed a dome-shaped highly reflective lesion (Fig. 292). A-scan demonstrated high, regular internal reflectivity (Fig. 293) that was very consistent with a choroidal hemangioma. The patient was referred for photodynamic therapy (PDT) by a retina specialist with a good response and resolution of the visual distortion.

Occasionally, a hemangioma will show an atypical pattern of internal reflectivity. This makes the distinction from a metastatic lesion much more difficult.

# Case Study 162
## Metastasis to Choroid

GS is a 61-year-old man with a history of colon cancer who presented with a shadow just below the center in his left eye for a month. He presented to his optometrist who found vision of 20/20-1 OD and 20/25-2 OS. Fundus examination revealed an orange coloration of the paramacular area, but a distinct mass was not appreciated. The patient was referred for fluorescein angiography that demonstrated diffuse leakage from the choriocapillaris.

A-scan demonstrated mostly medium high spikes with some irregularity (Fig. 294). No spontaneous vascularity was noted. The differential diagnosis included metastatic tumor to the choroid and choroidal hemangioma. The patient was referred to his primary care doctor for systemic evaluation. Repeat colonoscopy showed no recurrence of the primary tumor and the metastatic workup was negative. The lesion was followed for several months without evidence of growth. He ultimately opted for treatment with PDT.

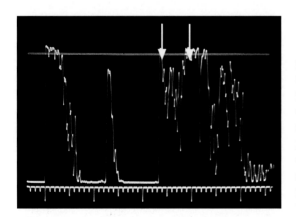

FIG. 294. A-scan of an irregular choroidal hemangioma (*arrows*)

Another orange-pigmented lesion included in the differential diagnosis of metastatic tumor is amelanotic melanoma. Choroidal melanomas are usually darkly pigmented but about 10% have lesser degrees of pigment that can result in their clinical confusion with other lesions. Echography is very valuable in distinguishing these entities from each other. The B-scan appearance is about the same for choroidal hemangioma, metastatic tumor, and amelanotic melanoma, but the internal reflectivity patterns on A-scan are very distinctive. The following table compares these reflectivity patterns:

| Hemangioma | Metastatic tumor | Amelanotic melanoma |
|---|---|---|
| High | Low to high | Low to medium |
| Regular ("sawtooth") | Irregular | Regular |
| No vascularity | No vascularity | Spontaneous vascularity |

Systemic non-Hodgkin's lymphoma can rarely present as an intraocular tumor. It may invade the choroid as a solitary orange mass or as diffuse choroidal thickening. Central nervous system (CNS) lymphoma has a much higher probability of ocular and orbital involvement than the systemic form. It usually causes multiple punctate white dots in the choroid with vitreous cells, but may also invade the optic nerve with fulminate disc and peripapillary edema. An older patient with chronic vitritis should always be evaluated for the possibility of CNS lymphoma with neuroimaging studies.

# Case Study 163
## Optic Nerve Lymphoma

RT was an 82-year-old man who noted blurred vision in both eyes for several weeks. He was seen by an optometrist who documented vision of 20/80 OD and 20/100 OS. Slit-lamp examination was unremarkable except for mild nuclear sclerotic cataracts. Fundus examination showed bilateral optic disc edema (Fig. 295). The patient was referred for neurological workup and an MRI scan was obtained. It showed no abnormalities in the brain, but some enhancement of both optic nerves with gadolinium injection (Fig. 296).

Echography showed thickening of the both optic nerves, with the right measuring 4.73 mm and the left 6.98 mm (Fig. 297). There was a negative 30° test bilaterally that ruled-out increased optic nerve sheath fluid and was suggestive of cellular infiltration of the nerves.

Lumbar puncture was performed and a few large B cells were found on microscopic examination of the spinal fluid. The diagnosis of CNS large cell lymphoma was made and the patient was referred for radiation therapy. His vision improved to 20/30 OD and 20/40 OS with almost total resolution of the optic disc swelling. Repeat echography verified reduction of the optic nerve thickness. He remained in remission for several months but then the lymphoma recurred and he expired shortly afterwards.

It is much less common for systemic non-Hodgkin's lymphoma to involve ocular tissue, but infiltration of the uveal tract is the usual route of invasion when it does invade the eye.

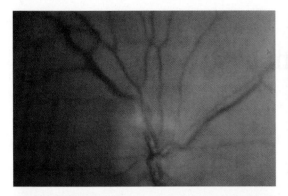

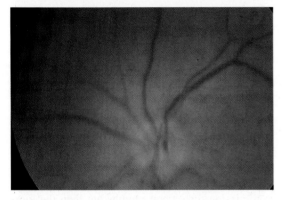

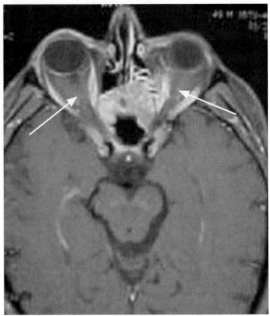

FIG. 296. Magnetic resonance imaging of lymphoma of optic nerves (*arrows*)

FIG. 295. Optic disc edema. Top: Right disc. Bottom: Left disc

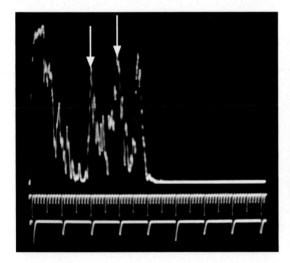

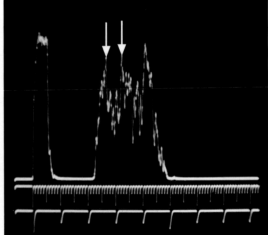

FIG. 297. Left: A-scan of lymphoma of right optic nerve (*arrows*). Right: A-scan of left optic nerve (*arrows*)

# Case Study 164
## Ocular Lymphoma

KE is a 62-year-old man who presented to his ophthalmologist with the complaint of decreased vision in his right eye over several weeks. He had a history of systemic lymphoma that had been treated 18 months previously, resulting in remission. Examination found the visual acuity in his right eye to be 20/100 and his left eye 20/30. The slit-lamp examination was unremarkable but evaluation of the fundus demonstrated a yellow-orange diffuse thickening of the posterior pole.

Echography revealed choroidal thickening (Figs. 298 and 299). He was diagnosed as having posterior scleritis and started on high-dose oral prednisone. His vision improved and the echographic findings

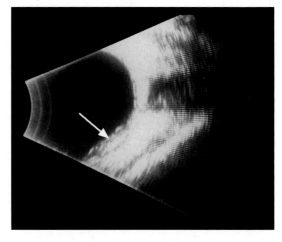

FIG. 299. B-scan of the lesion (*arrow*)

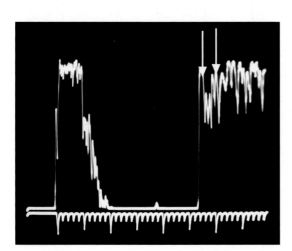

FIG. 298. A-scan of lymphoma of the choroid (*arrows*).

showed resolution of the thickening. However, the symptoms and signs of infiltration of the posterior pole recurred in a few weeks and he was found to have infiltration of the liver and spleen on CT scan. A lumbar puncture was performed and was negative for malignant cells. He died shortly after and autopsy demonstrated non-Hodgkin's lymphoma.

Inflammatory infiltrates, such as in posterior scleritis, can simulate amelanotic neoplastic lesions. The sclera becomes thickened with edema of adjacent tissue, such as the choroid and subtenon's space. This condition is usually quite painful but in cases with lesser degrees of pain, the lesion can be confused with a tumor.

# Case Study 165
## Posterior Scleritis

DF is a 26-year-old man who complained of mild aching behind his left eye and some blurring for several weeks. He presented to an optometrist who documented vision of 20/20 OD and 20/30+2 OS. Slit-lamp examination revealed mild injection of the conjunctiva of the right eye and a clear anterior chamber without flare or cells. Fundus examination revealed a creamy yellow lesion temporal to the macula. Echography demonstrated a dome-shaped lesion on B-scan with low-to-medium irregular reflectivity on A-scan with some high reflective scleral thickening (Figs. 300 and 301). The differential diagnosis included an inflammatory choroidal edema secondary to posterior scleritis. He was treated with topical

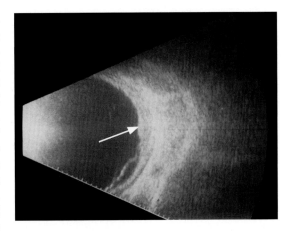

FIG. 301. B-scan of the same area (*arrow*)

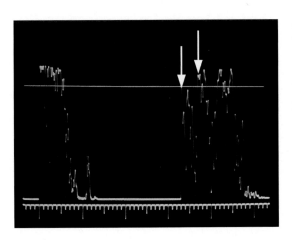

FIG. 300. A-scan of nodular postscleritis (*arrows*)

steroids and systemic nonsteroidal anti-inflammatory medication with resolution of his symptoms and the fundus lesion over 2 weeks.

Another nonpigmented malignant tumor of the fundus is retinoblastoma. The average age of patients with this lesion is under 2 years but they have been reported in adults. Even though it is rare, the differential diagnosis of an amelanotic mass in an adult should include retinoblastoma. Biswas et al.[62] reported on three cases of adults with retinoblastomas and summarized 20 cases from the literature. Two of their cases were noncalcified. Most of the patients reported in the literature had posterior lesions but this tumor can rarely present peripherally.

# Case Study 166
## Retinoblastoma in an Adult

AH is a 35-year-old man who presented to his ophthalmologist with the complaint of floaters and reduced vision in his right eye for several months. Examination documented vision of 20/40 in that eye and 20/20 in the left eye. Slit-lamp examination revealed trace cells in the anterior chamber and an inferior sector cataract. Fundus examination showed 1+ vitreous cells and what appeared to be inflammatory debris near the 6:00 pars plana.

B-scan demonstrated a probable mass in the inferior peripheral fundus (Fig. 302). Internal reflectivity was difficult to characterize because of the very peripheral location of the lesion. Several probable calcium flecks were detected within the lesion on B-scan. The differential diagnosis included melanoma, medulloblastoma, and other solid tumors.

A needle biopsy was performed and malignant cells consistent with retinoblastoma were documented on cytological analysis. The patient elected to have his eye enucleated and a retinoblastoma was confirmed. Although retinoblastoma is rare in adults, it is the most common malignant ocular tumor in children, where it often presents as leukocoria.

The role of echography in the workup of leukocoria is invaluable. The various entities in the differential diagnosis that can be elucidated by echography include retinoblastoma, medulloepithelioma, toxocara, Coats' disease, retinal detachment (including that seen in incontinentia pigmentosa and Norrie's disease), persistent hyperplastic primary vitreous (PHPV), and retinopathy of prematurity (ROP).

The most serious entity in the differential of leukocoria is retinoblastoma, which is a potentially life-threatening tumor for which timely diagnosis and treatment are mandatory. The prognosis for survival has improved dramatically with modern treatment, including radiation and chemotherapy, with a survival rate approaching 95% in developed countries. Unfortunately, these tumors are a significant cause of mortality in developing countries because many patients are not seen for medical care until relatively late in the progress of the disease. The incidence of retinoblastoma is about the same in blacks and Asians as among Caucasians. This is opposed to choroidal melanomas that are much more common among fair-skinned populations in a ratio of 18:1.[63]

Ultrasound has made the challenging evaluation of leukocoria a much easier task than in the past.

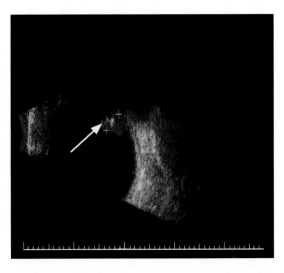

FIG. 302. B-scan of peripheral retinoblastoma in an adult (*arrow*)

371

The ability of echography to detect calcium is the major differential feature that enables the diagnosis of retinoblastoma with a 98% degree of accuracy when calcification is present. It is estimated that about 90% to 95% of these tumors contain calcium that is often scattered in clumps within the tumor.

# Case Study 167
## Retinoblastoma

ML is a 2.5-year-old girl who was included in a family photo sent out as a Christmas card. An ophthalmologist acquaintance received one of the cards and noticed that the child had a bilateral white pupillary reflex caught in the camera flash. He contacted the parents and suggested they seek immediate consultation. The girl was seen the next day by a pediatric ophthalmologist who verified bilateral leukocoria and made a tentative diagnosis of retinoblastoma.

She underwent an examination under anesthesia the next day and echography was performed. Bilateral subretinal masses were detected with the one in the right eye almost filling the globe (Figs. 303

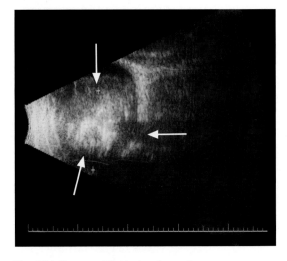

FIG. 304. B-scan of the lesion (*arrow*)

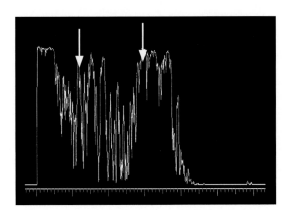

FIG. 303. A-scan of retinoblastoma (*arrows*)

and 304) and the left measuring just over 8 mm. High reflectivity on A- and B-scan consistent with calcium deposits was documented in both lesions. The right eye (with the larger tumor) was enucleated and the left was treated by radiation. This was standard treatment for retinoblastoma at the time, but current therapy usually includes chemotherapy with an attempt to reduce the tumor mass.

The presence of calcium in an intraocular mass in a child is almost pathognomonic of retinoblastoma; however, about 5% to 10% of these malignant tumors do not contain calcium.

# Case Study 168
## Retinoblastoma with Fine Calcification

TC is a 4-year-old girl who was noted by her parents to "not focus on things" with her right eye. She was examined by her pediatrician, who could not see a red reflex in that eye and referred her to a pediatric ophthalmologist, who noted a paramacular mass. B-scan demonstrated a subretinal mass with an irregular surface. A-scan revealed medium and regular internal reflectivity (Fig. 305). Calcium was not detected by either modality. The lesion was assumed to be a noncalcified retinoblastoma and treatment with chemotherapy was begun. She was followed with monthly examination under anesthesia and a small calcified lesion was noted in the left eye 6 months later. This was highly consistent with retinoblastoma. Another course of chemotherapy was instituted and the lesion was noted to regress.

Fine calcium deposits within a retinoblastoma are not detectable by MRI scan, and may even be missed on CT scan. Echography can often detect them in such cases.

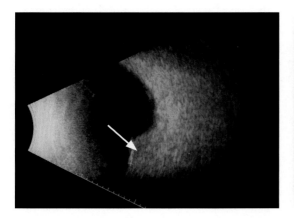 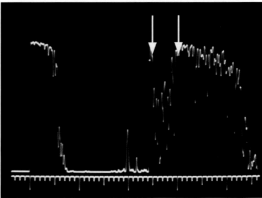

FIG. 305. Left: B-scan of retinoblastoma without calcium (*arrow*). Right: A-scan of lesion (*arrows*)

# Case Study 169
## Retinoblastoma

DH is a 3-year-old child who was brought in to see the ophthalmologist because her parents noted drifting of her left eye. Clinical examination by an ophthalmologist found vision in her right eye of 20/30 on the picture chart and 20/100 in her left eye. The anterior segment examination of both eyes was normal, but fundus exam of the left eye was difficult because of diffuse vitreous opacities. There was the impression of a possible mass lesion in the posterior and temporal aspect of the globe.

Computed tomography scan revealed a probable subretinal mass without evidence of calcification (Fig. 306). The child was referred for

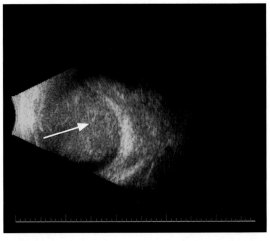

FIG. 307. B-scan of retinoblastoma with faint calcification (*arrow*)

echography and B-scan documented a temporal lesion with a few scattered calcific flecks (Fig. 307). The diagnosis of retinoblastoma was made on this basis and treatment with chemotherapy was initiated.

A variant of retinoblastoma is the diffuse infiltrating type. This lesion occurs in older children (average age, 6 years old) and is more common in males. There is no family history of tumor, as opposed to typical solid retinoblastoma in which 5% to 8% of patients have a relative with the neoplasm. The majority of these tumors do not contain calcium. Bhatnagar and Vine[64] reported that only 4 out of 28 cases were calcified. These children commonly present with symptoms and signs of inflammation compared to typical patients, who are first detected on the basis of a white pupil.

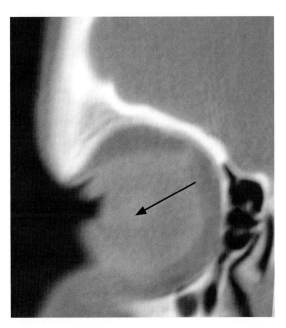

FIG. 306. Computed tomography of retinoblastoma failing to show calcium (*arrow*)

# Case Study 170
## Infiltrating Retinoblastoma

TB is a 7-year-old boy who was brought to an ophthalmologist because the parents noted a red left eye in their child, who complained that it "hurt a lot of the time." He was taken to an ophthalmologist and examination documented visual acuity in the right eye of 20/25 and the left eye of 20/200. Slit-lamp examination revealed 1+ cells and flare in the left anterior chamber, and fundus examination found 3+ vitreous cells and a hazy view of the fundus with a vague impression of retinal elevation temporal to the macula. The differential diagnosis included Coat's disease.

Echography was performed and B-scan demonstrated moderate vitreous cells with a subretinal mass temporally. No calcium was detected in the lesion. A-scan showed medium internal reflectivity (Fig. 308). The differential diagnosis included a noncalcified retinoblastoma and was reported to the referring ophthalmologist with the statement, "a subretinal mass in a child is a retinoblastoma until proven otherwise." An anterior chamber tap was performed and cytology was consistent with retinoblastoma. The child was treated with chemotherapy with regression of the tumor.

The second most common tumor in children that may present as leukocoria is medulloepithelioma or dyktioma. This lesion is most often found in the anterior segment, where it arises within the ciliary body, but it can rarely occur in the optic nerve because it originates from the primitive medullary epithelium (inner layer of the optic cup).

It has malignant potential and can recur locally after resection with invasion of adjacent tissues.

Echographic findings include heterogeneous reflectivity that correlates to the variable pathological structure of medulloepithelioma (Fig. 309). Broughton and Zimmerman[65] divide these tumors into nonteratoid dyktioma, which is a dense proliferation of cells and is low-to-medium reflective on A-scan. The teratoid type can have a number of tissue elements including skeletal muscle, cartilage, and brain, with resultant heterogeneous A-scan reflectivity. Clinically, these foci of cartilage in a teratoid medulloepithelioma appear as chalky opacities within the tumor. Shields describes the presence of neuorepithelial-lined cysts filled with a hyaluronic acid matrix seen clinically in 60% of his cases. Such cysts would create additional interfaces for sound reflection augmenting the heterogeneity of the A-scan spikes.

The mean age of presentation is 4, but there are reported cases in adulthood. Shields et al.[66] describe two characteristic clinical findings associated with medulloepithelioma. One of these is a notch in the lens, called a lens coloboma, that may be the earliest sign of this tumor if not associated with a uveal coloboma. The second sign is the formation of a cyclitic membrane. The authors recommend that an unexplained cyclitic membrane in a child should be cause to eliminate a medulloepithelioma. This lesion can present in a child with leukocoria, reduction of vision due to cataract formation, or pain and redness suggesting intraocular inflammation.

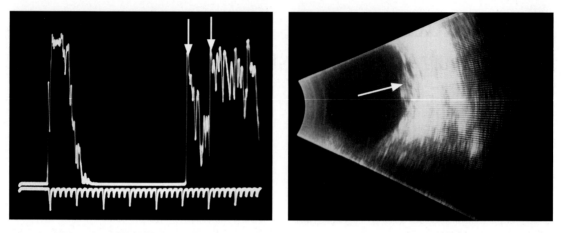

FIG. 308. Left: A-scan of a mildly elevated mass in a child (*arrows*). Right: B-scan of the lesion (*arrow*)

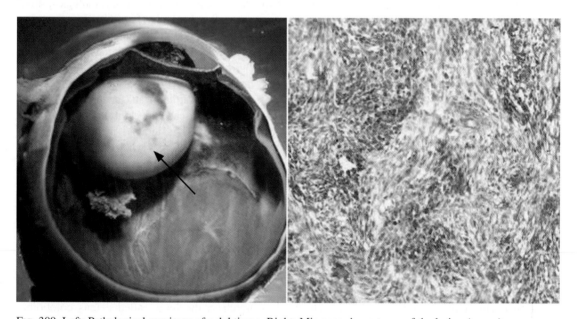

FIG. 309. Left: Pathological specimen of a dyktioma. Right: Microscopic anatomy of the lesion (*arrow*)

# Case Study 171
## Medulloepithelioma

AH is a 13-year-old girl who complained of reduction of vision in her right eye. She was seen by an ophthalmologist, who documented vision of 20/50-2 OD and 20/20 OS. Slit-lamp examination found a sectorial cataract and mild vitreous reaction. Careful examination of the fundus periphery suggested inflammatory debris near the ciliary body adjacent to the lens opacity. She was diagnosed with pars planitis and treated with subtenon's triamcinalone injections on two occasions. The peripheral lesion increased in size, so she was referred for echography.

Ultrasound demonstrated a peripheral lesion by directing the probe in an extreme longitudinal direction toward the 1:00 position. It was too peripheral to allow differentiation, but there was the impression of high internal reflectivity. Immersion scan was performed with a 10-MHz probe and a distinct mass lesion was imaged (Fig. 310). The irregular internal reflectivity in an anterior tumor was consistent with medulloepithelioma and the eye was enucleated with pathological confirmation of the diagnosis.

The other leukocoria-related disease entities in which the diagnosis can be facilitated by echography include Coat's disease. This is usually a unilateral condition found in males two thirds of the time in the 8-month to 18-year-old age group. It is the result of excessive permeability of retinal capillaries causing subretinal lipid exudation. Echography often demonstrates a convectionlike movement of cholesterol deposits under the retina. The various pathological entities resulting in leukocoria can be subtel and be missed on gross examination by the non-ophthalmologist. Mothers often have an innate sense of when something is wrong with their

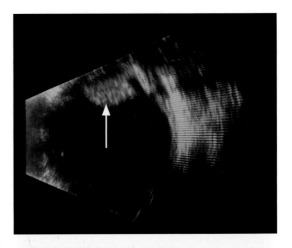

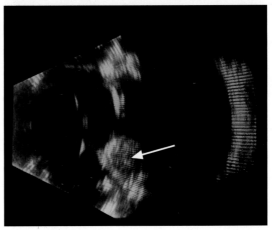

FIG. 310. Top: Peripheral B-scan view of a dyktoma (*arrow*). Bottom: Immersion B-scan of the lesion (*arrow*)

child's eye and the pediatrician is will advised to take her concerns very seriously.

381

# Case Study 172
## Coat's Disease

CG is a 10-year-old boy who was noted by his mother to have a "glassy-eyed" appearance in his left eye in certain lighting conditions. He had not complained about problems with this eye, but was unable to see the television when his mother covered the normal eye. He was seen by his ophthalmologist, who documented vision 20/20 OD and 20/400 OS. The slit-lamp examination was normal, but the fundus examination on the left showed an elevated yellowish subretinal "mass" temporally and into the macula.

Echography revealed subretinal exudation with the slow spontaneous convective flow consistent with cholesterol (Fig. 311). No mass lesion was noted and the opposite eye was normal without evidence of retinal elevation.

Leukocoria is a frequent presenting sign of persistent hyperplastic primary vitreous or PHPV. This condition is due to persistence of the fetal hyaloid artery and the presence of retrolental material with a vitreous stalk attaching to the posterior pole. It usually occurs unilaterality in a microophthalmic eye.

Echography is useful in demonstrating the retrolental material, the vitreous stalk, and the microophthalmia.

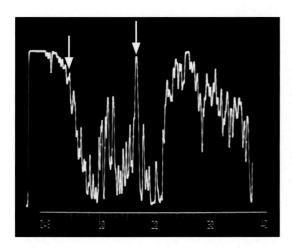 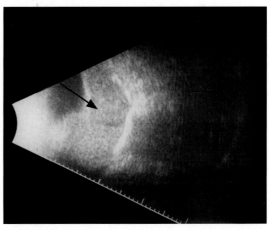

FIG. 311. Left: A-scan probe directly over lesion of Coat's disease with cholesterol (*arrows*). Right: Transocular B-scan of the subretinal space (*arrow*)

# Case Study 173
## Persistent Hyperplastic Primary Vitreous

RS is a 3-month-old baby boy who was noted by his mother to have a white pupil in the left eye while she was nursing him. The family comprehensive ophthalmologist thought he had a congenital cataract and scheduled him for cataract surgery. The child's mother sought a second opinion from a pediatric ophthalmologist who referred him for an ultrasound evaluation.

Echography revealed dense retrolental material with a high reflective stalk attaching near the macula (Fig. 312). The axial length of the right eye measured 22 mm and the left eye measured 19.5 mm. The diagnosis of persistent hyperplastic primary vitreous (PHPV) was made and a vitreoretinal specialist was consulted, anticipating the need for vitrectomy in conjunction with lensectomy. The parents were informed that the prognosis for useful vision was guarded.

The spectrum of PHPV extends from mild retrolental tissue with a thin stalk extending towards the optic nerve to severe posterior segment pathology.

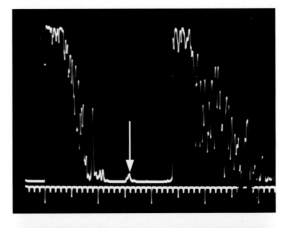

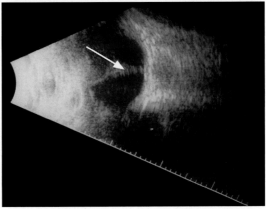

Fig. 312. Top: A-scan of persistent hyperplastic primary vitreous with stalk (*arrow*). Bottom: B-scan of the stalk (*arrow*)

# Case Study 174
## Optic Nerve Coloboma

RH is a 6-month-old baby who was noted by his mother to have a white pupillary reflex in the left eye. He was referred to a pediatric ophthalmologist, who suspected PHPV and suggested surgical removal of the lens with the parents. The child was then referred for ultrasound to eliminate significant vitreous pathology that would require the assistance of a vitreoretinal surgeon.

B-scan showed possible retrolental opacity but also demonstrated a colobolatous appearance to the optic disc (Fig. 313). The diagnosis of a probable "morning glory" optic nerve coloboma was made and the parents were informed that anterior surgery would probably not result in useful vision because of the optic nerve pathology. They elected to cancel the surgery.

Leukocoria in the setting of a premature infant who received supplemental oxygen therapy is most often due to retinopathy of prematurity. This

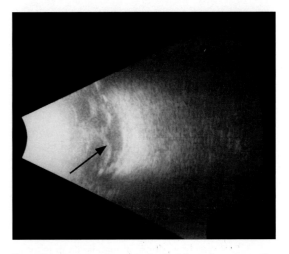

FIG. 314. B-scan of anterior retinal loop in retinopathy of prematurity (*arrow*)

condition is generally bilateral and usually occurs in an infant less than 1500 g in birth weight and less than 32 weeks of gestational age. Advanced forms of this condition can result in retinal detachment due to fibrovascular traction. Echography may demonstrate anterior peripheral loops of the detached retina, which can present as a white pupil (Fig. 314).

Another cause of leukocoria is toxocara. This is transmitted to humans by contact with fecal material from puppies and is the result of the interruption of the normal life cycle of the larvae form of the parasite *Toxocara canis*. It is usually unilateral and occurs in the 6- to 8-year-old age group. A positive ELISA test is diagnostic in the clinical setting of a child with intraocular inflammation with a history of contact with puppies.

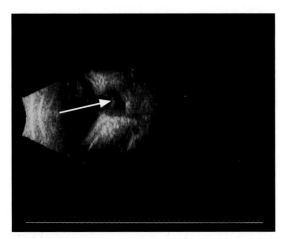

FIG. 313. B-scan of optic nerve coloboma (*arrow*)

Wan and colleagues[67] described the echographic findings of a peripheral calcified granuloma with a vitreous membrane extending from the lesion towards the posterior pole (Fig. 315).

The sensitivity of echography in detecting calcification is applicable to other fundus lesions. Choroidal osteoma or osseous choriostoma is a choroidal tumor with dense bone formation. A series of cases were originally published by Don Gass et al. in 1978.[68] A case study appeared with

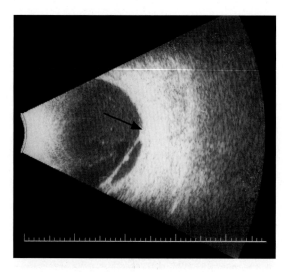

FIG. 315. B-scan of a peripheral granuloma in toxocara (*arrow*)

a pathological description in 1981 by Williams and colleagues.[69] They report a patient who was examined with a choroidal tumor that was suspicious for a malignant melanoma. A P32 (radioactive phosphorous) test was performed with uptake of the radioactive nucleotide consistent with melanoma. The eye was enucleated and microscopy demonstrated a heavily ossified tumor consistent with a choroidal osteoma.

A number of case reports describing this entity have since been published. It generally is found in women in the 20 to 40 age group and is unilateral in about 75% of cases. It may result in reduction of visual acuity if the macula is involved. It has no malignant potential but can be associated with subretinal neovascularization that can be a cause of visual loss and is amenable to laser treatment.

Plain film radiograpy and CT scan can detect the bone in this tumor. Echography is a highly accurate, readily accessible, and cost-effective method to evaluate this lesion. The extremely high reflectivity is most evident when the gain is reduced to display the lesion in comparison to the adjacent normal choroid. It appears in a flat plaquelike configuration, as opposed to the lumpier, irregular appearance of optic disc drusen. Choroidal osteomas tend to markedly shadow the sclera and orbital tissue posterior to the lesion. Dystrophic calcification is not as thick and is located superotemporally versus the more central location of choroidal osteoma.

# Case Study 175
## Choroidal Osteoma

TD is a 28-year-old woman who presented to her ophthalmologist with the complaint of distortion of the vision in her left eye over several months. Examination found visual acuity in the right eye of 20/20 and in the left of 20/50. Fundus examination demonstrated a reddish-orange lesion just above the macula with sharply defined borders. Fluorescein angiography revealed diffuse leakage from the tumor and an area of subretinal neovascularization at the temporal border.

Echography was performed and a very high reflective lesion was demonstrated on both B- and A-scan (Fig. 316). The thickness was difficult to determine because of the high spike on A-scan that shadowed out the sclera and made exact measurements impossible. Basal dimensions were 5.2 mm by 6.1 mm on B-scan. These findings in conjunction with the clinical appearance were highly consistent with a choroidal osteoma. The patient was referred to a retinal specialist for the application of photocoagulation to the neovascularization.

Choroidal melanomas rarely contain calcium. This usually appears on B-scan as one or two focal calcium deposits (Fig. 317). It is easily missed on A-scan because of its localization to a small area of the tumor. The majority of the lesion will meet the A-scan criteria of low-to-medium and regular internal reflectivity.

A relatively common cause of calcium deposits in the eye is calcified drusen of the optic disc that are easily detectable by ultrasound. They are reported to occur in 0.34% to 3.7% of the general population. They are bilateral in up to 75% of cases and there is a family history in approximately 3% to 4%.[70] Large drusen can compress optic nerve fibers with resultant visual field defects. They

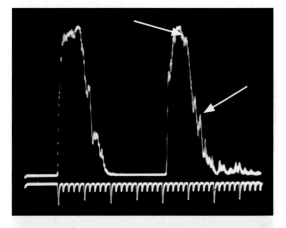
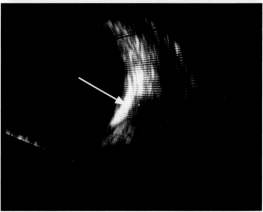

FIG. 316. Top: A-scan of a choroidal osteoma (*first arrow*) and orbital shadowing (*second arrow*). Bottom: B-scan of the lesion (*arrow*)

are often mistaken for papilledema when buried beneath the surface of the nerve. It is important to recognize these lesions as the cause of apparent

389

optic disc swelling to avoid an extensive and costly neurological workup.

B-scan is more sensitive than A-scan in their detection. The probe is placed temporally on the globe with the white dot superiorly (transverse view) and angled anteriorly or posteriorly until the optic nerve shadow is displayed. The tip of the optic nerve is imaged and the gain is decreased. Any bright reflections are carefully analyzed (Fig. 318). To insure that this reflection is not an artifact, the nerve is reexamined in either a horizontal view, with the probe perpendicular to the temporal limbus and the white dot nasally, or in a longitudinal view, with the probe on the superotemporal globe and the white dot directed downward toward the optic nerve (Fig. 319). The high reflectivity should also be visible in this view and its absence is evidence against the presence of drusen.

A common scenario in many communities is the presentation of a teenage girl to her primary care doctor with the complaint of increasing headaches. She is referred to an eye doctor who notes blurred

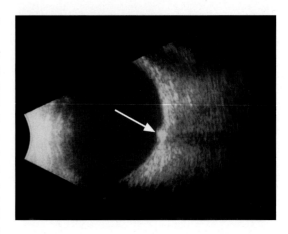

FIG. 318. Transverse B-scan of optic nerve drusen (*arrow*)

optic nerve heads and orders an MRI scan, not uncommonly followed by a neurological consultation and a spinal tap. A timely demonstration of calcified drusen by echography would obviate an otherwise expensive and uncomfortable workup.

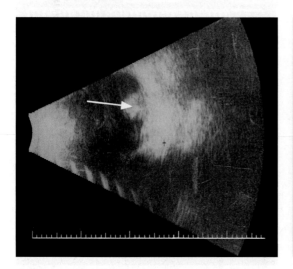

FIG. 317. B-scan of calcium deposits within choroidal melanoma (*arrow*)

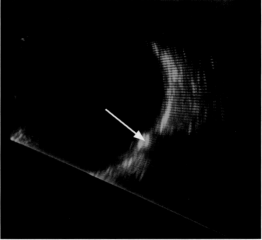

FIG. 319. Longitudinal B-scan of optic nerve drusen (*arrow*)

# Case Study 176
## Optic Nerve Drusen

BC is a 13-year-old girl who saw an optometrist with the complaint of headaches and difficulty in seeing the board in school. She was found to be slightly myopic, but he noted swelling of the optic nerves on examination and referred her for an MRI scan and scheduled a neurology consultation. The MRI scan was reported to be normal, as was the neurological examination. The neurologist made a presumptive diagnosis of pseudotumor cerebri and performed a spinal tap, which showed a slightly elevated opening pressure. She was begun on oral diamox but discontinued it after a week due to the side effects. Another carbonic anhydrase inhibitor was tried with the same result. She was then given Lasix without improvement of her headaches and no change in the optic nerve elevation. She was finally seen by a neuro-ophthalmologist who requested an ultrasound.

Echography revealed small calcified drusen in the right optic disc and medium drusen in the left (Fig. 320). The optic nerve diameters in both orbits were normal with OD measuring 2.6 mm and OS 2.7 mm without evidence of increased optic nerve sheath fluid. The Lasix was stopped and she was told to follow up in a year.

Other calcified lesions include dystrophic calcification of the choroid. This is generally an idiopathic and harmless deposition of calcium usually found in the temporal fundus near the equator. The other eye should be carefully examined with the B-scan in the corresponding area of the fundus as this process is often bilateral (Fig. 321). Rarely such calcium deposition is the result of parathyroid dysfunction, chronic renal failure, or vitamin D intoxication with so-called malignant calcification

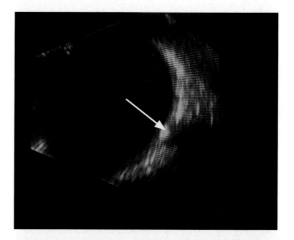

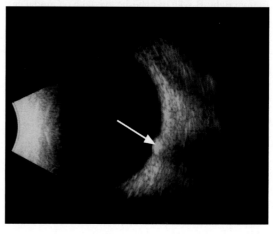

FIG. 320. Top: B-scans of right optic disc drusen (*arrow*). Bottom: B-scan of left optic disc drusen

with widespread deposition of calcium in ocular and distant body tissues.

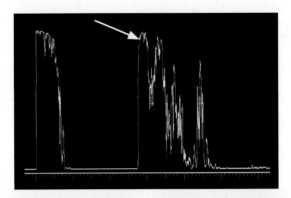

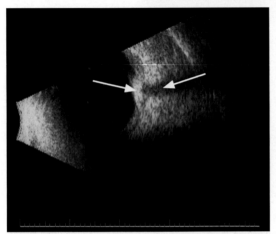 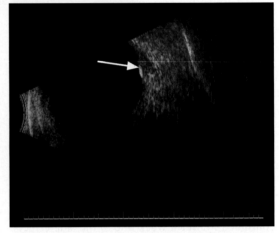

FIG. 321. Top: A-scan of choroidal calcification (*arrow*). Bottom left: B-scan of eye with focal calcification (*arrow*). Bottom right: B-scan of opposite eye with choroidal calcification (*first arrow*). Orbital shadowing (*second arrow*)

# Case Study 177
## Idiopathic Choroidal Calcification

MT is a 72-year-old man who saw his optometrist for a routine eye examination. His best corrected visual acuity was 20/25 in both eyes with mild cataract formation. Fundus examination found a partially pigmented lesion in the right fundus superior temporal to the macula. The patient was told he may have a malignant tumor and he was referred for echography.

B-scan revealed a highly reflective lesion of the choroid in the right superior temporal fundus that measured just over 5 mm in basal dimensions. The left eye was carefully scanned and a small high reflective area was found in the superior temporal quadrant (Fig. 322). A-scan showed a high foreign body-type signal. The diagnosis of idiopathic choroidal calcification was made. It was suggested to the referring optometrist that serum calcium be obtained to rule out the remote possibility of a systemic calcium disorder. This was later reported to be normal.

Choroidal and retinal calcification can be a non-specific finding in prephthisical or phthisical eyes from any cause, including trauma, chronic iritis, or neovascular glaucoma. This process usually occurs in an extensive platelike calcification of most of the choroid or unevenly in one or more areas of the fundus (Fig. 323). Tumors of the anterior regment are generally, uncalcified with the rare exception of retinoblastoma. The most common neoplasms in this part of the globe are melanomas of the conjunctiva, iris, and ciliary body. Conjunctival melanomas tend to be invasive and can penetrate the globe, which makes surgical excision impossible with rare exceptions.

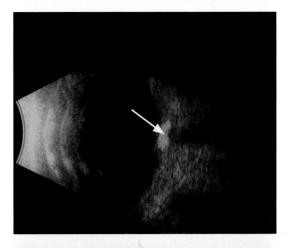

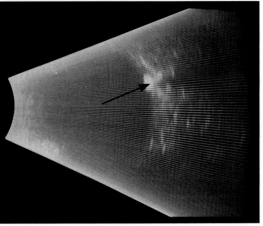

Fig. 322. Top: B-scan of right eye dystrophic calcification (*arrow*). Bottom: B-scan of left eye with dystrophic calcification

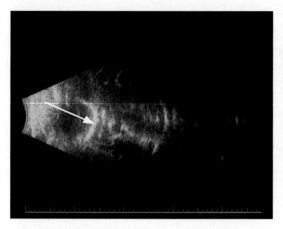 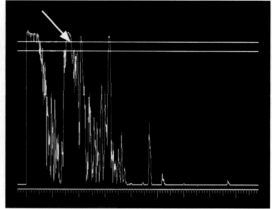

FIG. 323. Left: B-scan of choroidal calcification in a phthisical eye (*arrow*). Right: A-scan of calcium (*arrow*)

# Case Study 178
## Conjunctival Melanoma

WN is a 53-year-old woman who noticed a pigmented area on her right eye. She neglected it for several months because of other health problems but finally consulted an ophthalmologist. On examination she was found to have a darkly pigmented conjunctival lesion next to the temporal limbus. He diagnosed conjunctival melanoma and recommended enucleation pending evidence of intraocular extension.

Echography was performed with 20- and 50-MHz immersion scanning. There was an obvious demarcation line over halfway into the sclera where the lesion invaded, but there was not evidence of intraocular invasion (Fig. 324). Microscopic invasion of the sclera could not be eliminated. The options were discussed with the patient and she elected to undergo a lamellar resection with cryotherapy to the bed of the lesion. Pathology found an epitheloid conjunctival melanoma with clear scleral margins She has been free of recurrence of tumor for more than 2 years.

Conjunctival nevi are relatively common and rarely convert to malignant melanoma. Shields et al.[71] found the average age of initial manifestation of the lesion of 32 years, but the lesions can appear in early childhood and sometimes in the elderly. They are more common in Caucasians with brown irises and are often found on the bulbar conjunctiva (72%), caruncle (15%), and plica semilunaris (11%). They most frequently occur in the horizontal meridian (temporally in 46% and nasally in 44%). Biomicroscopic examination with the slit lamp reveals cystic changes in 65%. Immersion high-frequency echography can be quite helpful in detecting these cystic changes (Fig. 325).

An iris nevus is a solid lesion of the iris that can have a fusiform or focal nodular shape as imaged by immersion (Fig. 326). Occasionally, disruption of the iris pigment epithelium or pigment deposition can be seen. These lesions can safely be followed over time with slit-lamp photographs and high-frequency immersion ultrasound. If growth is observed then an iris melanoma must be suspected. Clinically suspicious findings include iris distortion, ectropion uveae, and sector cataract. If these changes are observed in an actively growing lesion, then treatment options, such as sector iridectomy, should be offered to the patient. The ciliary body must be carefully imaged with ultrasound biomicroscopy (UBM) to eliminate macroscopic invasion that would necessitate iridocyclectomy. The overall mortality rate for melanoma of the iris is 4% to 8%, according to Harbour et al.[72]

Diffuse and ring melanomas are rarer presentations of iris melanomas and have a higher metastatic potential.

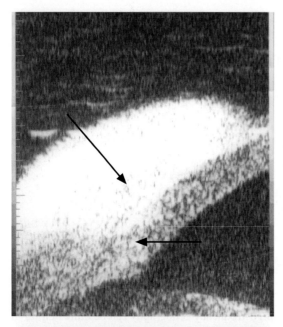

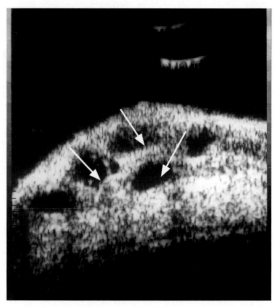

FIG. 325. Ultrasound biomicroscopy of cystic changes in conjunctival nevus (*arrows*)

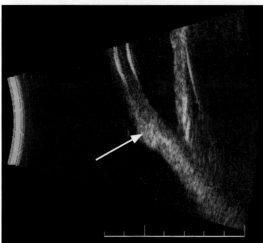

FIG. 324. Top: Ultrasound biomicroscopy of conjunctival melanoma (*large arrow*) with scleral invasion (*small arrow*). Bottom: Immersion scan of lesion with 20-MHz probe (*arrow*)

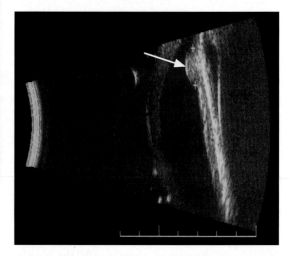

FIG. 326. Immersion scan (20-MHz) of iris nevus (*arrow*)

# Case Study 179
## Ring Melanoma

AT is a 26-year-old man who was noted to have a pigmented lesion of his right iris on examination 2 years previously. UBM had been performed on his initial visit and was consistent with an iris nevus of the temporal iris (Fig. 327). He was instructed to return for follow-up in 6 months but came back 2 years later when he noted increased iris pigmentation. At this time slit-lamp examination demonstrated pigmentary deposition in the angle from the 4:00 meridian around to 12:30. Some pigmented cells were noted in the anterior chamber. His intraocular pressure in that eye was 26 mm versus 17 mm in his left eye.

Immersion scanning with a 20-MHz probe demonstrated thickening of the iris root in the area of the pigmentary changes (Fig. 328). This finding was consistent with a ring melanoma and the patient was referred to an oculoplastic surgeon for enucleation after a systemic workup for metastases was performed.

The prognosis for ciliary body melanomas is worse than in any other part of the uveal tract. This is due to the undetected growth of these tumors in this symptomatically silent area and their proximity to emissary canals, which can allow extraocular egress of malignant cells. These tumors are suspected clinically if iris bulging, sector cataracts, lens displacement, or sentinel vessels (engorged episcleral vessels) are noted.

A- or B-scan echography can usually image at least the posterior part of these lesions if the probe is placed on the sclera against the orbital rim and rotated anteriorly towards the ciliary body. Internal reflectivity by A-scan may be more medium reflective and somewhat more irregular than posterior choroidal melanomas. This is due to the normal "bumpy" surface of the ciliary body. These lesions can sometimes be found to have cystic spaces internally that correspond to empty cavities or fluid-containing spaces. UBM is quite useful in displaying the entire tumor with its most anterior extension.

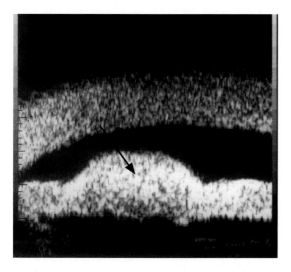

FIG. 327. Ultrasound biomicroscopy (50 MHz) of iris nevus (*arrow*)

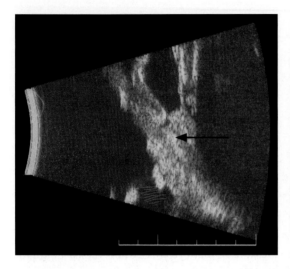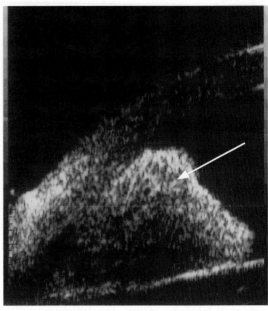

FIG. 328. Left: Immersion scan of diffuse melanoma (*arrow*). Right: Ultrasound biomicroscopy (50 MHz) of diffuse spread of lesion (*arrow*)

# Case Study 180
## Ciliary Body Melanoma

EH is a 61-year-old man followed annually at the Veteran's Administration Hospital for a mild cataract. Different ophthalmology residents on each examination usually saw him as they rotated through the eye clinic. He came in for his annual exam and the resident noted an injected episcleral vessel on the inferotemporal right globe. The visual acuity was 20/40 in this eye, compatible with a moderate degree of nuclear sclerosis and peripheral cortical opacity. Fundus examination was unremarkable but the periphery could not be well visualized because of the peripheral cataract. The patient was referred to the university hospital for echography.

Ultrasound revealed a solid lesion in the area of the inferior ciliary body. The tumor could not be imaged in its entirety because of the peripheral location and the difficulty in angling the probe in the direction of the inferior periphery because of the interference by the superior orbital rim. It was also partly visualized by placing the probe directly at the 6:00 limbus and examining the globe just under the probe, although part of it was hidden in the initial spike (Fig. 329). The reflectivity on A-scan was medium and regular with moderate spontaneous internal vascularity.

Immersion scanning was performed with a 10-MHz probe and a solid lesion of the inferior ciliary body measuring 5.5 mm in height by 16 mm in basal diameter was visualized (Fig. 330). The diagnosis of a ciliary body melanoma was made and the patient elected to undergo radioactive plaque therapy after a systemic workup showed no evidence of metastatic tumor.

The differential diagnosis of anterior segment tumors includes such entities as ciliary body cysts,

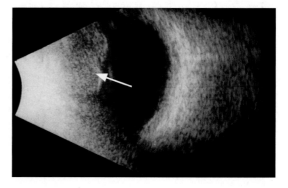

FIG. 329. Contact B-scan of ciliary body melanoma directly under probe (*arrow*)

medulloepitheliomas, leiomyomas, and adenomas of the nonpigmented ciliary epithelium.

Cystic lesions are the most common of these entities and are readily detected on immersion imaging

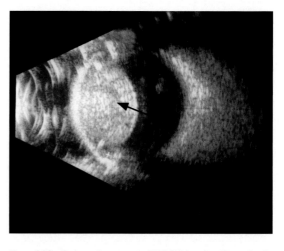

FIG. 330. Immersion scan (10 MHz) of ciliary body melanoma (*arrow*)

by high-frequency ultrasound. Primary cysts are of neuroepithelial origin and are usually located at the iridociliary junction. They are often detected on routine slit-lamp examination as a focal bulge in the iris. Single cysts are most common, but multiple cysts (Fig. 331) are found in over 1/3 of the cases according to Marigo et al.[73] Immersion ultrasound scanning with a standard 10-MHz B-scan probe can detect cysts over 1 mm in diameter. The resolution is much better with higher frequency probes (20, 35, and 50 MHz), with the ability to detect very small cysts in the 30-μm range.

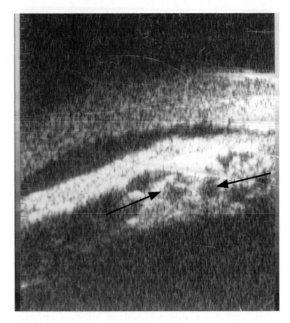

FIG. 331. Ultrasound biomicroscopy of multiple iris/ciliary body cysts (*arrows*)

# Case Study 181
## Iris Cysts

RP is a 22-year-old woman who was seen by her optometrist for a routine eye examination. She was noted on slit-lamp inspection to have a bulge in the left temporal iris. Her pupil was dilated and no retroiridial or ciliary mass could be detected. Transillumination was performed and no pigmented lesion was seen.

Immersion echography was performed with both a 20- and 50-MHz probe. One larger and several smaller iris cysts were seen (Fig. 332). The patient was reassured that this was a benign lesion without any evidence of malignancy.

Large pigment epithelial cysts may displace the iris anteriorly resulting in angle closure glaucoma. They mechanically push the iris forward and narrow the angle. Marigo et al. state that when multiple cysts involve more than 180° of the iris, then angle closure with elevated intraocular pressure may develop.[73] This occurs in about 10% of patients with these cysts.

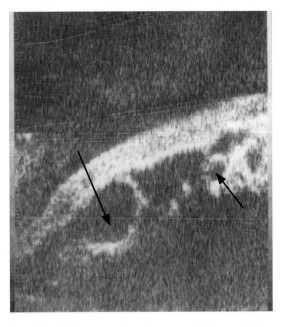

FIG. 332. Ultrasound biomicroscopy of large ciliary body cyst (*large arrow*) and several smaller cysts (*small arrow*)

# Case Study 182
## Iris Cyst with Angle Closure

TA is a 43-year-old man who presented to his ophthalmologist with complaints of intermittent pain and blurred vision in his right eye. The visual acuity was 20/20 in both eyes and intraocular pressure was measured to be 21 mm in the right eye and 16 mm in the left. Slit-lamp examination showed narrowing of the temporal angle of the right eye and gonioscopy confirmed a closed angle temporally but a 2+ open angle superiorly, nasally, and inferiorly. The opposite eye had a 2 to 3+ open angle for 360°.

Immersion ultrasound using a 50-MHz probe demonstrated large ciliary and retroiridial cysts that bowed the iris anteriorly and closed the temporal angle (Fig. 333). Because of the chronic nature of the problem in this patient, it was elected to treat him with topical medication to lower the pressure and defer surgical intervention pending uncontrollable pressure from further angle closure.

Focal angle closure can also be a result of epithelial "pearl" formation and retained cortex in the capsular bag. This can create a mass effect with mechanical pressure on the iris that bows it forward and narrows the angle.

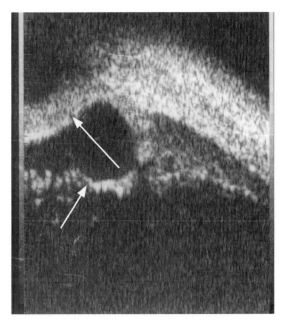

FIG. 333. Ultrasound biomicroscopy of ciliary body cyst (*bottom arrow*) with iris bowing (*top arrow*)

# Case Study 183
## Epithelial Cyst of Posterior Capsule

JE is a 43-year-old man who was born with congenital cataracts. He underwent bilateral lens needling procedures as a teenager. He had vision in the 20/80 range in both eyes until a few months before presentation to an ophthalmologist with complaints of a reduction of vision in his right eye. Examination showed vision of 20/100 in that eye and 20/80 in the left eye. The pupils were under 3 mm, updrawn, and minimally reactive to direct light. Slit-lamp examination showed a bulge in the temporal iris with the appearance of a pigmented mass on transillumination. The posterior pole could be visualized on fundus examination but the peripheral retina and ciliary body could not be seen.

Echography demonstrated the posterior lens capsule with the appearance of a solid lesion arising from it and bowing the iris forward by direct pressure (Fig. 334). This image was consistent with lens epithelium and cortex organized into a retroiridial mass with focal angle closure, but a neoplastic process, such as melanoma, could not be totally eliminated. The patient was instructed to return for repeat immersion scanning in 4 months.

Rare tumors of the anterior segment include adenoma of the iris pigment epithelium that can erode through the stroma and become visible on slit-lamp examination. According to Shields et al.,[74] these lesions can be differentiated from ciliary body melanomas on the basis of transillumination and careful slit-lamp examination with gonioscopy. They have a solid appearance on echography.

Other lesions, such as adenoma and adenocarcinoma of the nonpigmented ciliary body epithelium (NPCE), are acquired, versus medulloepitheliomas, which are congenital tumors derived from the NPCE. Shields states that they can be distinguished from ciliary body melanomas by a complete lack of pigment, lack of setinal vessels, and a generally smaller size than melanomas. The echographic findings are nonspecific.

Rarely, leiomyomas can involve the ciliary body and peripheral choroid. Shields[75] reports that they are most common in women in the third decade of life. An important echographic feature in some cases is a normal choroidal layer, suggesting that this tumor is located in the suprauveal space. This fact is significant in the surgical treatment of these lesions. They could potentially be removed from the suprachoroidal space without disruption of the adjacent choroid with a good visual result.

Anterior segment tumors can be simulated by very peripheral views of a cataractous lens. When the B-scan probe is placed on the temporal sclera and angled very anteriorly, the opacified crystalline lens can be imaged with the artifactual appearance of a tumor.

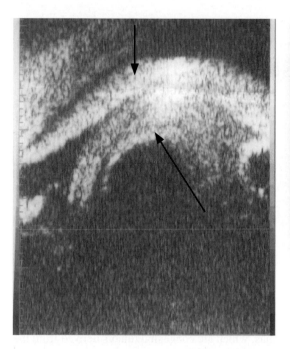
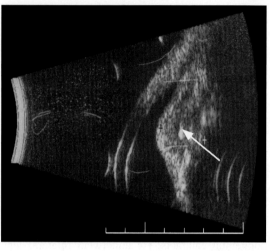

FIG. 334. Left: Immersion scan with 50-MHz probe of posterior capsule pearls (*bottom arrow*) with iris bulge (*top arrow*). Right: 20-MHz image of the same lesion (*arrow*)

# Case Study 184
## Pseudomelanoma and Cataract

AM is a 75-year-old woman who was scheduled for cataract surgery on a 4+ nuclear sclerotic lens. The ophthalmologist had difficulty visualizing the fundus and performed a B-scan examination. When the probe was placed on the posterior temporal sclera against the orbital rim and aimed towards the cornea, a dome-shaped mass was imaged (Fig. 335). The diagnosis of a probable ciliary body melanoma was made and the patient was referred to an oncologist to be evaluated for systemic metastases. The workup was negative for tumor and a discussion was instituted regarding treatment options, including enucleation. This greatly concerned the patient and she sought a second opinion.

Immersion echography was performed and a dense cataractous lens was imaged but no mass lesion was identified (Fig. 336). The diagnosis of a lens artifact simulating a tumor was discussed with the patient to her great relief.

This situation is relatively common with different appearances of the lens/tumor artifact (Fig. 337). Helpful clues to eliminate a tumor include the inability to image the lesion when the probe is placed on the sclera directly over the area of the "tumor," the symmetrically round shape, and the absence of subretinal fluid. If the diagnosis remains in doubt, then an immersion scan can be performed that will

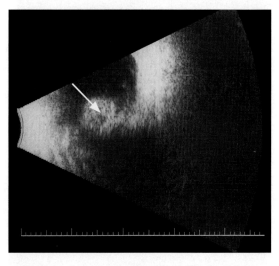

FIG. 335. B-scan with peripheral view of cataractous lens (*arrow*)

demonstrate a cataractous lens and the absence of a tumor.

Another lens tumor-simulating artifact is a dislocated cataractous lens that rests on the posterior retina. This can be particularly deceiving in a patient with opaque media, such as a cloudy cornea in which the presence or absence of the lens in its normal retroiridial position cannot be determined on slit-lamp examination.

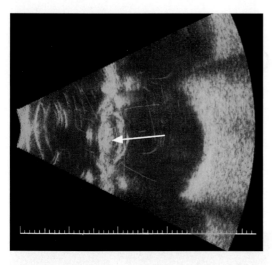
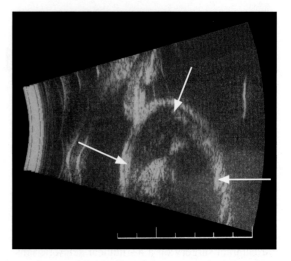

FIG. 336. Left: Immersion scan of cataractous lens with 10-MHz probe (*arrow*). Right: Immersion scan of lesion with 20-MHz probe (*arrows*)

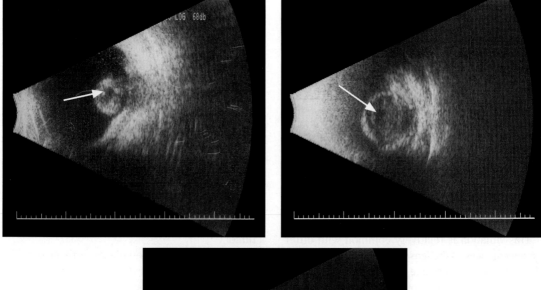

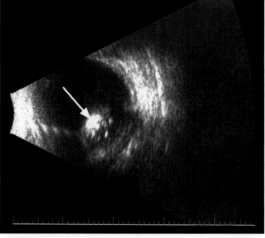

FIG. 337. Top left and right: Three B-scans of peripheral views of cataractous lenses (*arrow*). Bottom: Simulates a retinoblastoma

# Case Study 185
## Pseudomelanoma and Dislocated Lens

CD is a 43-year-old man with a history of a serious infection in his left eye years ago that resulted in some decreased sight in that eye. His vision had decreased slowly since that time and was very poor at the time of presentation to an optometrist. Examination found vision in that eye of counting fingers at 1 m and 20/30 in the right eye. Slit-lamp examination showed scarring of the right corneal stroma with a poor view of the anterior chamber and lens.

The fundus could not be visualized, so B-scan was performed with the appearance of a mass near the inferior equator. There was substantial shadowing of the globe and orbital tissue directly behind the lesion (Fig. 338). This lesion was solid with low internal reflectivity on A-scan (Fig. 339).

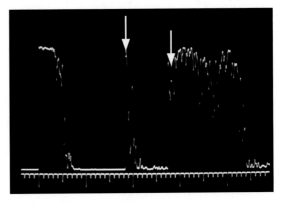

FIG. 339. A-scan of dislocated cataractous dislocated lens (*arrows*)

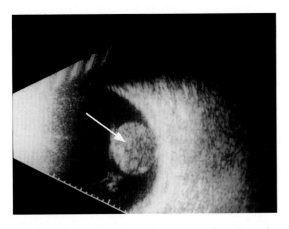

FIG. 338. B-scan of dislocated cataractous lens (*arrow*)

However, when the patient was asked to move his eye the lesion rolled along the fundus to a new position with the resultant diagnosis of a dislocated lens and the patient was reassured that he did not have cancer. It was elected to defer treatment unless he decided at some point to undergo penetrating keratoplasty. A combined procedure with a fragmatome lensectomy and vitrectomy would then be the operation of choice.

Echography plays a very important role in the evaluation of various intraocular and peribulbar lesions. It can detect and differentiate various lesions with greater accuracy than any other imaging modality. The performance of this technique by a properly trained examiner will prove invaluable in the clinical setting.

# Part VII
## Echography in Developing Countries

Ophthalmic echography can play a unique role in the clinical practice of ophthalmology in emerging and developing countries. These areas often have limited access to imaging techniques, such as computed tomography (CT) and magnetic resonance imaging (MRI) scanning. The multiple obstacles to utilization of these modalities for the average patient include cost, waiting time, travel distance, and cultural barriers. The availability of echography in the eye clinic can directly impact the quality of care in these countries.

Ocular and orbital pathology usually is not very different from that seen in more developed parts of the world, but it often presents at advanced stages that render diagnosis and treatment more difficult. It is common to encounter mature "white" cataracts, large corneal scars, advanced glaucoma, end-stage vitreoretinal pathology, and marked proptosis. Such conditions have often been present without treatment for long time periods because of the lack of medical resources in the local area.

Eye trauma with concussive or penetrating injuries is frequently not treated in a timely fashion, which can result in globe abnormalities that preclude adequate visualization of the posterior segment. The potential to enhance the patient's quality of life with available resources is inversely proportional to the complexity of the pathology. Ultrasound can rapidly screen out those who are not realistic candidates for therapeutic intervention. The patient can be advised as to his prognosis after an echographic examination that takes only a few minutes to perform.

# Part VII
## Demography in Developing Countries

# Case Study 186
## 'T' Retinal Detachment

JG is a 25-year-old Honduran man who was struck in the eye during a machete fight when he was 18 years old. He had been taken to the emergency room of the government hospital in a city that was several hours driving distance from his village. It was a Friday evening and the emergency room had closed and he was left at the doorway until Monday morning when he was admitted in shock after losing over half of his total blood volume. He was taken to surgery where his facial lacerations were repaired and he was given several units of blood donated by his relatives. No primary repair was performed of a central corneal laceration.

He presented to the eye department of the same hospital 7 years later when he heard that a visiting team from the United States was conducting free eye screening. He had traveled for half a day by bus and walked several miles to reach the clinic. He stated that his extended family had offered to try to raise the money to pay for surgery if the American team would perform it.

He complained of intermittent aching pains around his right eye. The eye was evaluated and found to have visual acuity of bare light perception with 20/30 in the left eye. Slit-lamp examination with a portable instrument showed 1+ conjunctival injection and a dense central corneal scar with the appearance of iris to the wound. The anterior chamber could not be adequately visualized. Intraocular pressure measured 7 mm OD and 14 mm OS. The fundus could not be seen.

Echography demonstrated a high reflective, funnel-shaped membrane inserting at the optic disc. A bridging membrane was also seen anteriorly connecting the sides of the funnel (Fig. 340). The diagnosis of a total retinal detachment was made and he was informed that his vision could

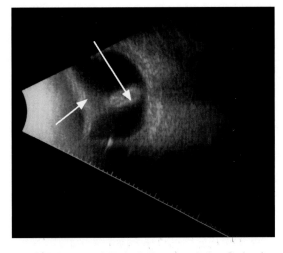

FIG. 340. B-scan of 'T-sign' (*first arrow*) detached retina (*second arrow*)

not be restored and he should not waste the time and expense to seek care at the main government hospital. He was started on prednisolone acetate and atropine drops and offered enucleation if the pain became too severe. He was educated to seek immediate attention if the opposite eye showed inflammatory symptoms indicative of sympathetic ophthalmia, such as pain and redness.

A major advantage of echography in such conditions is the potential to avoid the unnecessary utilization of precious resources in hopeless situations. Many patients with treatable eye problems in these countries are denied treatment because of the lack of medical and surgical supplies. Ultrasound can help to screen out those patients with irreversible pathology who would otherwise draw from a pool of limited supplies and professional expertise.

# Case Study 187
## Retinopathy of Prematurity and Retinal Detachment

MA is a 9-month-old Mongolian girl was born prematurely with 1.7 kilogram birth weight. She received supplemental oxygen for an extended period of time. Her mother stated that her daughter would not look at her face and that her eyes "wandered back and forth." She had been told at the government hospital that cataract surgery could be attempted but "there might be some complications," so she sought another opinion when she heard that some Japanese eye doctors were visiting a local clinic.

Examination showed an absent red reflex bilaterally and a poor view of the fundi. Lens opacities were noted bilaterally. The child had a moderate searching pendular nystagmus and would not fixate to light with either eye.

B-scan revealed membranous loops in the right eye consistent with an anterior retinal detachment (Fig. 341). Echography of the left eye showed a high reflective "funnel" inserting into the optic

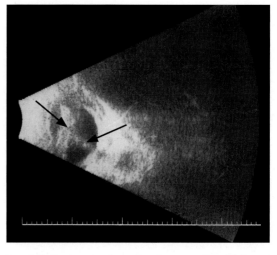

Fig. 342. B-scan of retinopathy of prematurity with funnel retinal detachment (*arrows*)

disc that was typical for a total retinal detachment (Fig. 342). The mother was told that the prognosis was poor for vision, but the doctors promised to discuss the child's case with a vitreoretinal specialist when they returned to Japan.

Echography can help to identify those cases that may be benefited by the latest surgical instrumentation in expert hands. Patients can be advised to seek such care if available in their own country or to travel to other areas if they have the resources. A number of nongovernmental organizations (NGO), such as ORBIS, send teams of ophthalmic specialists to developing countries and this can provide a resource to refer appropriate cases.

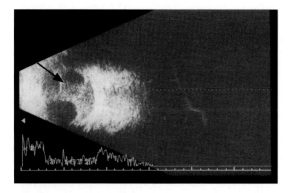

Fig. 341. B-scan of retinopathy of prematurity with anterior retinal detachment (*arrow*)

# Case Study 188
## Macular Detachment

A 34-year-old Mongolian man presented with a dense cataract in his left eye. There was a history of some sort of systemic infection 5 years previously to which he ascribed the onset of visual problems in the eye. The visual acuity in this eye was measured at light perception while uncorrected vision in his right eye was 20/80. There was a 2+ afferent defect of the left pupil. Slit-lamp examination showed a white cataract OS and a clear lens OD. Cycloplegic retinoscopy revealed a refractive error in the right eye of −3.00 +5.00 × 90.

Echography of the left eye demonstrated a partial posterior vitreous detachment with moderately dense intravitreal opacities. There was a shallow retinal detachment of the posterior pole with an area of vitreoretinal traction near the macula (Fig. 343). He was informed that cataract surgery would restore only 5% to 10% of the vision in that eye. He was given the option to go to Russia where vitreoretinal surgery was available, but informed that the prognosis for central vision was poor. He was discouraged from trying to find the resources to make the trip and undergo surgery because the

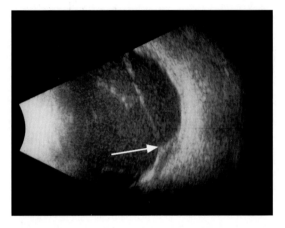

FIG. 343. B-scan of vitreoretinal traction (*arrow*)

vision in his other eye could be improved with spectacle correction. A pair of glasses was obtained for him that improved the vision in his right eye.

Echography can be a useful guide to those cases in which surgery might not only be futile for visual recovery, but would pose significant risk for the loss of a future opportunity to improve vision.

# Case Study 189
## Advanced Persistent Hyperplastic Primary Vitreous

JH is a 23-month-old Bolivian boy who had never "used his eyes" since birth, according to his parents. Examination found no fixation to light with the phthisical right eye but there was some intermittent fixation with the left. A local self-proclaimed pediatric ophthalmologist was planning to do cataract surgery on the left eye but the parents heard that a team of doctors was visiting from the United States and brought the child for consultation.

Echography confirmed a phthisical right eye with a total retinal detachment. B-scan of the left eye showed dense retrolental opacification and a high reflective tract inserting into the fundus just below the optic disc (Fig. 344). The retina appeared attached without evidence of traction. The axial length of the eye was about 21 mm. The findings were highly consistent with advanced persistent hyperplastic primary vitreous (PHPV). The parents were advised against the planned cataract surgery, but told to travel to La Paz and consult with a vitreoretinal surgeon who had experience in such cases.

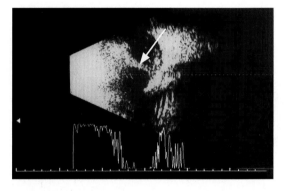

FIG. 344. B-scan of persistent hyperplastic primary vitreous (*arrow*)

Medical history in these patients is often sketchy at best. They may show up with an ocular problem that is the end result of previous trauma or unsuccessful medical/surgical therapy.

# Case Study 190
## Dislocated Lens

AV is a 63-year-old Peruvian man with a red, painful right eye and moderately dense lens opacity in his left. He had undergone some sort of surgery in his right eye several years previously by a group of doctors on an outreach program from a regional government hospital and had never seen very well with progressive loss of vision and increasing discomfort over the past several months. Examination found vision in the right eye of bare hand motions at 1 m and 20/80 OS. There was 3+ corneal edema of the right cornea with poor visualization of the anterior chamber, and no view of the fundus on that side.

Echography revealed 1 to 2+ vitreous opacities and a high reflective surface suspended in midvitreous, apparently enmeshed in vitreous membranes. It was somewhat mobile and drifted slowly as he moved his eye back and forth. The macula appeared thickened (Fig. 345) with a partial posterior vitreous detachment. The impression was that of a dislocated lens resulting from his previous surgery. The echographic findings suggested that his prognosis for significant improvement in vision was limited due to chronic cystoid macular edema.

His intraocular inflammation was treated with intensive topical steroids, atropine cycloplegia, and systemic anti-inflammatory drugs. Vitreoretinal surgery was only available at the main teaching (social security) hospital in Lima and because he

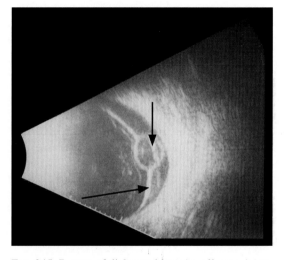

FIG. 345. B-scan of dislocated lens (*small arrow*) suspended by vitreous membrane (*large arrow*)

was unemployed, he was not eligible for services at that hospital. He was informed that he could apply for care at one of the charity hospitals, since there was over a year waiting period for consultation with a vitreoretinal team visiting from Germany.

Retained intraocular foreign bodies are not uncommonly encountered in patients with a history of activities at risk for small particles striking the eye at high velocity.

# Case Study 191
## Intraocular Foreign Body

A 25-year-old man from Myanmar presented with a history of poor vision in his right eye for 2 years. He had been hammering a piece of pipe and felt a sharp pain in that eye that improved over the next several hours. Several months later he noted that the vision in the eye was a little blurry and this became progressively worse.

Examination revealed visual acuity OD of 20/200 and OS of 20/30. There was no afferent pupil defect. Slit-lamp examination showed a small inferior corneal scar and a normal anterior chamber without reaction. Intraocular pressure was 15 mm OU. The right lens was densely cataractous and the fundus could not be visualized. He brought a report of an x-ray that had been read as normal.

B-scan showed a few vitreous membranes without traction on the retina. As the eye was systematically scanned, a strongly reflective signal was noted in the inferior vitreous. This was confirmed on both transverse and longitudinal views with the probe (Fig. 346). A high spike (100% compared to the initial signal) was detected on the A-scan, which confirmed the impression of an intraocular foreign body. The patient was unable to identify the

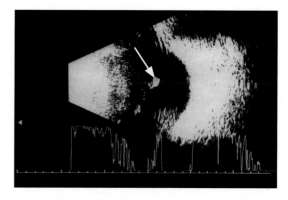

Fig. 346. B-scan of intraocular foreign body (*arrow*)

type of metal of which the pipe was composed. It was recommended to the surgeon that the cataract be removed and an attempt made to remove the particle with a magnet. Vitreoretinal surgery was not available so the particle would be left in the eye if it were not magnetic.

Foreign bodies in the anterior chamber can be a source of infection or chronic inflammation. These are usually more accessible to surgical removal in developing areas and echography can be valuable in localizing them.

# Case Study 192
## Foreign Body in Anterior Chamber

GA is a 34-year-old native of Vanuatu who was hammering a piece of metal when he suddenly felt pain in his right eye with blurry vision that worsened over the next several days. He made his way to a local medical outpost and was given a bottle of antibiotic eye drops. This helped a little but over the next several weeks his vision deteriorated. A team from Surgical Eye Expeditions (SEE) International was coming to the capital, Port Villa, and screening volunteers were working through the main islands to find patients for the visiting doctors. He was seen by one of them and referred to Port Villa for the SEE team because his vision was down to hand motions in the right eye. Their examination found 2+ corneal edema and a significant anterior chamber reaction that prevented a view of the posterior segment.

They had access to a 20-MHz probe with their ultrasound unit and found a high reflective foreign body–like signal in the area of Descemet's membrane with multiple signals (Fig. 347). The diagnosis of a retained foreign body in the anterior chamber was made and the patient underwent successful surgical removal after the epithelium was scraped off and topical glycerol was used to deturgese the stroma. He was treated with topical antibiotics and steroids with gradual improvement in his vision to 20/50.

Blunt trauma to the eye is more common among men than women and is often due to ocular injuries sustained in fighting. Echography is very useful in evaluating the globe to stage the type and extent of injury.

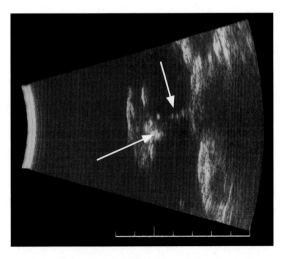

FIG. 347. Immersion 20-MHz B-scan of a foreign body in the anterior chamber horizontal (*arrow*) with multiple signals (*second arrow*)

# Case Study 193
## Lens in Anterior Chamber

GQ is a 45-year-old Peruvian man who was hit in the right eye with a fist the previous week. He had been intoxicated and had not realized the severity of his injury until several days later. The vision in that eye was cloudy and became increasingly painful over the next several days. He presented at a local outreach clinic manned every other week by ophthalmology residents in fulfillment of their requirements to work in rural areas during their training. The patient was examined and found to have vision in the right eye of counting fingers at 1 m and OS of 20/30. Intraocular pressure was 55 mm OD and 18 mm OS by Schiotz tonometry. External examination with a portable slit lamp showed 3+ corneal edema. He was diagnosed with closed angle glaucoma and given pilocarpine eye drops to use four times a day. He returned the next day without any improvement and increased pain in the eye. He was told nothing could be done except to remove the eye.

He made his way to a larger city and was seen at a government hospital. Echography was available and B-scan demonstrated the presence of the crystalline lens in the anterior chamber (Fig. 348). It was concluded that the blow had expulsed the lens forward. The posterior segment appeared normal except for mild vitreous opacities.

He was scheduled for lens removal. He was given topical beta blockers and intravenous (IV) mannitol prior to surgery to reduce the chance of an expulsive choroidal hemorrhage. The lens with its capsule was simply expressed from the eye in an intracapsular method. A Weck cell sponge anterior vitrectomy was performed. His vision

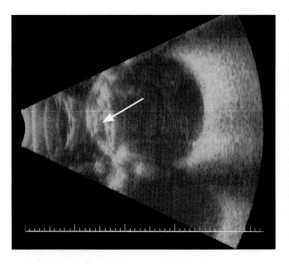 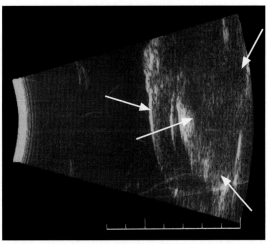

FIG. 348. Left: Immersion scan with 10-MHz probe of lens in the anterior chamber (*arrow*). Right: Immersion scan with 20-MHz probe of cornea (*first arrow*) and lens (*arrows*)

later improved to 20/100 with 2+ residual corneal edema and intraocular pressure of 20 mm. An intraocular lens was not implanted because the vision potential was limited and an anterior chamber lens would potentially further compromise the cornea.

# Case Study 194
## Disrupted Lens Capsule

JB is a 23-year-old Mexican man who fell into a metal pipe at work and struck his left eye and immediately noted loss of vision with severe pain. He was taken to the emergency room and was diagnosed as having a ruptured globe. An ophthalmology resident at the government hospital did a primary closure the next day. He told the patient he had a cataract and would need surgery the following week. One of the staff ophthalmologists in the residency program had an interest in echography and had recently taken a course in anterior segment techniques and offered to examine the patient before surgery.

The finger of a sterile glove was cut off and filled with balanced salt solution with the B-scan probe inserted into it. Methylcellulose was applied to the tip of the glove and gently applied to the closed lids. There was some vitreous hemorrhage and a possible inferior retinal detachment. The crystalline lens could not be visualized and there was amorphous material in the anterior vitreous (Fig. 349). This was interpreted as a disrupted lens capsule and the patient was referred to a vitreoretinal surgeon.

Trauma can cause various degrees of vitreoretinal pathology, from a partial posterior vitreous detach-

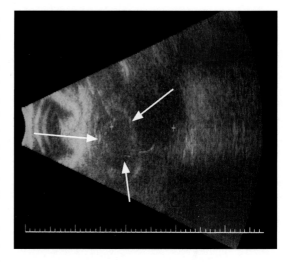

Fig. 349. Immersion scan of disrupted lens capsule (*arrows*)

ment to a giant tear and retinal detachment. A severely ruptured globe can usually be readily diagnosed with such clinical signs as hemorrhagic conjunctival chemosis, light perception vision, and hypotony. However, focal occult rupture can be more difficult to diagnose. Echography is a valuable resource to detect disruption of the wall of the globe.

# Case Study 195
## Ruptured Globe

YS is a 56-year-old Egyptian man who had been struck in the face with the end of a shovel as he stood behind a fellow worker on a construction site. His left eyelids were swollen shut and there was significant bruising that involved the paraocular area and into the upper cheek. He presented to the eye clinic at the local hospital 2 weeks later with resolution of the eyelid edema, but had blurred vision, floaters, and mild discomfort in that eye.

Examination showed vision in the right eye of 20/25 and in the left of 20/60. The intraocular pressure was 15 mm OD and 13 mm OS. Slit-lamp examination showed mild anterior chamber reaction and some vitreous cells in the left eye with an adequate view of the fundus, but a poor view of the inferior temporal periphery because of some residual hemorrhagic debris in that area.

B-scan revealed a vitreous membrane inserting at the 4:30 position with focal thickening of the retinochoroid layer suspicious for an occult rupture (Fig. 350). Vitreoretinal surgery was considered, but was not locally available. The clinical situation was felt to be stable and careful observation was planned. The patient was advised to return in 2 weeks for

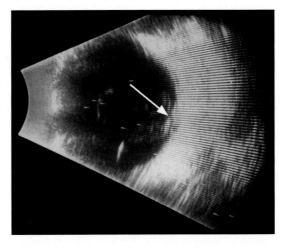

FIG. 350. B-scan of vitreous incarceration in occult rupture site (*arrow*)

reevaluation and referral for surgery if evidence of a traction retinal detachment was seen.

There are often limited therapeutic options in more remote areas of developing countries. Echography can assist in identifying those individuals in whom intervention may be worthwhile.

# Case Study 196
## Intumescent Lens and Angle Closure

A 72-year-old native of Vanuatu lived on one of the remote islands. He lost his left eye as a child due to injury and had gradually experienced reduction in the vision in his right eye with a rapid decline over the past several weeks with some discomfort. He heard that a volunteer group from Australia was taking people from his island by sailing vessels to the capital city of Port Villa on the island of Efate for the treatment of eye problems. He and many of the inhabitants had never left their island and were afraid to make such a journey over open ocean to be treated by strangers. However, his vision was almost gone and he felt he had no choice but to go.

Examination showed vision in the right eye of light perception and a phthisical left eye. There was 2 to 3+ corneal edema with a hazy view of the anterior chamber. There appeared to be a dense cataractous lens and no view of the fundus. The intraocular pressure was measured to be 50 mm by Schiotz tonometry.

Echography using an immersion technique revealed a large cataractous lens measuring over 6 mm with a shallow anterior chamber (Fig. 351). The posterior segment appeared unremarkable. The diagnosis of an intumescent lens with secondary angle closure was made and he underwent lens removal by extracapsular extraction the next day. His pressure was measured at 20 mm and he could see at the 20/200 level. The plan was to supply him with a pair of donated +12.0 aphakic spectacles. The optic

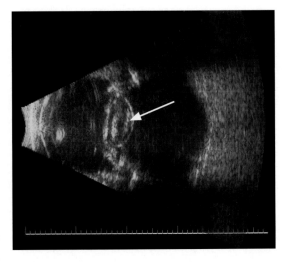

FIG. 351. B-scan of intumescent lens (*arrow*)

nerve showed 8/10 cupping and he had moderate constriction of his visual field on confrontation testing. He was very happy with the result and returned to his island. He encouraged his visually impaired friends to make the journey to the capital the following year when the volunteer team would return.

Diabetes is often undetected or undertreated in many less advanced areas of the world. The ocular complications of this disease include cataract formation and vitreous hemorrhage, which can obscure the fundus. Echography allows visualization of the posterior pole and the patient can be advised on the prognosis for visual recovery.

# Case Study 197
## Vitreous Hemorrhage

HA is a 32-year-old Peruvian woman who had been diagnosed with diabetes and started on insulin after several years of excessive thirst, frequency of urination, and spontaneous weight loss. She had never had an eye exam. She stated that her left eye had become quite blurry over several weeks and she saw many tiny spots.

Examination found vision in the right eye of 20/40 and the left eye of 20/200. There was a questionable afferent pupil defect in the left eye. Slit-lamp examination was normal and intraocular pressures measured 13 mm in both eyes. The right fundus examination showed moderate proliferative diabetic retinopathy with dot and blot hemorrhages and several foci of intraretinal vascular abnormalities. The optic disc was documented to be covered by greater than 50% neovascularization. The left fundus could not be visualized due to vitreous opacities.

Echography of the left eye revealed 3+ pointlike vitreous opacities consistent with moderate subhyaloid hemorrhage (Fig. 352). The retina was attached and no areas of vitreoretinal traction could be identified. She was instructed to minimize heavy lifting and to elevate her head at night when sleeping.

A portable laser had been donated to the clinic and panretinal photocoagulation was applied to the right eye. She was instructed to return in a month to institute laser treatment in the left eye with the anticipation that the hemorrhage would clear enough to allow some laser treatment. She was informed that there was a good chance of visual improvement once the blood was gone from the eye.

Eyes with a history of trauma are sometimes subject to increased intraocular pressure with resultant optic nerve damage. The B-scan can be

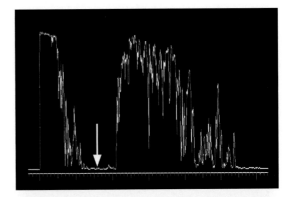

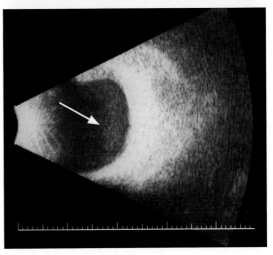

FIG. 352. Top: A-scan of vitreous hemorrhage (*arrow*). Bottom: B-scan of subhyaloid hemorrhage (*arrow*)

helpful in detecting optic nerve cupping when it is moderately severe (greater than 0.7 cup-to-disc ratio). It is helpful to view the nerve head in different probe positions (vertical, horizontal, and longitudinal) to find which best displays the optic cup.

# Case Study 198
## Advanced Optic Nerve Cupping

A 52-year-old Ethiopian woman gave a vague history of some sort of injury to her left eye several years ago. She had intermittent episodes of pain in this eye and the vision had gradually dropped to light perception. Examination found vision in the right eye of 20/30 and in the left of bare light perception. Her intraocular pressure was difficult to measure in the left eye because of corneal edema and scarring. This prevented a view of the fundus.

B-scan with a horizontal axial view showed marked cupping of the optic nerve consistent with advanced glaucomatous nerve damage (Fig. 353). She was informed that there was no hope for vision in that eye.

Intraocular tumors may present in late stages with severe morbidity. Some intraocular tumors have a different incidence in developing countries than those in the Western nations. Malignant melanoma is the most common intraocular tumor in Caucasian races and is rare in people of darker skin pigmentation. Poorer areas of the world have a higher rate of ocular invasion by metastatic and secondary neoplasms due to failure to treat the primary tumors at early stages when their spread can be more readily controlled. Retinoblastoma is the most common intraocular tumor of children throughout the world, but it presents in more advanced stages in less technologically developed areas.

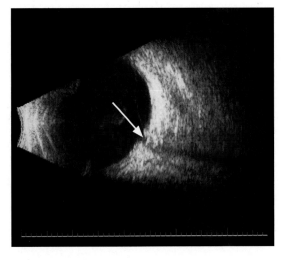

FIG. 353. B-scan of advanced cupping of the optic nerve (*arrow*)

# Case Study 199
## Retinoblastoma

TY is a 2-year-old Bolivian child who was noted by her parents to progressively cross her eyes since she was 6 months old. A local health station nurse told them that she would "grow out of it." Her left eye later became red much of the time and the "pupil began to appear a different color than the other eye." She was seen at the local clinic and the parents were given some eye drops for infection and told to bring her back if things got worse.

She was brought into a screening clinic set up by a group of volunteer ophthalmologists from the United States. Her left eye had an esotropia of 50 prism diopters and would not fix on a picture target. The pupil had a white reflex and she was suspected to harbor an intraocular mass.

Echography of the right eye revealed a large mass lesion that filled most of the globe and calcium deposits were detected on A- and B-scan (Fig. 354). A small peripheral calcified mass was noted in the temporal periphery of the left eye (Figs. 355 and 356). The diagnosis of a bilateral retinoblastoma was made and the child was scheduled for enucleation of the right eye with the intent to remove as much of the optic nerve as possible. MRI imaging was not available to evaluate the nerve or CNS for invasion by tumor. A-scan measurements of the optic nerve were performed and were within normal limits, but microscopic invasion by tumor could not be ruled out. She was referred to the oncology center of a government hospital for chemotherapy in an attempt to preserve the left eye. She was told to return in 6 months for repeat clinical examination and ultrasound of the left eye to evaluate the status of the tumor.

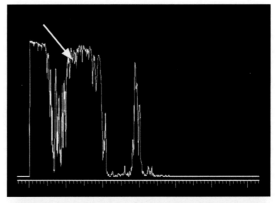

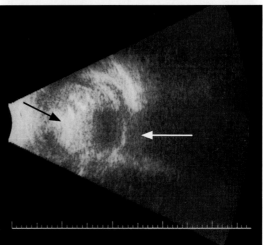

FIG. 354. Top: A-scan of large retinoblastoma (*arrow*). Bottom: B-scan of tumor (*first arrow*) with scleral and orbital shadowing (*second arrow*)

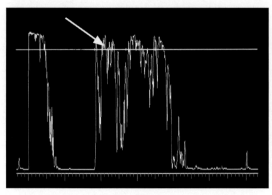

FIG. 355. A-scan of small retinoblastoma (*arrow*).

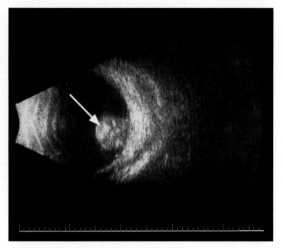

There is a long differential diagnosis of lesions besides retinoblastoma that can cause leukocoria. Several of the more important ones can only be accurately diagnosed by echography. The correct

FIG. 356. B-scan of tumor (*arrow*)

diagnosis can direct appropriate treatment and spare a child unnecessary surgery in such cases.

# Case Study 200
## Persistent Hyperplastic Primary Vitreous

MA is an 18-month-old Honduran male who was noted to have a white pupil reflex in the right eye when a photograph was taken by a visiting relative. He was taken to the local clinic where a probable tumor in the eye was diagnosed and he was referred to the eye department of a government hospital in the capital city, 100 miles away.

He was seen in the eye clinic and the diagnosis of retinoblastoma was made and the child was scheduled for enucleation the next day by one of the ophthalmology residents. A visiting team from an international volunteer group was asked to see the child just prior to surgery. Echography revealed a retrolental opacity with a moderate stalk going back to the optic disc (Fig. 357). The diagnosis of persistent hyperplastic primary vitreous (PHPV) was made and it was suggested that enucleation be cancelled and a lensectomy/vitrectomy be performed instead. The parents were told that this eye would never see well, but without surgery it would probably become blind and painful and have to be removed.

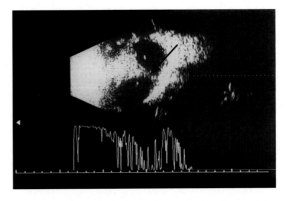

FIG. 357. B-scan of persistent hyperplastic primary vitreous with stalk (*arrow*)

The limited clinical signs in orbital disease make it difficult to be certain about a specific diagnosis. Often only a long differential diagnosis is possible. Patients may present in advanced stages of orbital disease. Treatment options are usually limited based on what is locally available, such as basic antibiotics, prednisone, and topical beta blockers.

# Case Study 201
## Graves' Disease

A 34-year-old Indonesian man had a 2-year history of prominence, redness, and irritation of his right eye. He had been treated with prednisone during this time with doses varying from 80 mg a day initially to 20 mg when the process seemed less severe. He had not been evaluated for osteoporosis, ulcers of the stomach, tuberculosis, or diabetes during this time. He had a striking Cushinoid appearance to his facies. Ocular examination showed exophthalmometry measurements of 25 mm OD and 21 mm OS. There was moderate conjunctival injection and chemosis of the right eye. His vision was 20/40 OD and 20/25 OS with a 2+ posterior subcapsular cataract noted on the right. Intraocular pressure measured 21 mm OD and 20 mm OS. Fundus examination showed a cup to disc ratio of 5/10 OD and 4/10 OS. Various ophthalmology residents had followed him in the clinic over the 2-year period with the diagnosis of orbital pseudotumor. A plain film skull x-ray had been obtained at one time that was interpreted as normal by the radiologist.

A diagnostic echography unit was donated to the hospital and a training course was set up. This patient was brought in for echographic examination. The A-scan revealed marked thickening of all of the extraocular muscles bilaterally with medium-to-high irregular reflectivity (Fig. 358). B-scan revealed abnormal thickening of the superior rectus/levator complex bilaterally.

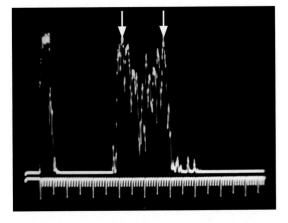

FIG. 358. A-scan of thickened extraocular muscle (*arrows*)

The diagnosis of Graves' disease was made and the patient was sent for thyroid testing. His basic thyrotropin level was normal but antithyroid antibody testing was not done. He was advised to begin tapering his prednisone with the goal to lower the dose to physiologic levels within 3 months. He was given the treatment options of orbital radiation or an injection of kenalog into the orbital tissue.

There are often very limited resources to address paraocular and orbital problems. CT and MRI scanners may be found in the major cities with limited access by much of the population because of expense and travel distance. Plain film x-rays are more readily available but are of limited value in orbital diagnosis.

443

# Case Study 202
## Orbital Pseudotumor

A 41-year-old man was seen as part of the ultra-sound-training course given by a visiting volunteer team to the university hospital in Jakarta, Indonesia. He gave a history of "a big right eye with some aching for several weeks." Examination showed 8 mm of proptosis of that eye with 3+ conjunctival injection and chemosis. The vision was measured at 20/70 OD and 20/25 OS. The left eye appeared normal on clinical examination. A plain film x-ray of the orbits was read as normal. He was diagnosed with an orbital tumor and was in the process of being referred to another city for orbital biopsy.

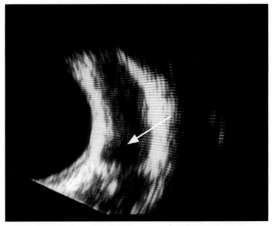

FIG. 360. B-scan of lesion (*arrow*)

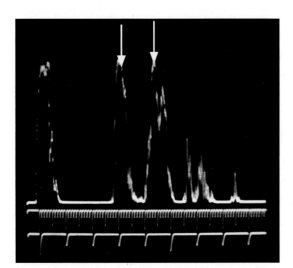

FIG. 359. A-scan of orbital pseudotumor (*arrows*)

Echography revealed low reflective thickening of several extraocular muscles, increased subtenon's lucency, and a well-outlined low reflective lesion in the mid-orbit (Figs. 359 and 360). These findings were consistent with orbital pseudotumor and high-dose steroids were started after a chest x-ray and blood glucose tests were performed. He responded with rapid improvement in the proptosis and inflammatory signs.

Inflammatory conditions of the orbital and periorbital area are often not treated by anti-inflammatory medications in the early stages and can progress to painfully debilitating problems.

# Case Study 203
## Orbital Myositis

A 43-year-old Mongolian woman who had intermittent pain and swelling around her left eye for over a year. The symptoms had recently increased to the point that she was constantly in pain. She slept poorly at night and was not able to perform her household and childcare chores during the day. She had taken aspirin intermittently without relief of her symptoms. She presented to the government hospital outpatient clinic and was given a supply of ibuprofen. This lessened her pain somewhat, but she was generally incapacitated and sought help at a facility in another city. Examination in the eye department showed marked temporal conjunctival and episcleral injection of the left eye with mild lid swelling. The vision was reduced to 20/60 in that eye while the right eye was measured at 20/30. She had a 10-prism diopter left esotropia with increased pain on looking to the left. Slit-lamp examination of the left eye showed a clear cornea and a deep anterior chamber with mild flare but no cells. Fundus examination showed a clear vitreous cavity and some possible thickening of the temporal retinochoroidal layer.

Echography revealed moderate thickening of the sclera and some increased lucency of subtenon's space. The left lateral rectus muscle was thickened near its attachment to the globe and posteriorly (Fig. 361). The diagnosis of a lateral rectus myositis with adjacent scleritis was made and she was started on high-dose oral steroids with rapid resolution of her symptoms.

Some orbital problems, such as cystic lesions, are amenable to simple surgical incision and drainage. These procedures often do not require the technology and trained personnel as would be necessary for more complex procedures. Ultrasound

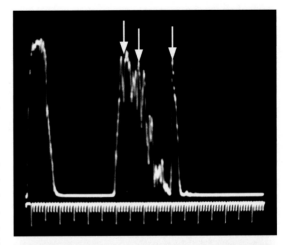
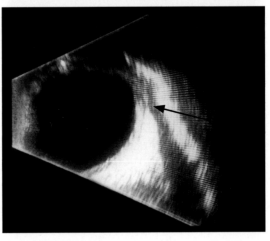

FIG. 361. Top: A-scan of thickened sclera (*first arrow*) and muscle belly (*second* and *third arrows*). Bottom: B-scan of tendon (*arrow*)

may be useful in such situations both by enabling a correct diagnosis and by guiding needle aspiration of the lesion.

447

# Case Study 204
## Orbital Lymphangioma

A 10-year-old child presented at a large teaching hospital with the sudden onset of painful proptosis of her left eye that started several days previously. The parents gave a history of several episodes of less extreme protrusion of the globe that had occurred several times over the past 2 years but had always resolved spontaneously without any medical treatment. Examination found 7 mm of proptosis of that eye with moderate subconjunctival hemorrhage and several hemorrhagic cysts under her upper eyelid. There was firm resistance to retropulsion of the globe. The vision was normal as was the intraocular pressure. The fundus examination was unremarkable. Extraocular movements were full.

Echography demonstrated a diffuse multicystic orbital lesion with large retrobulbar low reflective cysts (Figs. 362 and 363). The findings were

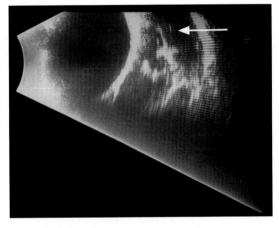

FIG. 363. B-scan of lesion (*arrow*)

consistent with a spontaneous bleed into an orbital lymphangioma. The tumor was too extensive for a total resection, but the largest cyst appeared amenable to needle aspiration under ultrasound guidance.

The aspiration was performed the next day and 5 cc of blood were removed with marked reduction of the proptosis. The parents were instructed that this procedure could be repeated if the symptoms recurred.

Pathology of the paranasal sinuses is common in developing areas. It is often untreated and can reach advanced stages before care is sought. This can be a source of significant morbidity. Plain film x-rays can be of some value, but significant problems can be missed because of the limited resolution.

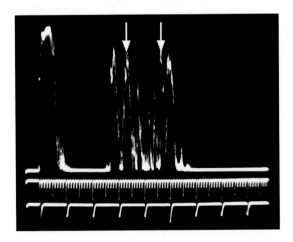

FIG. 362. A-scan of bleed into lymphangioma (*arrows*)

# Case Study 205
## Mucocele

CA is a 43-year-old woman with a history of progressive proptosis and downward displacement of her right eye over several years. She complained of minimal discomfort and was not aware of double vision. Clinical examination found proptosis of that eye of 7 mm and hypoglobus of 5 mm compared to the left. She brought a copy of an x-ray with her that had been obtained about a year previously, but it did not demonstrate the cause of her problem. There was mild opacification of her right maxillary sinus but no other evident sinus abnormalities.

A-scan revealed a low reflective orbital lesion in the right superior nasal orbit with a sudden drop-off in the orbital bone spike consistent with a bone defect. The echo signals behind this defect were low to medium and slightly irregular (Fig. 364). These findings were highly consistent with a frontal ethmoidal mucocele. The patient was informed that a team of otolaryngologists would be in the area in 9 months and that arrangements would be made for them to remove the mucocele if that was her desire.

Sinus-related paraocular problems can be easily detected by echography with appropriate treatment by inexpensive antibiotics that are available in even the poorest of areas.

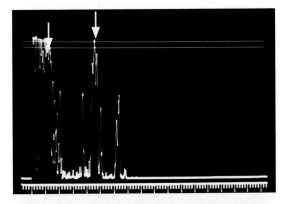

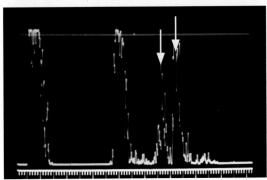

FIG. 364. Top: Paraocular A-scan of orbital component of mucocele (*arrows*). Bottom: Transocular A-scan of mucocele with bone defect (*arrows*)

# Case Study 206
## Sinusitis

TI is a 13-year-old girl who presented to a screening clinic with moderate swelling of her right upper and lower eyelids. She was quite uncomfortable and had gotten worse over 2 weeks. Examination found 2+ lid edema and erythema on the right with normal appearance of the globe and a full range of extraocular movements.

A-scan revealed marked signals from the right ethmoid and maxillary sinuses with less significant spikes on the left side (Fig. 365). The diagnosis of acute sinusitis was made and she was started on keflex and Sudafed with resolution of her symptoms over several days.

Sinus infections can have serious sequelae if not properly treated. They have the potential to be the source of intracranial infections. They can be the source of abscess formation subperiosteally or within the orbit.

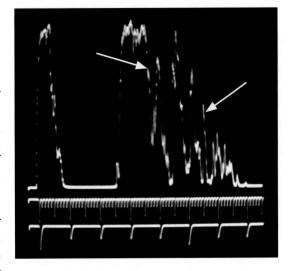

FIG. 365. A-scan of ethmoid sinus signals (*arrows*)

# Case Study 207
## Subperiosteal Abscess

MH is a 15-year-old Honduran girl who complained of headaches and pressure around her eyes for more than a year. Her parents noted intermittent lid swelling that resolved spontaneously but the episodes of pain and swelling were lasting longer and seemed more severe. She had been taken to the local clinic and given penicillin tablets by a health worker. This had provided some relief for a few weeks, but the symptoms recurred.

She complained of severe pain around her left eye that was made worse when she looked left and right. She was taken to a government hospital and referred by the triage nurse to the eye clinic. Examination found moderate lid edema on the left and nasal conjunctival injection. Visual acuity was normal in both eyes with unremarkable slit-lamp and fundus examinations.

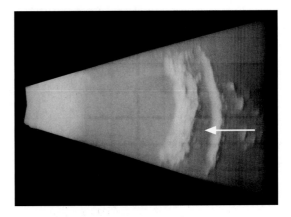

FIG. 367. B-scan of abscess (*arrow*)

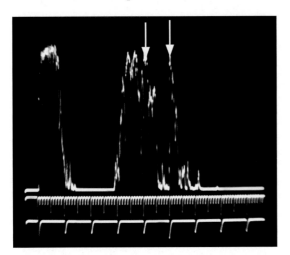

FIG. 366. A-scan of subperiosteal abscess (*arrows*)

Plain film x-rays were read as normal. Echography revealed a sharply outlined low reflective area in the superior orbit (Figs. 366 and 367). This was interpreted as consistent with a subperiosteal abscess. She was taken to the operating room with a surgical team comprised of an ophthalmologist and otolaryngologist for drainage of the abscess. IV antibiotics had been started preoperatively and were continued for several days afterwards. Repeat ultrasound showed resolution of the subperiosteal infiltrate.

Some benign orbital lesions do not result in functional problems and are best left untreated because potentially serious complications can occur from surgical intervention.

# Case Study 208
## Lipodermoid

A 23-year-old Mongolian woman noted a yellow lesion in the outer corner of her right eye. It was soft to the touch and caused no symptoms except for a possible vague aching feeling. She was concerned and sought attention at the university hospital. An ophthalmology resident examined her and diagnosed an orbital tumor. She was scheduled for excisional biopsy in the following week. The only available CT scanner was down for repairs. A plain film x-ray was read as normal.

A visiting oculoplastics team from the United States was asked to evaluate her as part of a teaching conference. The lesion was felt to be consistent clinically with a lipodermoid and echography was done for confirmation.

Ultrasound revealed a soft high reflective lesion that extended into the anterior orbit (Fig. 368). The border was poorly defined and it was uncertain as to how far posteriorly it went. The echographic impression was consistent with lipodermoid.

The consulting group of doctors recommended that surgery be cancelled because the lesion was benign and posed no danger to the eye. It was felt

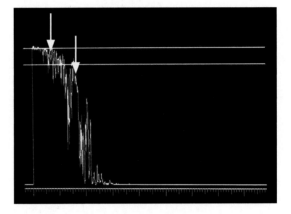

FIG. 368. A-scan of lipodermoid (*arrows*)

that the complications of "chasing the tumor" back into the orbit posed significant risk of damage to the extraocular muscles or optic nerve.

In developing countries, ultrasound has the dual benefit of screening out ocular problems before limited resources are depleted in their evaluation and directing the most appropriate and cost-effective therapy.

# Part VIII
## Orbital Imaging

Tristan F.W. McMullan, MA, PhD, FRCOphth*
H. Christian Davidson, MD†

## Introduction

This section aims to provide a guide to orbital imaging as related to orbital disease. Imaging of the visual pathway as a whole will not be covered; this is covered in several excellent neurophthalmological texts. However, in the context of some diseases (e.g., optic nerve meningioma, trauma, etc.), the assessment of extraorbital pathology and structural change must be considered.

## Anatomical Considerations

The bony orbit is simplistically divided into a floor, roof, and medial and lateral walls. More posteriorly, however, the floor and medial wall do not have much more than an artificial separation and it is a mistake to consider the orbit as having a boxlike cross-section (Fig. 369). The rim or arcus marginalis defines the orbit's anterior extent. The septum that arises from the arcus marginalis is used to define the anterior limits with preseptal structures thought of as eyelid and postseptal structures pertaining to the orbit.

The floor is comprised of the orbital plates of the maxilla zygoma, with a negligible contribution from the palatine bone. The roof is comprised of the frontal bone with a contribution from the lesser wing of the sphenoid. The lateral wall is provided by the zygoma

anteriorly and the greater wing of sphenoid posteriorly. The frontal process of the maxilla, the lacrimal bone, and the lamina papyracea of the ethmoid bone and the sphenoid provide the medial wall posteriorly. The apex of this bony pyramid is the optic canal that passes through the lesser wing of the sphenoid. It transmits the optic nerve and ophthalmic artery and associated sympathetic fibers. There are two main fissures, the superior orbital fissure between the greater and lesser wings of the sphenoid and the inferior orbital fissure between the maxilla and the greater wing of the sphenoid. The superior orbital fissure communicates with the cavernous sinus and middle cranial fossa. It transmits the lacrimal nerve (sensory CN V, joined by parasympathetic to lacrimal gland), frontal nerve (sensory CN V), trochlear nerve (motor CN IV), superior ramus of the oculomotor nerve (motor CN III), nasociliary nerve (sensory CN V, ciliary nerves join later), inferior ramus of the oculomotor nerve (motor CN III, parasympathetic), abducens nerve (motor CN VI), and ophthalmic vein. The inferior orbital fissure allows communication between the orbit and the pterygopalatine fossa and the masticator space. It transmits the maxillary nerve, with its branch the infraorbital nerve, and branches of the inferior ophthalmic vein.

## Radiological Investigations

Investigations of the bony orbit are best achieved with computerized tomography (CT), which is superior to magnetic resonance imaging (MRI) in delineating bone structure and abnormality. Axial scans are the most familiar and either direct or reformatted coronals are invaluable. Sagittal sections

*Tristan F.W. McMullan, MA, PhD, FRCOphth
Consultant Ophthalmic & Oculoplastic Surgeon, Department of Ophthalmology, Northampton General Hospital, Cliftonville, Northampton, United Kingdom
† H. Christian Davidson, MD
Associate Professor, Department of Radiology, University of Utah, Salt Lake City, Utah

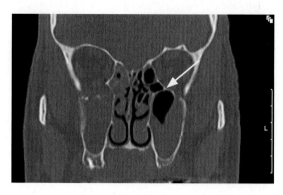

FIG. 369. Computed tomography coronal view showing 30° to 40° angulation of the floor relative to the horizontal

are useful in delineating the posterior extent of fractures. The two most common windows are bone (where the soft tissue is ill defined and the bone marrow and diploic spaces are easily seen) and soft tissue, where the reverse is true, with the bone having very high signal and little definition but allowing clearer discernment of the orbital contents. For many clinicians, CT is the investigation of choice for the quality of the bony imaging, cheap and easy acquisition, and lack of concern regarding metallic foreign bodies that might become ferromagnetic missiles in MR scanners, with resultant eye damage. The use of contrast is dictated by the relevant clinical setting; CT contrast material contains iodine and a history of iodine or contrast allergy should be excluded. Renal failure is a relative contraindication depending on the clinical setting. The relatively high dose of radiation should be considered in repeated imaging in children and pregnancy. Spiral CT scans allow for faster acquisition and reduced radiation exposure. Three-dimensional models can be simulated and used for surgical planning and also for the construction of stereolithographic models.

Magnetic resonance imaging is better for delineating soft tissues and the use of T1 fat suppression will allow orbital fat to be suppressed to delineate intraorbital structures. It will not necessarily pick out calcification and patients with ferromagnetic implants and intraocular or intraorbital foreign bodies cannot be routinely scanned. The acquisition times are longer and the process is noisier and more claustrophobiogenic. In general terms, T1-weighted scans are better for examining anatomy and T2-weighted scans are better for examining pathology. Short tau inversion recovery (STIR) sequences are helpful

in estimating water content in tissue, which is of relevance to estimating the inflammation in thyroid eye disease.[76] Other MRI scanning sequences, such as fluid inversion attenuation recovery (FLAIR) are more useful for the assessment of intracranial pathology. Likewise, diffusion-weighted scans and proton density scans are of less use in the orbit.[77,78]

## Liaison with the Radiology Department

As in any radiological evaluation, liaison with the radiologist and radiographer and obtaining a correct and timely investigation are likely to pay dividends. If a valsalva maneuver (suspected varix) is required it should be requested, etc. When obtaining radiological investigations, the referring clinician should always specify the differential diagnosis to the best of his or her ability to guide the radiologist. The purpose of the scan should also be born in mind if it is not merely being used to establish, confirm, or eliminate a diagnosis. For example, if thyroid-associated orbitopathy (TAO) is suspected, then an MRI with fat suppression or a STIR sequence will be much more valuable in assessing disease activity than a CT scan, but a CT will be more helpful in planning surgical decompression.

Other factors that should be considered when obtaining an investigation include the patient's weight and ability to fit inside the scanner, the patient's age or mental state (will they stay still or need sedation), claustrophobia, prior metallic intraorbital or intraocular foreign bodies, pregnancy, sensitivity to intravenous contrast, and the urgency of the investigation. Communication with the radiology department will help to address some of these issues.

## Interpretation

There are certain prerequisites before interpreting any investigation. The patient's name and date of birth or identity number must be confirmed and the laterality of the examination confirmed, with the normal protocol having the scans printed and displayed as though looking from the imaginary foot of the patient's bed, the patient's right being on the left as displayed. Different radiology departments have their own protocols for displaying sagittal images, but convention is normally to start with right (the first slice being through the right ear).

In the orbit thin cuts are essential to obtain meaningful information and 1- to 3-m cuts are standard.

The volume of the orbit is normally taken to be approximately 30 cc, with the orbital dimension about 4 cm in height, depth, and width. Within this 30 cc, the orbital contents are usually described by their relation to (1) the globe (anterior or retrobulbar) and (2) the muscle cone (intra- or extraconal or arising from the muscles). Within the muscle cone, the structures can be defined by their relationship to the optic nerve. Particular lesions can then be described as extraconal soft tissue mass (e.g., lymphoma) or intraconal lesion inseparable from the optic nerve (e.g., optic nerve glioma). The relative depth of the lesion has two important sequelae. An anteriorly placed extraconal lesion in region of the lacrimal gland fossa is going to be more accessible than an intraconal "peanut" at the orbital apex. The locations will also give clues as to the underlying pathology.

## Orbital Imaging in Orbital Disease

### Tumors

The prevalence of orbital tumors and simulating lesions is comprehensively reviewed by Shields et al.[79] In a case series of 1264 patients, the relative frequency of different pathology and the mean ages of the patients at presentation are described. Vasculogenic lesions comprised 17%, secondary involvement of the orbit was found in 11%, inflammatory lesions were found in 11%, lymphoid or leukaemic lesions accounted for 10%, the lacrimal gland accounted for 9%, and optic nerve or meningeal comprised 8% and metastases comprised 7%, which taken together comprised 73% of the series. A total of 56% of the lesions were biopsied. This series allows the clinician to assess which tumors are most common and aids in the construction of a differential diagnosis. Specific conditions have particular findings on MRI or CT imaging, which might be able to distinguish between the different pathologic entities. This series was constructed to allow a useful estimate of frequency in a large cohort, but when faced with an individual patient the diagnostic dilemma can be simplified to the following question: is the lesion structural in the context of congenital conditions or trauma, benign, malignant (primary or secondary), inflammatory or infective?

These broad categories are the most useful to the patient and clinician to allow a management plan to be adopted. Traumatic and structural lesions are best imaged with CT and in most cases the aim of the study is to define the relative anatomy rather than to arrive at a diagnosis. Infective cases are likewise usually imaged with CT to establish the extent of the infection, assess paranasal sinus involvement, and to confirm the diagnosis. This leaves the benign and malignant and inflammatory mass lesions. A recent article by Ben Simon and colleagues[80] has added some predictive characteristics of orbital mass lesions that are examined here.

The features that were assessed and found to have predictive value were location, content on CT or MRI, soft tissue characteristics, bone characteristics, and associated features. The authors provide a list of imaging features that were significantly different among the three groups (Table 1).

The features that are suggestive of a malignant process include irregular shape, molding around structures, diffuse lesions, perineural involvement, and bone erosion. Features more characteristic of a benign process include oval shape, hyperostosis, hyperintensity on T2, and hyperdensity or isodensity on CT. Orbital fat stranding (dirty fat) and pan orbital involvement are likely to be associated with inflammatory lesions. Primary bone lesions were likely to be benign in their series of patients.

When their patients with benign and malignant tumors were compared to each other (excluding inflammatory tumors), the various features were calculated to have a positive predictive value (proportion of patients who had the abnormal radiological feature and the disease compared to all patients who had the feature) where, for example, four patients had both perineural involvement and malignancy out of four patients with perineural involvement; perineural is 100% predictive for malignancy. They also assess negative predictive results (patients had neither radiographic feature nor disease relative to the number of patients without the feature). For example, absence of disease and absence of fat stranding was found in 65% of the total group of 100 patients, giving a negative predictive value of 65. When sensitivity and specificity are calculated, it was found to be absent in 65 patients, all of whom were negative for malignancy, giving a specificity of 100%, and in no patients with malignancy, giving a sensitivity

TABLE 1. Imaging Features with Significant ($p < 0.05$) Difference of Occurrence between Benign, Malignant, and Inflammatory Lesions among 131 Patients with Biopsy-Proven Orbital Tumors[*]

| Feature | Overall N | Overall % | Benign N | Benign % | Malignant N | Malignant % | Inflammatory N | Inflammatory % | p Value |
|---|---|---|---|---|---|---|---|---|---|
| Number of patients | 131 | | 65 | | 35 | | 31 | | |
| Panorbital | 9 | 7 | 2 | 3 | 0 | 0 | 7 | 23 | < 0.001 |
| Orbital fat | 6 | 5 | 0 | 0 | 0 | 0 | 6 | 19 | < 0.001 |
| Lacrimal fossa | 24 | 18 | 6 | 9 | 10 | 29 | 8 | 26 | 0.022 |
| Anterior orbit/preseptal | 41 | 31 | 13 | 20 | 19 | 54 | 9 | 29 | 0.002 |
| Sphenoid wing | 13 | 10 | 11 | 17 | 2 | 6 | 0 | 0 | 0.02 |
| Sinus opacity/frontal | 10 | 8 | 1 | 2 | 3 | 9 | 6 | 19 | 0.006 |
| Hyperostosis | 15 | 11 | 14 | 22 | 0 | 0 | 1 | 3 | < 0.001 |
| Primary bone | 14 | 11 | 13 | 20 | 1 | 3 | 0 | 0 | 0.002 |
| Erosion | 20 | 15 | 4 | 6 | 11 | 31 | 5 | 16 | 0.004 |
| Content[*] | | | | | | | | | |
| T2–isointense | 20 | 15 | 8 | 12 | 10 | 29 | 2 | 6 | 0.039 |
| T2–hyperintense | 34 | 26 | 25 | 38 | 4 | 11 | 5 | 16 | 0.005 |
| CT–hypodense | 7 | 5 | 7 | 11 | 0 | 0 | 0 | 0 | 0.033 |
| CT–hyperdense | 10 | 8 | 10 | 15 | 0 | 0 | 0 | 0 | 0.003 |
| Regular–oval | 19 | 15 | 19 | 29 | 0 | 0 | 0 | 0 | < 0.001 |
| Diffuse | 41 | 31 | 10 | 15 | 15 | 43 | 16 | 52 | < 0.001 |
| Molding | 12 | 9 | 2 | 3 | 10 | 29 | 0 | 0 | < 0.001 |
| Circumscribed | 80 | 61 | 48 | 74 | 19 | 54 | 13 | 42 | 0.007 |
| Irregular | 58 | 44 | 20 | 31 | 18 | 51 | 20 | 65 | 0.005 |
| Fat stranding | 5 | 4 | 0 | 0 | 0 | 0 | 5 | 16 | < 0.001 |
| Perineural involvement | 6 | 5 | 0 | 0 | 4 | 11 | 2 | 6 | 0.015 |
| Nerve distribution | 7 | 5 | 7 | 11 | 0 | 0 | 0 | 0 | 0.033 |

Abbreviation: CT, computed tomography.

*p* Values were calculated using Fisher exact test.

[*]Intensity (magnetic resonance imaging) and density (computed tomography) were graded relative to brain gray matter.

*Source*: Reprinted with permission from *Ophthalmology*, 112(12):2196–2207, Simon GJ, et al. Rethinking orbital imaging establishing guidelines for interpreting orbital imaging studies and evaluating their predictive value in patients with orbital tumors, Copyright (2005), with permission from American Academy of Ophthalmology.

of 0% (Table 2). The authors stated, "none of the features had a high sensitivity for diagnosing malignant versus benign processes."

The article also studied the associations between different features that would intuitively be expected, for example, opacity in the frontal and ethmoidal sinuses, and others that are less obvious, such as extraocular muscle atrophy and Meckel's cave involvement. The series of 135 lesions provides some clues as to radiologic features that are likely to be diagnostically useful, but the techniques have not been assessed prospectively to evaluate the accuracy of the predicted radiological diagnosis versus the eventual tissue diagnosis. A prospective study is required.

The radiographic features of the more common tumors and simulating conditions are tabulated in Table 3. The patterns of presentation vary considerably, but some broad generalizations can be made.

Inflammatory, infectious, and traumatic processes have unique features that are displayed on radiologic and echographic studies.

# Specific Disease Entities

## Thyroid Eye Disease

Dysthyroid orbitopathy can occur in the context of hyperthyroidism, hypothyroidism, and normal thyroid status. Prior radioiodine treatment and cigarette smoking are risk factors for disease and exacerbate disease severity. Thyroid orbitopathy is the most common cause of both unilateral and

TABLE 2. Positive Predictive Values, Negative Predictive Values, Sensitivity, and Specificity of Imaging Features in Evaluating Malignant versus Benign Processes (Excluding Inflammatory Lesions) in Patients with Orbital Tumors[*]

| | Benign vs. malignant (excluding inflammatory) | | | | | | | |
| | Positive predictive value[†] | | Negative predictive value[‡] | | Sensitivity[§] | | Specificity[#] | |
| Feature | n | % | n | % | n | % | n | % |
|---|---|---|---|---|---|---|---|---|
| Number of patients | | | | | 35 | | 65 | |
| Orbital fat | 0 | NA | 65 | 65 | 0 | 0 | 65 | 100 |
| Perineural involvement | 4 | 100 | 65 | 68 | 4 | 11 | 65 | 100 |
| Fat stranding | 0 | NA | 65 | 65 | 0 | 0 | 65 | 100 |
| Sinus opacity frontal | 3 | 75 | 64 | 67 | 3 | 9 | 64 | 98 |
| Panorbital | 0 | 0 | 63 | 64 | 0 | 0 | 63 | 97 |
| Moulding | 10 | 83 | 63 | 72 | 10 | 29 | 63 | 97 |
| Erosion | 11 | 73 | 61 | 72 | 11 | 31 | 61 | 94 |
| Lacrimal fossa | 10 | 63 | 59 | 70 | 10 | 29 | 59 | 91 |
| Nerve distribution | 0 | 0 | 58 | 62 | 0 | 0 | 58 | 89 |
| CT–hypodense | 0 | 0 | 58 | 62 | 0 | 0 | 58 | 89 |
| T2–isointense | 10 | 56 | 57 | 70 | 10 | 29 | 57 | 88 |
| CT–hyperdense | 0 | 0 | 55 | 61 | 0 | 0 | 55 | 85 |
| Diffuse | 15 | 60 | 55 | 73 | 15 | 43 | 55 | 85 |
| Sphenoid wing | 2 | 15 | 54 | 62 | 2 | 6 | 54 | 83 |
| Primary bone anterior orbit | 1 | 7 | 52 | 60 | 1 | 3 | 52 | 80 |
| Preseptal | 19 | 59 | 52 | 76 | 19 | 54 | 52 | 80 |
| Hyperostosis | 0 | 0 | 51 | 59 | 0 | 0 | 51 | 78 |
| Regular-oval | 0 | 0 | 46 | 57 | 0 | 0 | 46 | 71 |
| Irregular | 18 | 47 | 45 | 73 | 18 | 51 | 45 | 69 |
| T2–hyperintense | 4 | 14 | 40 | 56 | 4 | 11 | 40 | 62 |
| Circumscribed | 19 | 28 | 17 | 52 | 19 | 54 | 17 | 26 |

Abbreviation: NA, not applicable.

[*]Only features with significantly different occurrence between malignant and benign groups were included in the calculation.

[†]Rate of detecting disease among patients with positive test results equals number of patients with disease (malignant) and positive test results per number of patients with positive test results.

[‡]Rate of detecting nondisease among patients without positive test results equals number of patients without disease (malignant) and negative test results per number of patients with negative results.

[§]Rate of positive test results among patients with disease equals number of patients with disease (malignant) and positive test results per number of patients with disease (malignant).

[#]Rate of negative test results among patients without disease equals number of patients without disease (malignant) and negative test results per number of patients without disease (malignant).

Source: Reprinted with permission from Ophthalmology, 112(12):2196–2207, Simon GJ, et al. Rethinking orbital imaging establishing guidelines for interpreting orbital imaging studies and evaluating their predictive value in patients with orbital tumors, Copyright (2005), with permission from American Academy of Ophthalmology.

bilateral proptosis in adults. Imaging is useful to confirm the diagnosis and to monitor disease activity in some cases. MRI with fat suppression or STIR sequence can demonstrate extraocular muscle inflammation that confirms that the disease is in an active inflammatory stage that should respond to immunosuppression. The spent disease will not respond to immunomodulation and as such this distinction is clinically useful. Features of thyroid eye disease include enlarged extraocular muscles with sparing of the myotendinous insertions (Fig. 370), lacrimal gland enlargement, proptosis, and apical crowding. There may be dirty fat and increased orbital fat volume. There may be an association with sinus disease. In dysthyroid optic neuropathy, either the orbital apex is crowded to the extent that the optic nerve becomes compressed and an optic neuropathy ensues or the optic nerve may also lose its sigmoid shape and appear straight and the assumption is made that it is stretched by progressive proptosis with presumed microvascular sequelae (Figs. 371–373). If this were the suspected diagnosis, then CT would be a more appropriate investigation because bony

TABLE 3. Radiological and ultrasound features of common orbital disease

| Tumor | Figures | Age | Sex | Location | Shape/outline | MRI | T1 | T2 |
|---|---|---|---|---|---|---|---|---|
| **Intraconal** | | | | | | | | |
| Metastases, brain metastases in 2/3 | | Older except neuroblastoma | M=F | Intraconal > Muscle >Extra conal | Ill-defined mass | Variable | Variable | Variable |
| Cavernous hemangioma / Encapsulated | | Middle Age | F>M | Intraconal. Unilateral | Oval to round encapsulated | Well-defined mass, round or oval | Isointense to muscle | Hyperintense to muscle |
| **Optic nerve** | | | | | | | | |
| Optic nerve glioma (NF1) | | 90% <20 | F>M | Optic nerve. May be bilateral | Fusiform to globular | Lesion may be kinked | Isointense to brain | Mildly to strongly hyperintense |
| Optic nerve glioma (non NF1) | | 90% <20 | F>M | Optic nerve. Unilateral | Fusiform to globular | Fusiform lesion | Isointense to brain | Mildly to strongly hyperintense |
| Malignant optic nerve glioma | | Adult | M≥F | | Contoured | Enhancement in homogeneity and cystic areas | | |
| Optic nerve meningioma - may be assoc with NF2 | | Adult | F>M | Primary tumors arise from optic nerve meninges. Secondary tumors arise from e.g., sphenoidal ridge (Miller 2004) | Tubular lesion with tramtrack signs | Enhances with gadolinium. Doughnut sign on coronal MRI | Isointense to nerve or hypointense | Isointense to nerve or hyperintense |

| CT | Contrast enhancement | Bone involvement | Associated findings | Echography: Consistency | Spike height | Regularity | Vascularity | Attenuation |
|---|---|---|---|---|---|---|---|---|
| Bone destruction | Variable enhancement | Destruction | Breast, lung, stomach, thyroid, renal, melanoma | Very hard | Medium/high | Irregular V-pattern | 1+ to 4+ | Low |
| Homogenous Hyperdense legion. Ovoid legions. | Heterogeneous enhancement | Remodeling | No change with valsalva maneuver | Firm but decreases in size on compression | Medium/high | Regular | No | Medium |
| Irregular kinking of nerve | Variable enhancement | Optic canal may be enlarged | | Firm | Low/medium | Regular to 1+ irregular | 1 to 2+ | Low |
| Fusiform enlargement of nerve | Variable enhancement | Optic canal may be enlarged | | Firm | Low/medium | Regular to 1+ irregular | 1 to 2+ | Low |
| | | | | Firm | Low/medium | Regular to 2+ irregular | 1 to 3+ | Low |
| Calcification in 20-50%. Tram track sign after contrast | Uniform enhancement | Canal may enlarge. May be hyperostosis | | Firm | Medium/high | 1 to 2+ irregular | No | Low |

(continued)

TABLE 3. (continued)

| Tumor | Figures | Age | Sex | Location | Shape/outline | MRI | T1 | T2 |
|---|---|---|---|---|---|---|---|---|
| **Extraconal** | | | | | | | | |
| Lymphoma | | 50-70 | F>M | Any, extraconal, lacrimal. 75% unilateral | Range from well defined to ill defined infiltration | Moderate contrast enhancement | Isointense to muscle | Hyperintense to fat on T2, brighter than T1 (not universal) |
| Mucocele | | Adult | | Arises from paranasal sinus | Contoured round to oval | | Depends on protein content. Early: low signal. Late: high signal | Depends on protein content. Early: high signal. Late: low signal |
| Varix | | Any | M+F | May be assoc with intracranial venous abnormalities | Ill defined loculated mass | May collapse | Hypointense | Hypointense |
| Lymphangioma | | <10 | | Diffuse | Ill-defined or round and encapsulated with hemorrhage | | Hypo fat, hyper muscle | Hyper muscle and fat |
| Capillary hemangioma | | Infancy | | Superonasal. Usually extraconal | Diffuse to contoured | | Hypointense to fat, hyperintense to muscle | Hyperintense to fat and muscle |
| Dermoid | | <25 | | Superotemporal | Oval to round encapsulated | | Hypointense to fat | Isointense / hypointense to fat |
| Lacrimal gland tumors | | | | Lacrimal gland fossa. Orbital lobe of gland | Contoured | | | |

| CT | Contrast enhancement | Bone involvement | Associated findings | Echography: Consistency | Spike height | Regularity | Vascularity | Attenuation |
|---|---|---|---|---|---|---|---|---|
| Dense mass | Variable | Erosion and sclerosis uncommon | 1% of NHL pts get orbital disease | Hard/firm | Low/medium | Regular to 1+ irregular | 1 to 2+ | Low |
| Good visualization of bone anatomy | Margins enhance | Remodeling and thinning | Sinus disease | Hard | Low/medium | Regular to 2+ irregular | No | Low |
| Phleboliths | Patchy contrast enhancement | May rarely cause bone changes (islam et al.) | Rapid acquisition CT scan with valsalva | Soft | Baseline/low | Regular | No | Low |
| Irregular mass | Diffuse enhancement | No | May enlarge with valsalva on imaging but not clinically | Soft but becomes firm with hemorrhage | Low/medium | 3+ irregular but regular in hemorrhage into cyst | No | Low to medium |
| Irregular mass | Contrast enhancement | No | May have skin signs | Moderately firm | Medium/high | 2 to 3+ irregular | 3 to 4+ | Low to medium |
| | Capsule enhances on MRI | May mold bone | | Frim | Low/medium | Regular to 3+ irregular | No | Low to high |

(continued)

TABLE 3. (continued)

| Tumor | Figures | Age | Sex | Location | Shape/outline | MRI | T1 | T2 |
|---|---|---|---|---|---|---|---|---|
| Benign mixed tumor | | 30-40 | F=M | Benign mixed tumor | Well defined almond | | | Isointense to brain |
| Adenocystic | | 20-40 | F=M | Adenocystic | May be more nodular | | | |
| Rhabdomyo-sarcoma | | 90% < 16 | | Superonasal. Unilateral | Diffuse to contoured | | Isointense or hypointense to brain. Hypointense to fat, hyperintense to muscle | Hyperintense to fat and muscle. Hyperintense to brain. |
| Leukemia | | Adult CLL. Children AML | | UL or BL, may involve temporal fossa | Diffuse to contoured | | Isointense to muscle | Brighter on T2 |
| Schwannoma | | adult | | Extraconal | Oval to round encapsulated | Well defined fusiform | Hypointense to fat, isointense to muscle and brain | Hyperintense to fat |
| Neuro-fibroma solitary | | adult | | Localised: any, superior orbit | Oval to round well-outlined | Well defined on MRI. Fusiform | Hypointense to fat, isointense to muscle and brain | Hyperintense to fat |
| Neuro-fibroma Plexiform | | <10 | | Eyelid and contig-ous orbit | Ill defined mass | Infiltrative | Hypointense to fat | Hyperintense to fat |
| Hemangio-pericytoma | | Any, 5th decade | M=F | Superior | Oval to round well-outlined | | Isointense to brain | Isointense to brain |
| Fibrous Histiocytoma | | Adult | M=F | Anywhere, superior, nasal extraconal | Oval, well-outlined | | T1 intermediate signal | T2 high signal |

| CT | Contrast enhancement | Bone involvement | Associated findings | Echography: Consistency | Spike height | Regularity | Vascularity | Attenuation |
|---|---|---|---|---|---|---|---|---|
| | Enhances on MRI and CT | Bone molding | | Firm | Medium/high | Regular | 0 to 1+ | Medium |
| May calcify | | Bone erosion | | Firm | Low/medium | 2 to 4+ irregular | 0 to 1+ | Medium |
| Well defined isodense to muscle | Enhancement on MRI | Bone destruction | | Firm | Low/medium | Regular to 1+ irregular | 1 to 3+ | Medium |
| Irregular mass | | Subperiosteal with boney destruction = granulytic sarcoma (AML) | | Soft | Low/medium | Regular to 1+ irregular | No | Low |
| Homogenous isodense to brain | Heterogeneous Enhances on CT an d MRI | Bone remodeling | | Firm | Low/medium | 1 to 4+ irregular | 0 to 1+ | Medium |
| Homogenous isodense to brain. May calcify | Heterogeneous Enhances on CT an d MRI | Bone remodeling | | Soft to firm | Low/medium | Regular | 0 to 1+ | Low to medium |
| | Variable | Bone thinning may occur | NF1 | Soft | Medium/high | 3 to 4+ irregular | 1 to 2+ | Low |
| Homogenous lesion | | Possible bone erosion | | Firm | Low/medium | Regular | 0 to 1+ | Low to medium |
| | Moderate enhancement | Possible bone remodeling | | Firm | Low/medium | Regular | 2 to 3+ | Medium |

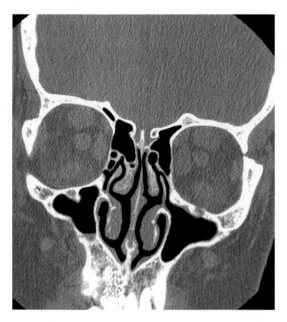

FIG. 370. Coronal computed tomography scan showing enlarged extraocular muscles (type 2 Graves' disease)

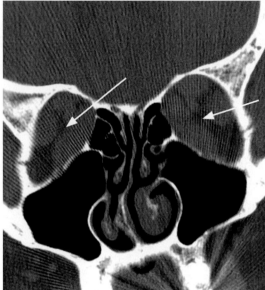

FIG. 372. Coronal computed tomography scan showing enlarged muscles filling the orbital apex in a patient with dysthyroid optic neuropathy (*arrows*)

decompression is a likely clinical outcome and CT is essential for surgical planning. Scans in patients with previous orbital decompression will show a mixture of findings depending on the nature of the

prior surgery. Prolapse of orbital contents into the paranasal sinuses is the desired result.

Idiopathic orbital inflammation (IOI) is a common disease of the orbit that has previously been

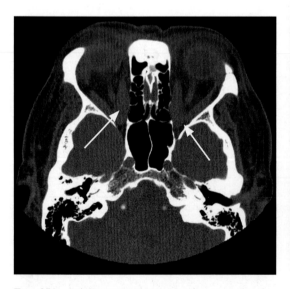

FIG. 371. Axial computed tomography scan showing enlarged muscles filling the orbital apex in a patient with dysthyroid optic neuropathy (*arrows*)

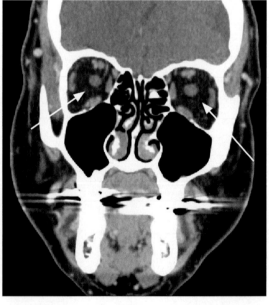

FIG. 373. Coronal computed tomography scan showing predominant enlargement of orbital fat volume (type 1 Graves' disease) (*arrows*)

described as orbital pseudotumor. It is usually but not always unilateral and may affect the lacrimal gland, the extraocular muscles, or the intra- or extraconal space. The diagnosis is one of exclusion, with lymphoma being an important differential, although lymphoma is not normally painful. In contradistinction to thyroid eye disease, IOI is said to affect the extraocular muscle tendons. Posterior scleritis can be detected by thickening of the sclera, but ultrasound is the preferred investigation to allow measurements of the scleral thickness to be made.

## Sarcoidosis

Sarcoidosis is rare in the orbit but may affect the lacrimal gland, the muscles, or the optic nerve. Radiologic features are nonspecific but imaging will assist with surgical planning for biopsy.

## Infection

Orbital cellulitis may be pre- or postseptal and as such can threaten to communicate infection with the cavernous sinus via the superior ophthalmic vein (SOV), which can be a devastating consequence. The most common scenario, however, is a subperiosteal abscess associated with contiguous sinus disease. Imaging is aimed at establishing that there is not some other pathology, such as rhabdomyosarcoma, and for possible surgical intervention as via an orbitotomy. The disease often presents in the younger age group and, as a result, sedation may be required to obtain images. Coordination between the pediatrician, radiologist, and anesthesiologist is crucial.

Mucormycosis is a disease of the immunocompromised and more frequently affects diabetics. The failure to manage this condition appropriately can be fatal. Imaging is aimed at assessing the orbit, paranasal sinuses, and cavernous sinuses, and disease extent.

## Trauma

The CT scan is the investigation of choice in most cases of trauma, particularly if there is even a vague suspicion of an orbital or intraocular foreign body.[81] Fracture of the orbital rim is less common but the floor and medial wall are susceptible to blowout fracture with the zygomatic complex often associated (Fig. 374). The purpose of the investigation is to establish the extent of the bony defect and the degree of soft tissue entrapment. The pediatric population can mislead the clinician with the white-eyed blowout, where a trapdoor greenstick-type fracture can entrap the inferior rectus and lead to rapid muscle necrosis; urgent imaging and intervention is required. A feature that should alert the referring clinician and radiologist is if the child is systemically unwell, with constitutional symptoms including fever and severe nausea associated with muscle necrosis.

Both bone and soft tissue windows should be obtained with either direct or reformatted coronal views. The corresponding sinuses are usually opaque due to blood that may manifest as a fluid level seen on axial scans. Air inside the orbit is a telltale sign of communication between the orbits and the sinuses and surgical emphysema may also be seen. The CT equivalent of the teardrop sign seen on plain films should alert the clinician to a small fracture.

Orbital foreign bodies should be sought and excluded as far as is possible (Fig. 375). A more devastating consequence of trauma is optic nerve canal damage and or traumatic optic neuropathy. Traumatic optic neuropathy may be associated with fracture of the optic canal that can be seen on CT or may be a localized pressure effect with vascular consequences that are best seen on high-resolution MRI.

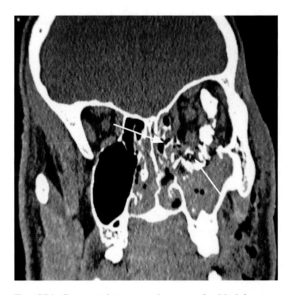

Fig. 374. Computed tomography scan of orbital fracture (*arrows*)

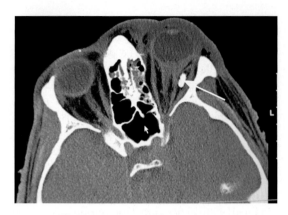

FIG. 375. Computed tomography scan of orbital foreign body (*arrow*)

## Pediatric Disease

The most common reason for obtaining a CT scan in children is in the context of orbital infection that is addressed above. It is worth noting that children can present with orbital cellulitis and a white eye and that other conditions can mimic orbital cellulitis.

The most common benign tumor in children is the capillary hemangioma. The most common orbital malignant tumor in children is a rhabdomyosarcoma, which has a variety of presentations that can mislead the clinician. A painless proptosis or a cellulitic picture can be the first sign of disease.

## Caroticocavernous Fistulas

Caroticocavernous fistulas may be evaluated with an MRI, although selective carotid angiograms remain the gold standard but are not without risk. CT, MRI, and orbital ultrasound will show an enlarged SOV and proptosis. Orbital color Doppler can demonstrate aterialization of the SOV. The fistulae are categorized by the anatomy of the feeder vessels and the flow rate. A history of trauma (not necessarily), a bruit and blood in Schlemm's canal, and an elevated intraocular pressure with conjunctival arterialization should prompt the diagnosis, which can be confirmed and characterized by imaging studies.

## Summary

When presented with orbital disease, the clinician can aid diagnosis and plan appropriate surgical intervention with the judicious use of orbital imaging—CT, MRI, and ultrasonography. In general terms, CT is best for bony disease, for example, fractures, and for planning decompression. MRI is more useful for soft tissue interpretation. Ultrasound is an extremely useful adjunct. The location of the tumor and the imaging and associated features are helpful in reaching a differential diagnosis and in determining the likelihood of benign versus malignant disease.[82]

# Part IX
## References

1. American Academy of Ophthalmology basic and clinical science course Section 3. San Francisco: San Francisco American Academy of Ophthalmology, 2005.
2. Ossoinig KC. Quantitative echography—the basis of tissue differentiation. J Clin Ultrasound 1974;2:33.
3. Biswas J, Mani B, Shanmugam MP, et al. Retinoblastoma in adults: report of three cases and review of the literature. Surv Ophthalmol 2000;44:409–414.
4. Boldrey EE. Risk of retinal tears in patients with vitreous floaters. Am J Ophthalmol 1983;96:783–787.
5. Walker AE, Robins M, Weinfeld FD. Epidemiology of brain tumors: the national survey of intracranial neoplasms. Neurology 1985;35:219–226.
6. Auw-Haedrich C, Staubach F, Witschel H. Optic disc drusen. Survey Ophthalmol 2002;47:515–532.
7. Foroozan R, Savino PJ, Sergott RC. Embolic central retinal artery occlusion detected by orbital color Doppler imaging. Ophthalmology 2002;109: 744–748.
8. Bullock JD, Campbell RJ, Waller RR. Calcification in retinoblastomas. Invest Ophthalmol Vis Sci 1977; 16:252–255.
9. Wilson GA, Devaux A, Aroichane M. Retinoblastoma, microphthalmia and the chromosome 13q deletion syndrome. Clin Exp Ophthalmol 2004;32:101.
10. Hoffman RO. Personal communication, 2006.
11. Mundt GH Jr, Hughes WF Jr. Ultrasonics in ocular diagnosis. Am J Ophthalmol 1956;41:488.
12. Zaldivar R, Shultz MC, Davidorf JM, et al. Intraocular lens power calculations in patients with extreme myopia. J Cataract Refract Surg 2000;25:668–674.
13. Gabbert-McConkie W, Kachur KH. Diagnostic ultrasound in CPT expert. Salt Lake City: Ingenix, 2006.
14. Byrne SF. The echographic measurement and differential diagnosis of optic nerve lesions [review]. In: Ossoinig, KC, ed. Ophthalmic echography. Dordrecht: Dr W Junk; 1987.
15. Coleman DJ. Reliability of ocular and orbital diagnosis with B-scan ultrasound. 1. Ocular diagnosis. Am J Ophthalmol 1972;73:501–516.
16. Bronson NR. Development of a simple B-scan ultrasonoscope. Trans Am Ophthalmol Soc 1972;70:365.
17. Ossoinig KC. Standardized echography: basic principles, clinical applications, and results. Int Ophthalmol Clin 1979;19:127.
18. Byrne SF, Green RL. Ultrasound of the eye and orbit. 2nd ed. St Louis: Mosby; 2002.
19. McNutt LC, Kaefring SL, Ossoinig KC. Echographic measurement of extraocular muscles. In: White D, Brown RE, eds. Ultrasound in medicine. New York: Plenium Press; 1977.
20. Volpe NJ, Sbarbaro JA, Livingston K, et al. Occult thyroid eye disease in patients with unexplained ocular misalignment. Am J Ophthalmol 2006;142: 75–81.
21. Ossoinig KC, Cennamo G, Byrne SF. Echographic differential diagnosis of optic nerve lesions. In: Thijssen JM, Verbeek AM, eds. Ultrasonography in ophthalmology. Dordrecht: Dr W Junk, 1981.
22. Byrne SF, Green RL. Ultrasound of the eye and orbit. 2nd ed. St Louis: Mosby, 2002.
23. Mcguire P. Working with a tough patient? Try these strategies. ACP-ASIM Observer. 2002.
24. Chobanian AV, Bakris GL, Black HR et al. Seventh Report of the Joint National Committee on Prevention, Detection, Evaluation, and Treatment of High Blood Pressure: the JNC report. JAMA 2003;289:2560.
25. Reese AB. Expanding lesions of the orbit (Bowman lecture). Trans Ophthalmol Soc UK 1971;91: 85–104.
25. (a). Eye involvement in sarcoidosis. The Ophthalmology Newsletter 1982:3(1):1–3.
26. Gamel JW, Font RL. Adenoid cystic carcinoma of the lacrimal gland: the clinical significance of a basaloid histologic pattern. Hum Pathol 1982;13:219–225.

27. Shields JA, Augsburger JJ. Cataract surgery and intraocular lenses in patients with unsuspected malignant melanoma of the ciliary body and choroid. Ophthalmology 1985;92:823.

28. Peter J, Savino DF, McLean IW, Zimmerman LE. Posterior uveal melanomas in aphakic and pseudophakic eyes. Am J Ophthalmol 1986;101:458–460.

29. Shammas HF, Blodi FC. Prognostic factors in choroidal and ciliary body melanomas. Arch Ophthalmol 1977;95:63–69.

30. Kirk HQ, Petty RW. Malignant melanoma of the choroid; a correlation of clinical and histological findings. Arch Ophthalmol 1956;56:843–860.

31. Haimann NH, Burton TC, Brown CK. Epidemiology of retinal detachment. Arch Ophthalmol 1982;100:289–292.

32. Endophthalmitis Vitrectomy Study Group. Results of the endophthalmitis vitrectomy study. A randomized trial of immediate vitrectomy and of intravenous antibiotics for the treatment of postoperative bacterial endophthalmitis. Arch Ophthalmol 1995;113:1479–1496.

33. Gass JDM. Reappraisal of biomicroscopic classification of stage of development of a macular hole. Arch Ophthalmol 1995;119:752–759.

34. Corbett JJ, Thompson HS. The rational management of idiopathic intracranial hypertension. Arch Neurol 1989;46:1049–1051.

35. Doxanas MT, Anderson RL. Clinical orbital anatomy. Baltimore: Williams and Wilkins, 1984.

36. Ben Simon GJ, Annanziata CC, Fink J, Villablanca P, McCann JD, Golberg RA. Rethinking orbital imaging. Ophthalmology 2005;112:2196–2206.

37. Migliori ME. Determination of the normal range of exophthalmetric values for black and white adults. Am J Ophthalmol 1984;98:438–442.

38. Goder GJ. Tumors of the lacrimal gland. Orbit 1982;1:91–96.

39. Shields JA. Inflammatory conditions that can simulate neoplasms. In: Shields JA, ed. Diagnosis and management of orbital tumors. Philadelphia: Saunders, 1989.

40. Gorman CA. Pathophysiology of graves. In: Rootman J, ed. Orbital disease. Present status and future challenges. New York: Taylor and Francis, 2005.

41. Vaidya B, Imrie H, Perros P, et al. The cytotoxic T lymphocyte antigen-4 is a major Graves disease locus. Hum Mol Gen 1999;8;1195–1199.

42. Bessell EM, Henk JM, Wright JE, et al. Orbital and conjunctival lymphoma treatment and prognosis. Radiother Oncol 1988;13:237–244.

43. Coupland SE, et al. Lymphoproliferative lesions of the ocular adnexa. Ophthalmology 1998;105:1430–1440.

44. Knowles DM II, Jakobiec FA. Orbital lymphoid neoplasms: a clinicopathological study of 60 patients. Cancer 1980;46:576–589.

45. Garrity JA, Trautmann JC, Bartley GB, et al. Optic nerve sheath meningoceles. Ophthalmology 1990;97:1519–1531.

46. Cameron JD, Letson RD, Summers, CG. Clinical significance of hematic cyst of the orbit. Ophthalmolmic Plast Reconstr Surg 1988;4:95–99.

47. Dolman PJ, Rootman J. Malignant Graves' disease. In: Rootman J, ed. Orbital disease. Present status and future challenges. New York: Taylor and Francis, 2005.

48. Ferry AP. Lesions mistaken for malignant melanoma of the posterior uvea: a clinicopathological analysis of 100 cases with ophthalmoscopically visible lesions. Arch Ophthalmol 1964;72:463–469.

49. Collaborative Ocular Melanoma Study Group. Accuracy of diagnois of choroidal melanomas in the collaborative ocular melanoma study: COMS Report No.1. Arch Ophthalmol 1990;108:1268.

50. Trubo R. Current considerations in managing melanoma. Eyenet 2006(Sept):31–32.

51. Finger PT, Kurli M, Reddy S, Tena LB, Pavlick AC. Whole body PET/CT for initial staging of choroidal melanoma. Br J Ophthalmol 2005;89:1270–1274.

52. Singh AD, Kalyani P, Topham A. Estimating the risk of malignant transformation of a choroidal nevus. Ophthalmology 2005;112:1784–1789.

53. Shields CL, Shields JA, Kiratli H, DePotter P, Cater JR. Risk factors for growth and metastasis of small choroidal melanocytic lesions. Ophthalmology 1995;102:1351–1361.

54. Shammas HF, Blodi FC. Orbital extension of choroidal and ciliary body melanomas. Arch Ophthalmol 1977;95:2002–2005.

55. Shields JA. Diagnosis and management of intraocular tumors. Phildalelphia: Mosby; 1983.

56. Shields JA. Retinoblastoma. In: Shields JA, ed. Diagnosis and management of intraocular tumors. St. Louis: Mosby, 1983.

57. Shields CL, Shields JA, DePotter P, Carter J, Tardie D, Barrett J. Diffuse choroidal melanoma. Clinical features predictive of metastases. Arch Ophthalmol 1996;114:956–967.

58. Schlotzger-Scherhardt S, Junermann A, Naumann GOH. Mushroom-shaped choroidal melanocytoma mimicking malignant melanoma. Arch Ophthalmol 2002;120:82–84.

59. Nelson CC, Hertzberg BS, Klintworth GK. A histopathologic study of 716 unselected eyes in patients with cancer at the time of death. Am J Ophthalmol 1983;95:788–793.

60. Madhavi K, Finger PT. The kidney, cancer, and the eye: current concepts. Surv Ophthalmol 2005;50:508.

61. Shields CL, Shield JA, Gross NE, Schwartz GP, Lally SE. Survey of 520 eyes with uveal metastases. Ophthalmology 1977;104:1265–1276.

62. Biswas J, Mani B, Shanmugam MP, Patwardham D, Kumar KS, Badrinath SS. Retinoblastoma in adults: report of three cases and review of the literature. Surv Ophthalmol 2000;44:409–414.

63. Dan-ning HU, Guo-pei YU, McCormick SA, Schneider S, Finger PT. Population-based incidence of uveal melanoma in various races and ethnic groups. Am J Ophthalmol 2005;140:612–617.

64. Bhatnagar R, Vine AK. Diffuse infiltrating retinoblastoma. Ophthalmology 1991;98:1657–1661.

65. Broughton WL, Zimmerman LE. A clinicopathological study of 56 cases of intraocular medulloepithelioma. Am J Ophthalmol 1978;85:407–418.

66. Shields JA, Eagle RC, Shields CL, De Potter P. Congenital neoplasms of the nonpigmented ciliary epithelium (medulloepithelioma). Ophthalmology 1996;103:1998–2006.

67. Wan WL, Cano MR, Pince KJ, et al. Echographic characteristics of ocular toxocarasis. Ophthalmology 1987;94(Suppl):135.

68. Gass JDM, Guerry RK, Jack RL, Harris G. Choroidal osteoma. Arch Ophthalmol 1978;96:428–435.

69. Williams AT, Font RL, Van Dyk HJ. Osseous choristoma of the choroid simulating a choroidal melanoma. Arch Ophthalmol 1978;96:1874–1877.

70. Friedman AH, Beckerman B, Gold DH, et al. Drusen of the optic disc. Surv Ophthalmol 1977;21:375–376.

71. Shields CL, Fasiudden A, Mashayekhi A, Shields JA. Conjunctival nevi. Arch Ophthalmol 2004;122:167–175.

72. Harbour JW, Augsburger JJ, Eagle RC. Initial management and follow-up of melanocytic iris tumors. Ophthalmology 1995;102:1987–1993.

73. Marigo FA, Esaki K, Finger PT, et al. Differential diagnosis of anterior segment cysts by ultrasound biomicroscopy. Ophthalmology 1999;106:2131–2135.

74. Shields JA, Shields CL, Mercado G, Gunduz K, Eagle RC. Adenoma of the iris pigment epithelium: a report of 20 cases. Arch Ophthal 1999;117:736–741.

75. Shields JA. Observations on seven cases of intraocular leiomyoma. Arch Ophthalmol 1994;112:521–528.

76. Hoh HB, Laitt RD, Wakeley C, et al. The STIR sequence MRI in the assessment of extraocular muscles in thyroid eye disease. Eye 1994;8:506–510.

77. Aviv RI, Casselman J. Orbital imaging: part 1. Normal anatomy. Clin Radiol 2005;60:279–287.

78. Aviv RI, Miszkiel K. Orbital imaging: part 2. Intraorbital pathology. Clin Radiol 2005;60:288–307.

79. Shields JA, Shields CL, Scartozzi R. Survey of 1264 patients with orbital tumors and simulating lesions: the 2002 Montgomery Lecture, part 1. Ophthalmology 2004;111:997–1008.

80. Ben Simon GJ, Annunziata CC, Fink J, et al. Rethinking orbital imaging. Establishing guidelines for interpreting orbital imaging studies and evaluating their predictive value in patients with orbital tumors. Ophthalmology 2005;112:2196–2207.

81. Ta CN, Bowman RW. Hyphema caused by a metallic intraocular foreign body during magnetic resonance imaging. Am J Ophthalmol 2000;129:533–534.

82. Lee AG, Brazis PW, Garrity JA, White M. Imaging for neuro-ophthalmic and orbital disease. Am J Ophthalmol 2004;138:852–862.

# Index